Diagnostic Imaging
of the Chest

Diagnostic Imaging of the Chest

Paul R Goddard BSc, MBBS, MD, DMRD, FRCR

Consultant Radiologist, Bristol Royal Infirmary

CHURCHILL LIVINGSTONE
EDINBURGH LONDON MELBOURNE AND NEW YORK 1987

CHURCHILL LIVINGSTONE
Medical Division of Longman Group UK Limited

Distributed in the United States of America by
Churchill Livingstone Inc., 1560 Broadway, New York,
N.Y. 10036, and by associated companies, branches
and representatives throughout the world.

First published 1987

ISBN 0-443-03659-4

British Library Cataloguing in Publication Data
Goddard, Paul R.
    Diagnostic imaging of the chest.
    1. Chest——Diseases——Diagnosis
    2. Imaging systems in medicine
    I. Title
    617'.540754   RC941
    ISBN 0-443-03659-4

Library of Congress Cataloging in Publication Data
Goddard, Paul R.
    Diagnostic imaging of the chest.
    Bibliography: p.
    Includes index.
    1. Chest——Radiography.   2. Diagnostic imaging.
I. Title. [DNLM: 1. Thoracic Radiography. WF 975 G578d]
RC941.G59 1986   617'.54'07572   86-17163
ISBN 0-443-03659-4

Printed and bound in Great Britain by
Butler & Tanner Ltd, Frome and London

This book is dedicated to my wife and two sons

Contents

Foreword

In many developed countries of the world, the medical profession is currently facing the uncomfortable prospect of attempting to control burgeoning health costs, and there is no doubt that if the profession does not accept this responsibility, governmental agencies will, to our sorrow. Although diagnostic imaging receives more blame for increased costs than is justified, there is good evidence that the development of new, extraordinarily expensive diagnostic equipment in recent years has contributed a good deal to cost escalation. Accepting that, it is clear that it is the radiologist on whom the onus must fall to control costs by restricting examinations to those that reveal the maximum amount of information with the minimum amount of expense at the most propitious stage in an investigation. In the final analysis, control over the sequence in which complex, expensive investigations are performed should rest with those who possess the expertise—the diagnostic imagers—but that is not to say that a radiologist should not attempt to impart his imaging and nonimaging colleagues the knowledge he has gained through prolonged study and experience. That is what this book is all about.

With the remarkable profligation of medical books in recent years, it is a pleasure to pick up a new book that presents a unique approach. Dr Goddard lends a personal touch to the investigation of thoracic disease that is one of the special qualities of this eminently readable text. Recommendations are based largely on his own experience rather than that of others—the bibliography is highly selective and anything but exhaustive. His approach to investigation is logical and appropriate, the question he repeatedly asks being 'what do I do next' to arrive at a diagnosis that will permit effective therapy? The mechanism by which he answers that question is through the medium of case presentations, *preceded* by appropriate roentgenographic illustrations (which incidentally are of excellent quality). The reader is thus in a position to decide in his own mind what the roentgenograms show before the truth is revealed; further, he can suggest what procedure might be performed next to yield the most valuable information. This quiz format is one of the major attractions of the book. The discussions that follow the succinct clinical histories reveal the opinions of the author, and by and large are thoughtful and comprehensive. The differential diagnosis of virtually all roengenographic patterns is provided by tables or flow charts. There is a remarkably tight correlation of all possible investigative techniques including conventional and computed tomography, nuclear medicine, ultrasound, MRI, and even certain clinical procedures such as pulmonary function tests and bronchoalveolar lavage.

This monograph consists of a comprehensive dissertation on the protean roengenographic manifestations of pulmonary disease. It answers a multitude of questions but goes further than that by posing questions to which answers are not yet apparent; it thus serves as a point of departure for further investigations. The completed work stands as tangible evidence of splendid cooperation between the author and his clinical colleagues over a span of years, and he is to be congratulated for an outstanding final product.

Robert G Fraser, MD
Birmingham, Alabama, USA

Preface

The chest radiograph remains the most widely used method of imaging the chest. There has, however, been a revolution in imaging technology over the past ten years. The purpose of this book is to introduce the newer imaging techniques that are available for examining the chest and to focus attention on older methods that may not be new but are still useful. It is also pointed out that investigations not strictly performed with the chest in mind, may render useful information with regard to intrathoracic pathology.

Many larger and entirely laudable texts have been written regarding chest radiology with the major emphasis being the interpretation of chest x-ray findings. It is not the intention of this book to compete with such texts but rather to *illustrate the use of chest radiographs and of complementary techniques.*

The cases have been chosen to provide a forum for discussing the value of the different imaging modalities and the wide variety of ways in which they may be useful.

It has not been possible to be comprehensive and exhaustive on chest problems since that would require a textbook ten times the size of this small offering. This book is by nature a monograph and the idiosyncrasies of the author undoubtedly show through. Thus some subjects have been discussed in length, others in passing and some, probably important topics, not at all. However, it is hoped that an integrated approach to chest radiology and imaging will be gained from perusal of the information presented. No single technique can be expected to provide a diagnosis in every chest problem and it is for this reason that discussion about the gamut of investigations has been undertaken.

The book has been compiled to discuss problems of the chest and mediastinum. Cardiac problems have only been mentioned in passing since another book in the same series will be covering the subject in much greater depth.

Acknowledgements

The idea for this book originated with Professor E Rhys Davies and the author would like to record his gratitude for the Professor's considerable support.

The book would not have been possible without the help of the Bristol radiologists and radiographers who have provided many of the films and the chest physicians, surgeons and oncologists who referred the patients for examination. In particular I would like to mention Dr G Laszlo, Dr J Bell, Dr Jill Bullimore and Dr Elizabeth Whipp, all of whom, wittingly or unwittingly, assisted in the production of this offering.

The Medical Physics Department has assisted in much of the author's research, in particular the work on CT and emission CT has been conducted with the help of Peter Jackson, Adrian Sargood, Paul Stevens and Elizabeth Pitcher.

All the photographs were the work of the Bristol Royal Infirmary Department of Medical Illustration, the line drawings were prepared by Mr E Turnbull, and the secretarial work was done by Jayne Hugh.

I am also indebted to the radiologists from whom I received instruction and hospitality when I was on tour in Canada and the United States as the Kodak Scholar of the Royal College of Radiologists. I am especially grateful for the help of Professors Robert Fraser, Eric Milne and Mel Figley.

Previous publications

A number of the illustrations have appeared previously in articles.

Clinical Radiology
Figures G, H, I and J.
    Cases 52 and 53.

Journal of Clinical Pathology
    Case 58.

Hospital Doctor
    Cases 24, 28, 31, 37, 39, 41, 45, 84, 89, 94 and 109.

Respiratory Disease in Practice
    Case 5.

Bristol Medico-Chirurgical Journal
    Cases 27 and 103.

Introduction

The initial radiological examination performed when a chest abnormality is suspected is the chest radiograph. Moreover a large number of chest x-rays are taken for screening reasons, for example pre-employment or pre-operative chest radiographs. In many cases the radiograph is the only radiological examination that is necessary. However, there is a significant number of patients in whom the radiograph may show an abnormality but the nature or extent of the lesion is obscure. There are also patients in whom there is an important and potentially life-threatening pulmonary disease (e.g. pulmonary embolism or pulmonary emphysema) but changes on the chest x-ray are only minimal or indeed the radiograph appears normal.

In this book chest problems are presented in a 'problem-orientated' manner. The starting point for most of the discussion is the appearance on a chest radiograph, although conditions in which the chest x-ray is of limited value are also demonstrated.

Using only one sign as the starting point has weaknesses since most conditions will present with a variety of radiological and physical signs. It does, however, allow a forum for discussion and the chapters are linked by referral to similar cases described in chapters about different radiological appearances.

Quiz format

The cases can be used as quizzes by reading only as far as the figure, examining the illustration and asking the questions:

1 What abnormalities can be seen?
2 What causes must I consider?
3 What should I do next?

1 | Investigations of value with regard to the chest

The main radiological investigations used in the examination of the chest are outlined below. Brief indications for each examination are given. At the end of the description of each technique the page numbers are listed of the examples referring to the technique. Thus, although the book is mainly organized in a 'problem orientated manner', it is possible by following the listed page numbers to read through the book examining a technique at a time.

1 Chest radiography

Plain chest radiographs have been the main investigation of the chest ever since the discovery of x-rays by Roentgen at the end of the last century. The plain radiographs are usually performed in the erect position and in the PA projection (posteroanterior). Lateral films, AP, oblique and apical films are also performed on the chest. Chest radiographs are indicated in almost any condition in which pulmonary or mediastinal abnormality may be suspected. They are also used as a routine screening investigation.
(*Chest x-rays are used in most of the examples, therefore the page numbers have not been listed.*)

Figure A Chest radiography

2 Fluoroscopy

Fluoroscopy provides information with regard to the movement of the chest and is valuable in placing lesions. Fluoroscopy is not used to the same extent as it previously was but is still of value when examining the diaphragm, for example, when a subphrenic abscess is suspected, and in the localization of masses that may be intra- or extrathoracic. Fluoroscopy of the chest is nowadays mainly used when performing contrast medium studies and biopsy techniques.
(Pages 8, 103, 144.)

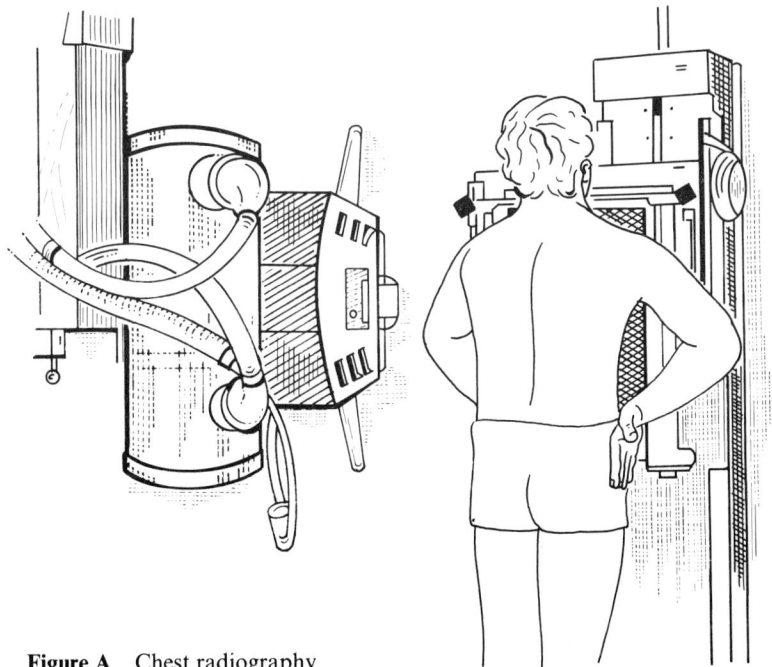

3 Linear tomography

Linear tomography has long been used in order to:

(a) accurately site lesions,

(b) determine whether there is cavitation,

(c) determine whether calcification is present in the lesion.

Its value lies in the ability to blur out overlying opacities and thus reveal the nature of lesions otherwise hidden by the skeleton or other structures.
(Pages 9, 45, 160.)

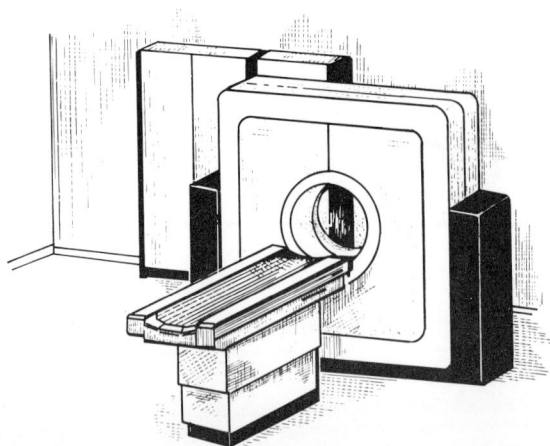

Figure B Whole-body computed tomography

4 Computed tomography

Computed tomography (CT) fulfils the same role as linear tomography but in addition will reveal much smaller pulmonary and pleural lesions. By virtue of the good soft tissue contrast it is of considerable assistance in the determination of mediastinal abnormalities. Skeletal and extrathoracic lesions are also well demonstrated by CT.

Computed tomography (CT) provides excellent anatomical information in the cross-sectional plane and good differentiation between tissues. In addition, contrast medium may be injected intravenously in order to further highlight vascular structures. CT can thus be used to look at any of the structures of the thorax, i.e.:

(a) the mediastinum and cardiovascular system,

(b) the lungs and pleura,

(c) the skeleton and extrathoracic soft tissues.

In the mediastinum the major indications are:

 (i) the analysis of mediastinal widening and masses,

(ii) the staging of malignancy by a search for enlarged lymph nodes.

In the lungs the main indications have been:

 (i) search for small pulmonary metastases (e.g. in teratoma),

(ii) staging of bronchogenic carcinoma.

In the skeleton and soft tissues the main indication has been staging of malignant disease.

Further indications for CT of the chest have, however, become apparent. These include:

(a) The assessment of cardiovascular lesions.
    This has become more valuable since the advent of rapid sequential scanning (repeated fast scanning). Aortic aneurysms, dissection of the aorta, and assessment of bypass graft patency are some of the uses that have been cited in the literature. Because of cardiac movement, there are better methods than CT for examining the heart.

(b) The detection and assessment of early or hidden pleuropulmonary disease including pulmonary emphysema, fibrosing lung diseases, radiation pneumonitis and fibrosis, and bronchiectasis.

(c) CT-guided needle biopsy—this is indicated when fluoroscopic guidance is unreliable.

(d) Assessment of spinal problems such as kyphoscoliosis and disc prolapse.

(Pages 12, 45–49, 125 and many other pages.)

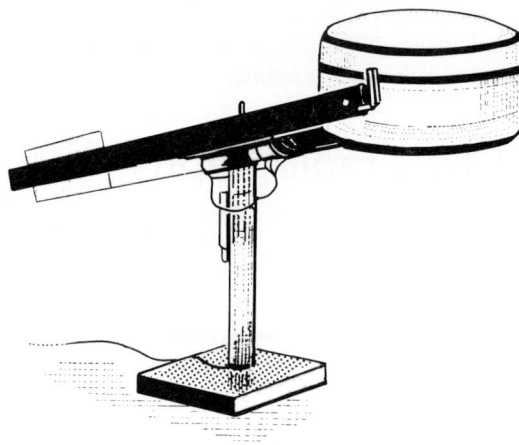

Figure C Gamma Camera

5 Radioisotopes

Radioisotope investigations of the thorax (excluding the cardiovascular system) fall mainly into two groups:

(a) Ventilation and perfusion studies—looking for defects of ventilatory or perfusion function

(b) Gallium scans and labelled white cell studies—looking for foci of infection, inflammation or neoplasia.

(Pages 29, 92–97, 128–131.)

Recently there has been considerable interest in positron emission tomography. Research has also been undertaken with permeability studies in adult respiratory distress syndrome.

Pulmonary secondary deposits may have some functional or metabolic properties of the primary—thus osteosarcoma metastases may ossify and take up bone scanning radiopharmaceuticals, and secondaries from thyroid carcinoma may sequester radioactive iodine.

6   Ultrasound

Because ultrasound, in the frequencies for diagnostic imaging, is not conducted through air, the use in the chest is limited to lesions with an acoustic window. Ultrasound has mainly been used in cardiac work but it is also useful in the evaluation of mediastinal masses. Pleurally based masses can be studied with efficacy—in particular the distinction between pleural effusion and pleural thickening can be made with ease.
(Pages 50, 103, 112, 139, 147.)

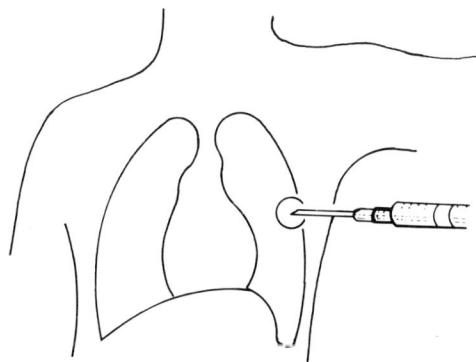

Figure D   Needle biopsy

7   Needle biopsy

The main indication for performing needle biopsy is an undiagnosed pulmonary mass or nodule. Percutaneous needle biopsy is a sensible investigation if the resultant diagnosis by cytology may result in a change in management of the patient. If the next step, such as thoracotomy, will be performed whatever the outcome of the test, there is little value in performing the biopsy. There must also be confidence in the cytopathology results. Thus close cooperation with the local chest physicians, thoracic surgeons and cytopathologists is essential.
(Pages 21, 50, 59, 61.)

8   Bronchography

Bronchography is used much less frequently than in the past. This is probably partly due to a change in disease prevalence (for example, decreased incidence of whooping cough and consequent bronchiectasis) but is also due to the advent of investigations that are better tolerated by the patient or provide greater information.

Bronchography at present still has a role in the investigation of patients who may have bronchiectasis causing unexplained haemoptysis or non-resolving chest infection. Fibreoptic bronchoscopy is nowadays used to demonstrate many of the causes of haemoptysis that would previously have been shown by bronchography, including endobronchial lesions such as adenomas. If it is felt that bronchography is still necessary, it may be used as an adjunct to bronchoscopy. Computed tomography is being used with increasing frequency to show bronchiectasis and even endobronchial lesions.
(Pages 50, 61, 64, 73, 89.)

9   Angiography and digital vascular imaging

Indications for pulmonary arteriography include the investigation of the following:

(a) Pulmonary embolism

(b) Pulmonary arteriovenous malformation

(c) Pulmonary artery aneurysm

Pulmonary angiography is also performed for a variety of cardiac conditions including congenital heart disease, acquired pulmonary valve lesions and wedge pressures in mitral valve disease. The investigation of cardiac abnormalities is, however, outside the scope of this book.

Superior vena cavography is done during the investigation of superior vena cava obstruction. Contrast medium is also frequently injected into the SVC via central venous pressure catheters in order to check the position of the tip.

Arch aortography is indicated in the investigation of a widened mediastinum following trauma in order to determine whether or not there is a traumatic aneurysm. It is also necessary when investigating a possible dissecting aneurysm. Arch aortography is also occasionally of assistance in unusual cases such as sequestrated segment. Selective bronchial artery catheterization and even embolization may be indicated

in a few patients, for example, haemoptysis due to a mycetoma.
(Pages 17, 133–137, 154, 163–165.)

Digital vascular imaging

This is a variation of angiography and the indications are the same as for angiography. By the use of digital subtraction it is possible to obtain clear images of arteries or veins either with a small injection of contrast medium or by the intravenous route.

10 Barium examinations

Barium examinations are usually performed because of symptomatology suggestive of alimentary tract abnormality. They can, however, be employed to assist in the elucidation of an abnormality shown on a chest radiograph. In particular a mass lesion posteriorly placed in the mediastinum may well involve the oesophagus. For example, carcinoma of the oesophagus, hiatus hernia and achalasia may all be detectable on a plain chest film and subsequently diagnosed by barium swallow. Chronic reflux and aspiration may result in a variety of changes on the chest x-ray ranging from pneumonia to fibrosis. Intermittent aspiration may cause symptoms that mimic asthma. Some conditions, such as scleroderma, cause pulmonary and oesophageal abnormalities.
(Pages 59, 90, 142, 153, 165.)

11 Myelography

Myelography is an occasional useful adjunct in chest investigation when a neurogenic origin for a thoracic mass is suspected or there is indication of neurological involvement.

12 Nuclear magnetic resonance imaging (magnetic resonance imaging)

Magnetic resonance imaging (MRI) is a method of obtaining images of the body using large magnetic fields and radiofrequencies. Originally known as nuclear

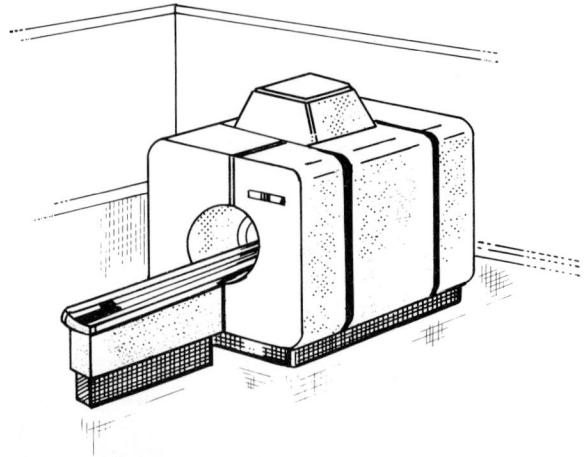

Figure E   Magnetic resonance imaging

magnetic resonance (NMR) the 'nuclear' has been dropped from the name because of confusion with nuclear medicine (radioisotope) scanning and because it is possible to obtain information from structures other than nuclei.

MRI provides images by a method completely different from any other imaging technique but at the same time they are readily interpretable by radiologists and clinicians experienced in sectional anatomy.

Magnetic resonance imaging (MRI) has rapidly become a technique of clinical significance. MRI has some unique properties complementing the diagnostic information available from other imaging modalities. The absence of ionizing radiation and of other known hazards is unquestionably a bonus.

MRI also has the ability to provide information on the processes occurring inside the cell and has great potential for spectroscopy, enabling the body chemistry to be studied in vivo.

MRI has been shown to be of value in the examination of patients with tumours by demonstrating the extent of neoplasia and sometimes enabling the distinction to be made between areas that are benign and those that are malignant without the necessity of biopsy. In the chest this would probably be most important in the mediastinum, although large pulmonary masses could also be assessed using magnetic resonance imaging. Early work has shown that in the mediastinum compression and invasion of vessels are more easily demonstrated on MRI spinecho images than on CT scan.

The technique is already being used for the assessment of cardiovascular disease and could in some cases replace investigations such as cardiac catheterization and angiography. There may also be a role for the technique in the evaluation of traumatic aortic rupture and in dissection of the aorta.

13 Digital chest radiography and the digital department

New methods of recording chest x-rays are being investigated in a number of places. At Birmingham, Alabama, digital chest radiography is being performed using a Picker machine. Under the direction of Professor Fraser the machine has been evaluated and modifications, such as dual energy scanning, have been suggested.

The study is of considerable importance since chest radiography accounts for between 25 and 40 per cent of all radiography. With the increasing importance of digital information such a unit may be essential apparatus in 10 years' time. Whereas it will never be suitable for all patients to have 'routine' CT scans of the chest, it may indeed be that the present plain film chest radiograph will be replaced by a digital image.

Various advantages and disadvantages have been identified:

(a) Good technical quality of image with no repeats being necessary.

(b) Manipulation of data enables lesions hidden in review areas (e.g. behind heart, at apices, overlying the diaphragm) to be seen more easily.

(c) Display of the image in a positive mode and alteration of the contrast may enable pulmonary nodules to be seen more easily. Seeing the black lesions against a white background may facilitate their detection as compared with display of grey nodules against a black background.

Potential advantages include ease of storage, retrieval and transmission.

Although manipulation of data may improve diagnosis it does, however, take longer than reading a standard chest film. At present, computation and storage are a problem rather than a benefit. Retrieval is also a problem at present. If one wishes to look at a series of chest radiographs, this is difficult. Digital systems cannot compare with a packet of films for ease of storage and access.

Technology is, however, changing at amazing speed.

Laser disk systems will allow thousands of images to be stored on one laser disk with millisecond retrieval time. Optical fibre transmission of digital information permits astonishingly fast transmission of images. Both the laser disk systems and the optical fibre techniques are available already and could be combined with the use of any digital apparatus. A 'juke box' system of laser disks has already been developed allowing 60 disks to be stored, each holding thousands of images, allowing a few seconds access time to any one image.

If finances permit, the hospital of the future will be organized such that computer terminals will be present in all wards, clinics and service departments. There will be almost immediate access to a patient's notes, pathology tests and display of digital radiological images. This should result in improved communication between doctors and a decrease in unnecessary or repetitive investigations. The computer links could also be available to the specialist's home often therefore obviating the necessity for emergency recall of a specialist to the hospital. Such systems would, as a spin-off, also expedite research.

If all x-ray examinations are to become digitized it will be necessary to employ the apparatus for mobile work in addition to departmental work. Filmless systems such as those presently being worked on by DigiRad and Fuji may well be the answer. (Page 31.)

Table 1 Non-radiological investigations

The main non-radiological investigations of chest conditions are listed below.

1	Pulmonary function studies
2	Serological and skin tests
3	Bronchoscopy
4	Transbronchial biopsy
5	Bronchoalveolar lavage
6	Mediastinoscopy
7	Mediastinotomy
8	Endoscopic examination of the pleural cavity (thoracoscopy)
9	Thoracotomy and open biopsy

2 | The pulmonary mass or nodule

The correct diagnostic procedure after the discovery of a pulmonary mass is a debatable question that arouses much controversy. Some surgeons may say that the only useful way to obtain a diagnosis and treat a patient with a pulmonary mass is by open surgery. The argument is based on the premise that 'all pulmonary masses require removal and even if the lesion is irresectable some removal is better than none'. This is, of course, a reiteration of that old surgical adage: 'If in doubt, cut it out.' The diametrically opposed view held by some clinicians is that the histological diagnosis and the staging of neoplasms is paramount and that all the possible investigations should be performed routinely before considering any treatment. The diagnostic radiologist and the discerning practitioner must carefully steer a course between such opposing views and provide a sensible scheme of investigation tailored to suit each individual patient.

There are many possible differential diagnoses when a patient presents with a pulmonary mass or nodule on the chest radiograph. Some of the important causes are listed in Table 2.

Clinical indications as to the nature of the mass are often extremely helpful. The history and physical examination may provide the diagnosis or at least give sensible indications as to which investigation to undertake. When the diagnosis is not immediately apparent an order of investigation is necessary. A flow chart of investigative procedure towards this aim is reproduced on page 7. Such a flow chart should not be used as a substitute for careful examination and thought but rather as an adjunct to assist in producing a sensible pattern of diagnostic imaging. No two patients are the same and a routine method of study in any clinical problem is liable to flounder. With these reservations in mind the flow chart may be examined.

The distinction between a pulmonary nodule and a mass is arbitrary. A nodule is basically a small mass, and conversely a mass is a large nodule. In the following discussion a pulmonary nodule is generally

Table 2   Solitary pulmonary mass or nodule

Common
1   Primary neoplasm, especially bronchogenic carcinoma
2   Metastasis, especially from sarcoma and neoplasms of colon, ovary, testis, kidney, thyroid
3   Granuloma, tuberculosis and, in the USA, histoplasmosis, coccidioidomycosis
4   Hamartoma
5   Bronchial adenoma
6   Abscess

Less common
1   Rheumatoid nodule
2   Pulmonary infarct
3   Arteriovenous malformation
4   Haematoma, contusion
5   Pneumoconiosis (progressive massive fibrosis)
6   Cyst, fluid filled (bronchogenic, bronchiectatic, hydatid)
7   Lymphoma
8   Neoplasm, benign (fibroma, lipoma, neurofibroma)
9   Fungus ball
10 Sequestrated segment

Lesions simulating a pulmonary mass
1   Loculated effusion
2   Pleural plaque, thickening or tumour (e.g. mesothelioma)
3   Chest wall lesion (skin tumour, nipple shadow, rib lesion)
4   Mediastinal mass
5   Artefact or film fault

This table does not list all the causes of a solitary mass. Conditions that cause multiple 'coin' lesions and many of the causes of pulmonary cavitation may also result in a solitary opacity. They are listed in Tables 3 and 6 pages 24 and 44.

used to describe an opacity that is less than 3 or 4 cm in diameter and an opacity larger than this is referred to as a mass. Discussion regarding nodules may also be relevant for lesions greater than 3 cm but the emphasis

Pulmonary Opacity on Chest X-Ray

Is it IMPORTANT?
Has it changed compared with previous films?
Is it calcified?

Previous films
available

Classical diagnostic
features

DIAGNOSIS

No previous films
available

Larger on latest
film

Smaller on latest
film - or no change
over a long period

Only action that
may be needed is
Follow up X-Ray

Is the lesion in the CHEST?

Lateral ± Tomography ± Fluoroscopy

Pleural
(see relevant
chapter)

Pulmonary

Are there clinical pointers?
Serology - Sputum - Cytology - etc -

Chest wall or -
outside chest (see -
relevant chapter)

DIAGNOSIS

Is the lesion single or multiple? Is there cavitation? Is the mediastinum involved?

CT/Linear Tomography (depending on availability)

Mediastinal involvement
(see relevant chapter)

Single lesion

Multiple nodules
(see relevant chapter)

Central

Peripheral

Bronchoscopy and
Transbronchial Biopsy

Negative

Needle Biopsy

Positive diagnosis

THORACOTOMY

Positive diagnosis

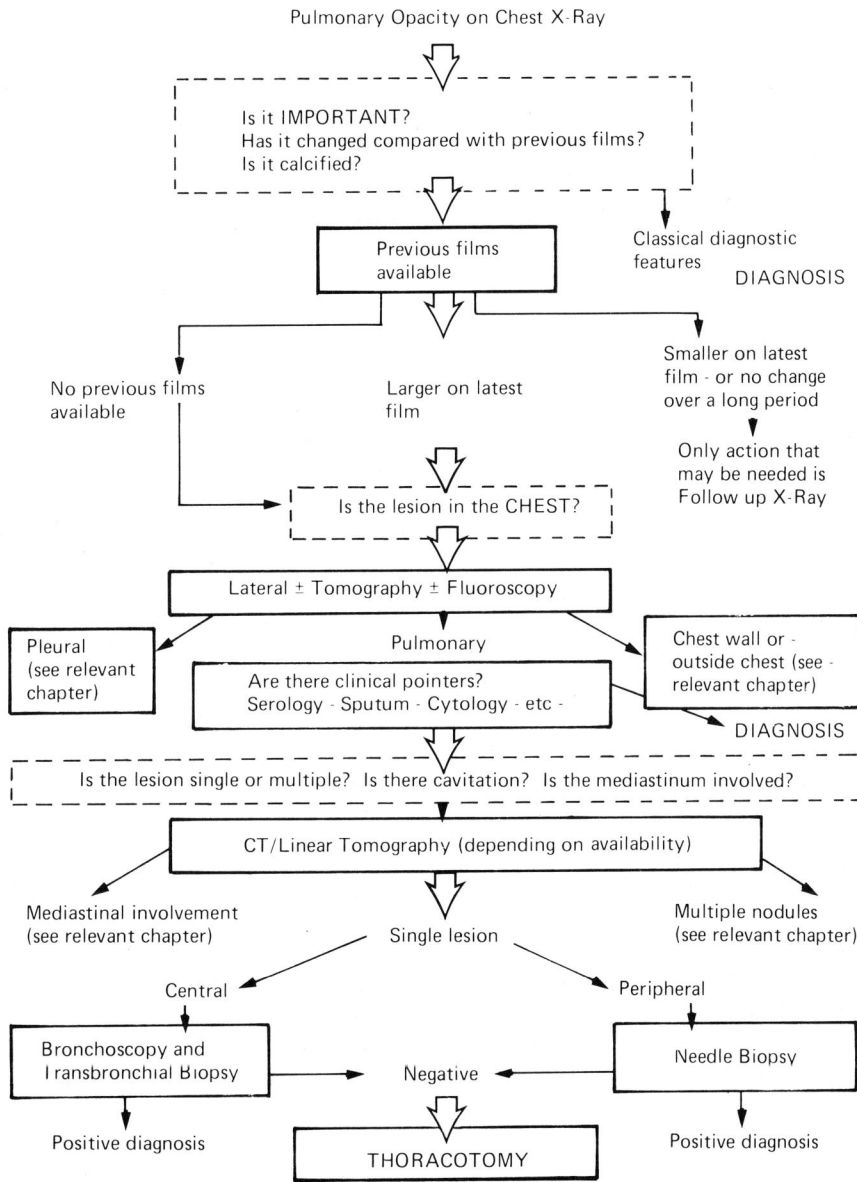

Figure F Pulmonary opacity on chest x-ray
Studying the flow chart.
Strict adherence to the flow chart is *not* recommended. At any stage of the investigation the diagnosis may become apparent and no further test may be required. In other cases, with the knowledge of the clinical condition, it may be prudent to perform the investigations in a different order. The flow chart should only be used to stimulate a logical pattern of thought with regard to a particular problem.

may well be different. For example with a very large pulmonary mass the diagnosis may commonly be made by sputum cytology, a method that rarely renders useful results with very small lesions.

Discovery of a nodule or mass

Most pulmonary nodules or masses are discovered by plain chest radiography. It is therefore vital that the chest x-ray should be of an optimal quality in order that lesions are not missed. Clearly, if a lesion is not suspected, the rest of the diagnostic armoury, however complex or technologically advanced, becomes of no value since it will not be brought into action. The high KV technique of chest radiography is a method which has gained wide acceptance throughout the world. The method is certainly a compromise insomuch that, in order to obtain images with sufficient latitude to show the lungs behind the heart and behind the diaphragm, there is a loss of contrast in the lung fields and of detail of the bones. Calcification in a nodule is more difficult to detect on high KV films than using the old low KV techniques. The high KV technique does, however, appear to be the best method of chest radiography that is presently widely available.

The most commonly employed KVp is 140 using a triple-phase generator. Some of the best standard PA chest radiographs are those obtained under the direction of Professor R Fraser (Birmingham, Alabama). His method employs a 10-ft FFD, 145 KVp, 6-in. airgap, automatic timer, and a brass filter on the x-ray tube [1]. The addition of a lateral film may increase pickup slightly and is definitely of value in determining the site of a lesion.

With the increasing use of CT for staging conditions such as teratoma or osteosarcoma, pulmonary nodules are also being discovered *de novo* using CT. Computed tomography is considerably more sensitive than chest radiography or whole lung tomography in detection of pulmonary nodules, being able to reliably detect lesions of 3 mm in diameter compared with 6 mm for whole lung tomography and 10 mm for plain chest radiography [2-7]. Pulmonary nodules may also be occasionally detected during scintigraphic examination (see pages 25-29).

Newer techniques in chest imaging, such as magnetic resonance imaging (MRI) and digital chest radiography, may be useful in the assessment of a pulmonary mass. MRI is able to provide information about pulmonary lesions only if they are fairly large. The Picker digital chest unit (discussed in Chapters 1 and 3) is able to show pulmonary nodules with greater ease than plain chest radiography [8].

The next step

Having discovered a pulmonary opacity it is important to plan the next step. If previous films are available, they may provide invaluable information. If, for example, the nodule was present on the previous films and is completely unchanged some months or years later it is reasonable to assume that the lesion is benign. No further action would be required in such a case. If, however, the nodule was not previously present or was previously much smaller, further investigation is warranted. It is thus mandatory that previous films are obtained if at all possible.

There may be clues in the patient's history regarding the aetiology of the pulmonary nodule, for example a known primary tumour or long-standing rheumatoid arthritis, a history of heavy smoking or a lifetime spent down the coal mines. The presence of a known primary malignant tumour increases the likelihood of a lesion being a secondary deposit. If the lesion is solitary and small, there is still, however, quite a high chance that it may be benign even if there is a known primary. This is particularly the case in the USA where granulomatous conditions such as histoplasmosis and coccidioidomycosis are common.

Clinical and laboratory tests will probably be undertaken at this stage. Sputum cytology is a non-invasive technique and is therefore certainly worth pursuing. With large masses a diagnostic result may be obtained in around 50 per cent of cases, but the yield in small pulmonary lesions is disappointingly low. The sputum should also be cultured for pyogenic organisms and, if there is any suspicion of tuberculosis, acid-fast bacilli should be sought and culture for tuberculosis undertaken. Other laboratory investigations such as haemoglobin, viscosity and ESR must also be considered as well as clinical tests such as the Kveim test for sarcoidosis and the Heaf test for tuberculosis. If hydatid is suspected, haemagglutination and indirect fluorescent antibody tests can be performed on serum. The Casoni skin test is no longer used [9].

The site and number of lesions will influence the choice of the next investigation. *Fluoroscopy* may be of value in order to:

1 Check the site of the lesion(s).
2 Perform low KV spot films in a variety of positions.

Fluoroscopy is useful in checking the position of a lesion and demonstrating it to be pulmonary rather than chest wall or extrathoracic in position. The lower KV of the spot films allows better tissue differentiation and demonstration of cavities, calcification etc.

At present in the UK, conventional *tomography* is one of the most commonly employed techniques for verification of the presence of a solitary opacity and for showing calcification, cavitation, and shape of a mass.

Case 1

Alfred W., aged 69, presented with haemoptysis.

The chest x-ray showed an ill-defined opacity in the right mid to lower zone overlying the posterior part of the right 9th rib. The lateral showed a dense opacity in the hilar region.

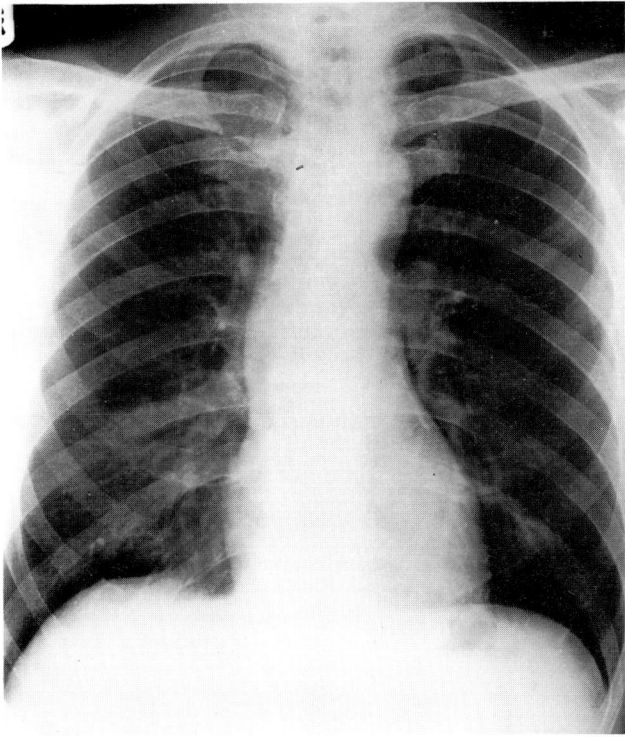

Figure 1a

Figure 1b

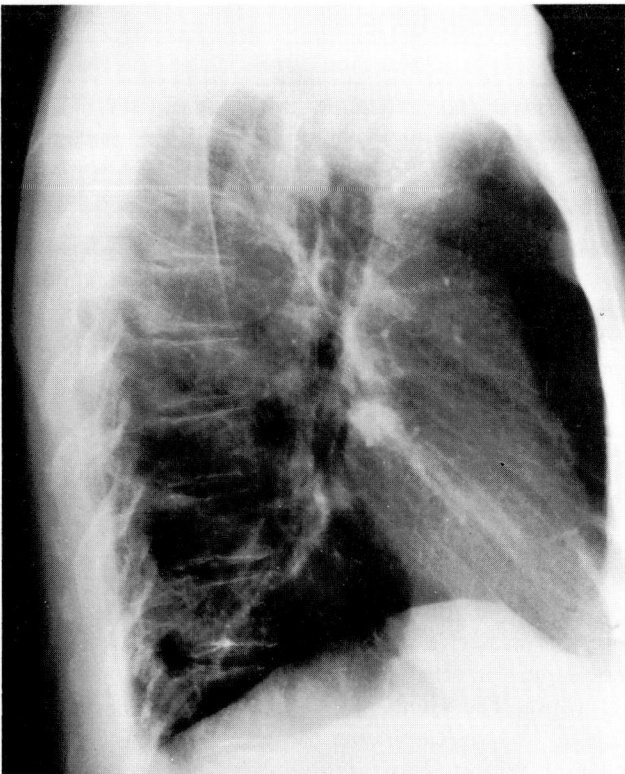

Linear tomography confirmed the presence of a 'cigar-shaped' opacity extending to the hilum. Bronchoscopy was performed and a small tumour was discovered plugging one of the secondary divisions from the right middle lobe bronchus. At surgery the tumour was removed and secretions were present in an area of segmental collapse beyond the tumour. Histology revealed carcinoid tumour. (Clinical details by courtesy of Dr J Harvey.)

Figure 1c

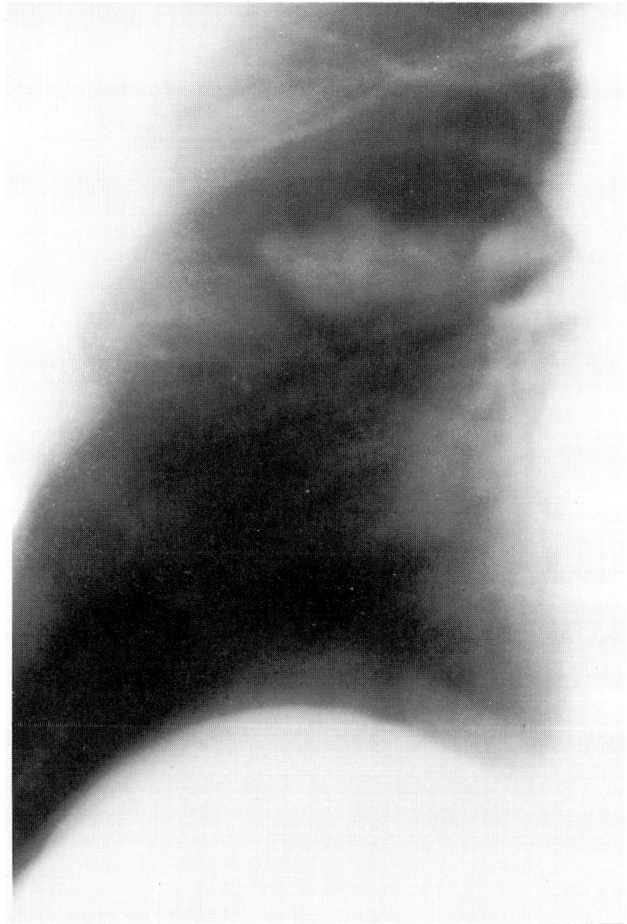

Case 2

An opacity was detected in the left lower zone on a routine staff chest x-ray. The mass had a well defined lower border but the upper margin was not clearly seen.

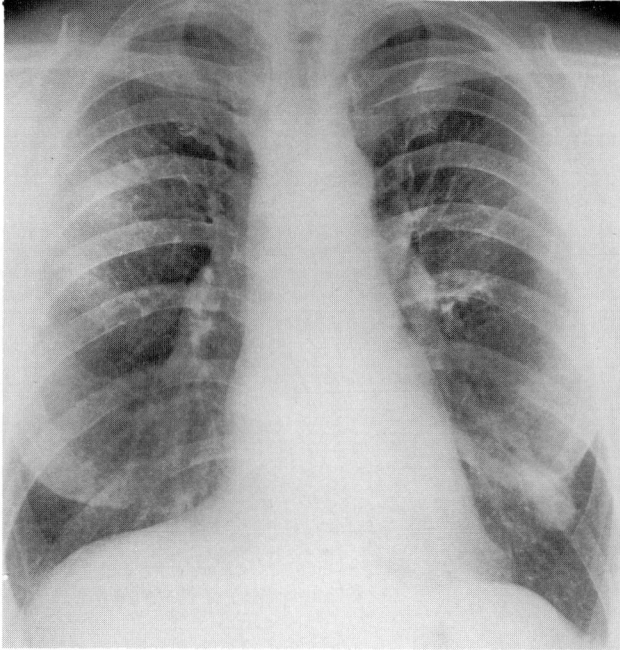

Figure 2a

Figure 2b

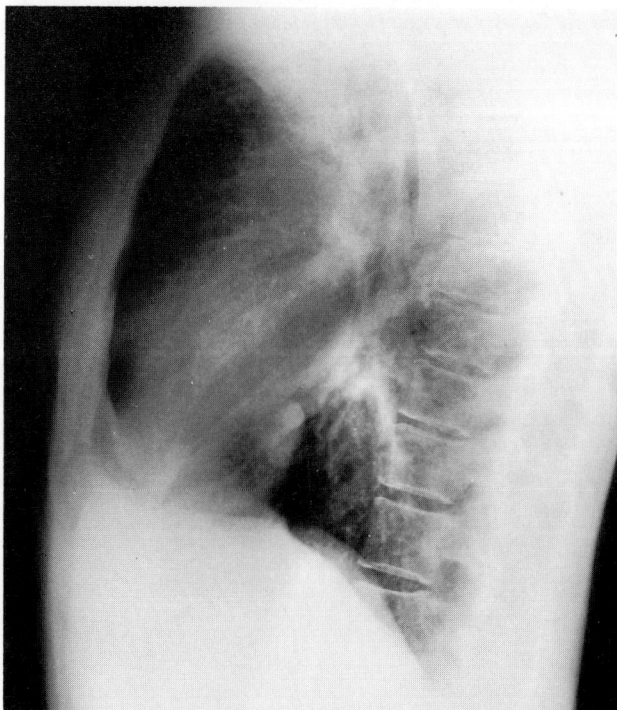

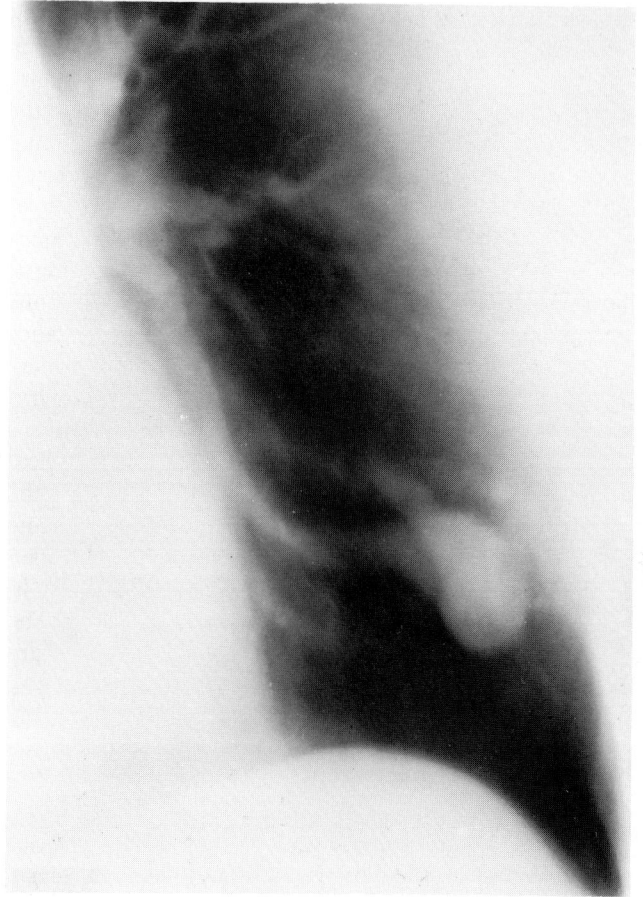

Figure 2c

The lateral (fig. 2b) showed the opacity to be intrapulmonary. Linear tomography (fig. 2c) was undertaken.

This clearly demonstrated large vessels entering and leaving the mass which was therefore diagnosed as being an arteriovenous malformation.

Arteriovenous malformations may be single or multiple. If they are large, they cause a thrill or murmur audible on auscultation. They are usually asymptomatic but can cause dyspnoea, cyanosis and haemoptysis. Many are associated with cutaneous or buccal telangiectasia.

In North America and increasingly in Great Britain, computed tomography (CT) is used in place of conventional tomography in the analysis of a pulmonary nodule or mass.

If one opacity has been detected, a search for other lesions is vital. If it is highly suspected or even proven that the mass is a primary carcinoma of the bronchus, the search for other lesions may be part of the staging procedure. The number of investigations undertaken in staging known carcinoma of the bronchus varies in different centres. Most centres with access to modern technology would agree that computed tomography of the chest is of considerable value, particularly in searching for enlarged mediastinal nodes or secondary pulmonary metastases. Some centres would continue the scanning downwards to include the liver and adrenal glands which are frequent sites of secondaries. Alternative techniques for the detection of liver metastases include ultrasound and scintigraphy. Since bone secondaries are common, isotope bone scanning is undertaken if there is any suggestion of bone symptomatology. In patients with finger clubbing and/ or joint pains radiographs of the wrists and ankles may be done to look for hypertrophic (pulmonary) osteoarthropathy.

In order to obtain cytological or histological specimens percutaneous needle biopsy may be undertaken. Non-radiological techniques to the same end include bronchoscopy, mediastinoscopy and open biopsy. All of the latter three techniques also assist in staging the tumour and determining the operability. The merits and demerits of most of these investigations are further discussed later in this chapter.

Case 3

Graham B, aged 58, presented with painful gynaecomastia, pain in the right side of his chest and clubbing of recent onset. The chest x-ray and a bone scan are shown.

Figure 3a

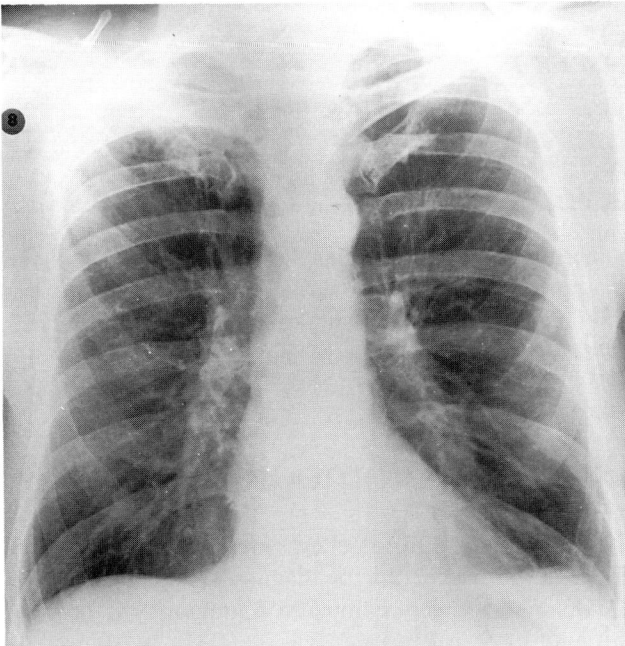

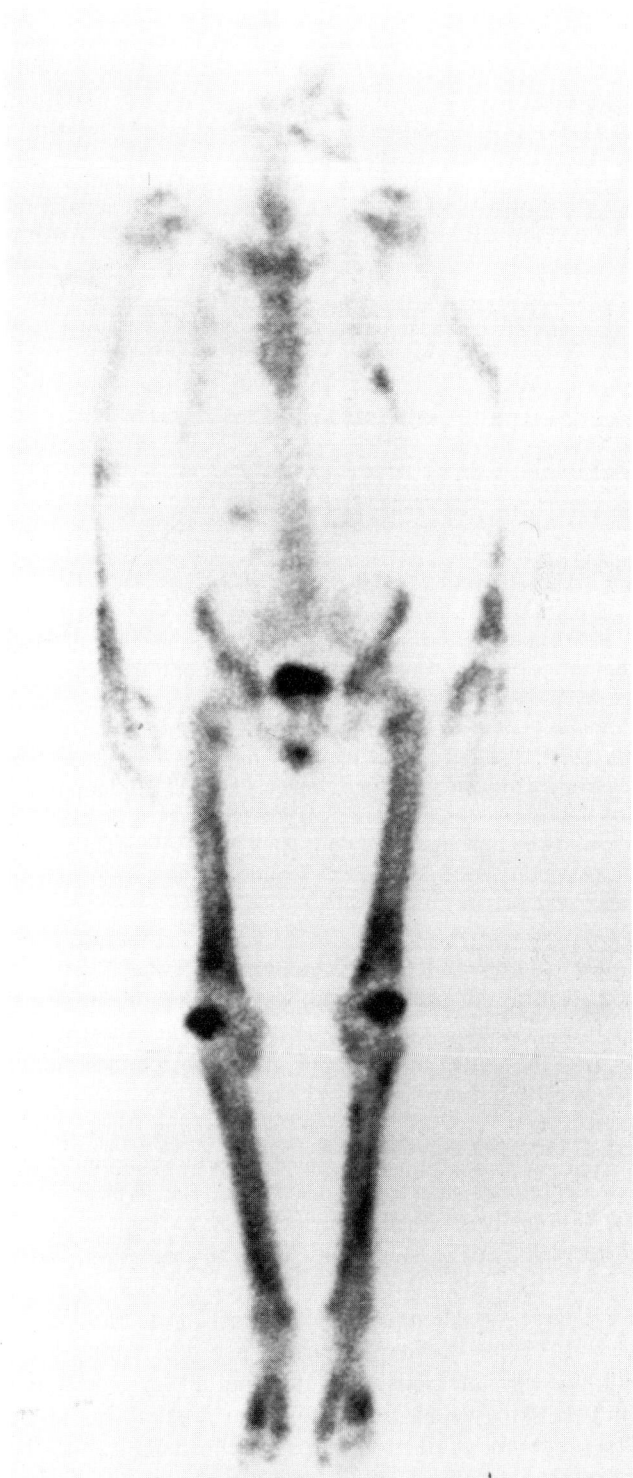

Figure 3b

The chest x-ray shows a radiolucent lesion in the left 8th rib and a small opacity in the lung adjacent to it. There is also slight opacification of the right apex.

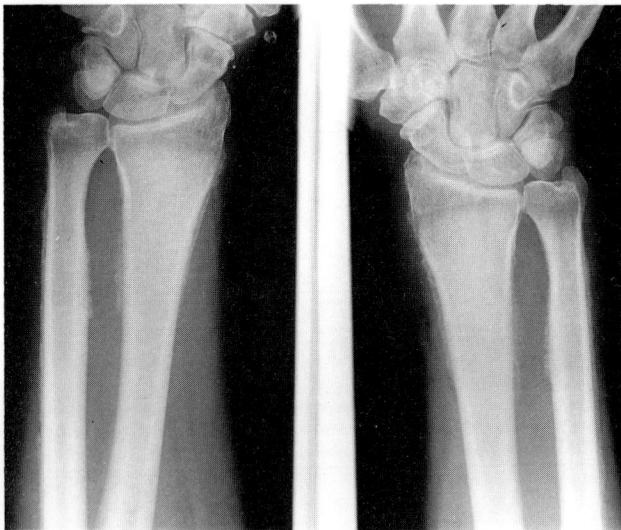

Figure 3c

Figure 3d

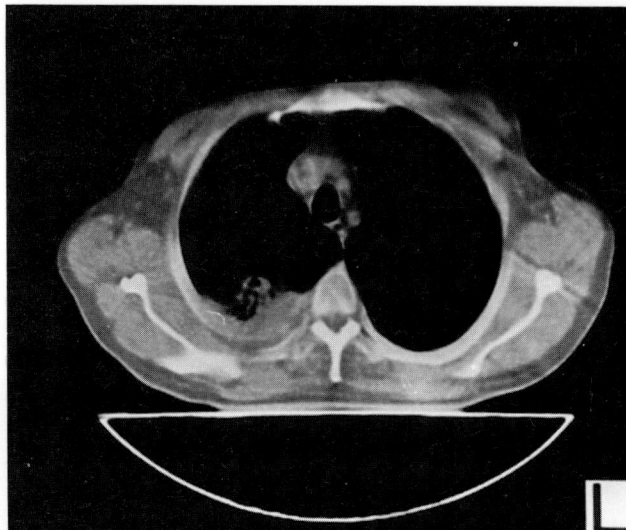

Figure 3e

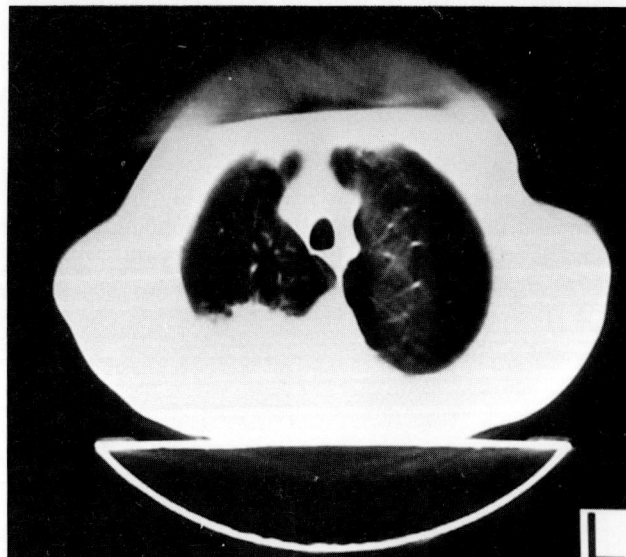

The bone scan shows uptake of radiopharmaceutical in the rib lesion and considerable uptake around the joints. An x-ray of the wrists (fig. 3c) shows periosteal new bone formation due to hypertrophic osteoarthropathy. Needle biopsy of the opacity in the left lung was performed and cytology of the aspirate revealed well differentiated squamous cell carcinoma. CT of the chest (figs. 3d and 3e) showed the opacity in the right apex to be a lobulated solid mass which was undoubtedly a primary 'Pancoast' tumour.

The likelihood of a diagnosis may change considerably if, rather than a single lesion, multiple nodular lesions are present. If nodules vary in size and shape, they are much more likely to be secondary deposits than due to a benign cause.

In Great Britain if there is a known malignant tumour and multiple pulmonary nodules greater than one centimetre in size are discovered, the likelihood of the lesions being metastatic becomes so high that no further diagnostic steps may need to be taken. With smaller lesions and when there is no known primary, the degree of diagnostic certainty is considerably less. Because biopsy techniques carry a risk of complications, non-invasive methods such as sputum cytology and culture, skin testing and serological studies should be first undertaken. If these prove ineffectual, it may be necessary to obtain either cytological or histological information by biopsy. Thoracotomy, percutaneous needle biopsy, bronchoscopic biopsy and mediastinoscopy are the main methods of obtaining the material.

If the nodules are less than 5 mm in size and too numerous to count, they may be referred to as 'miliary' in appearance. The differential diagnosis is then very different from that of a single nodule or mass and will accordingly be discussed in another section, pages 33–43.

Computed tomography

The value of CT in chest investigation has been discussed on page 2. In the diagnosis or management of a pulmonary opacity computed tomography is of value in a number of ways:

1 Analysis of the characteristics of the lesion itself, i.e. site, shape, radiodensity and vascularity (the latter may be assessed using contrast medium injection and rapid sequential scanning).

2 Detection of further unsuspected small pulmonary nodules. CT, as already discussed above, is far more sensitive than plain chest radiography or whole lung tomography in the detection of nodules.

3 Close examination of the mediastinum. Abnormal mediastinal nodes can now be detected with considerable accuracy. (See also below under Bronchoscopy and Mediastinoscopy.)

4 CT may also enable unsuspected pathology to be discovered. A severe degree of pulmonary emphysema may, for example, be present without being suspected on plain films. This may influence management [10].

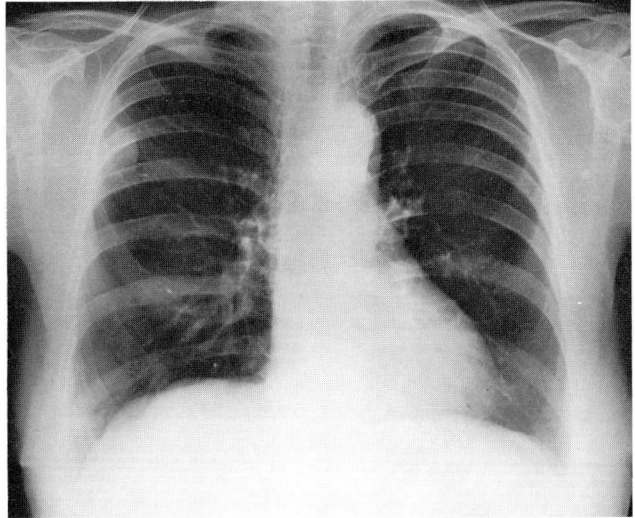

Figure 4a

Case 4

A peripherally placed opacity was discovered on routine staff chest radiography. Oblique views again indicated that it was peripherally positioned, probably involving the pleura. Computed tomography (CT) was done.

CT clearly showed the exact site of the lesion as sub-pleural with slight extension into the intercostal space. The density of the lesion was that of fat—the opacity in figures 4b and 4d should be compared with the subcutaneous fat. (Mean density of −102 HU.) The diagnosis of pleural

Figure 4b

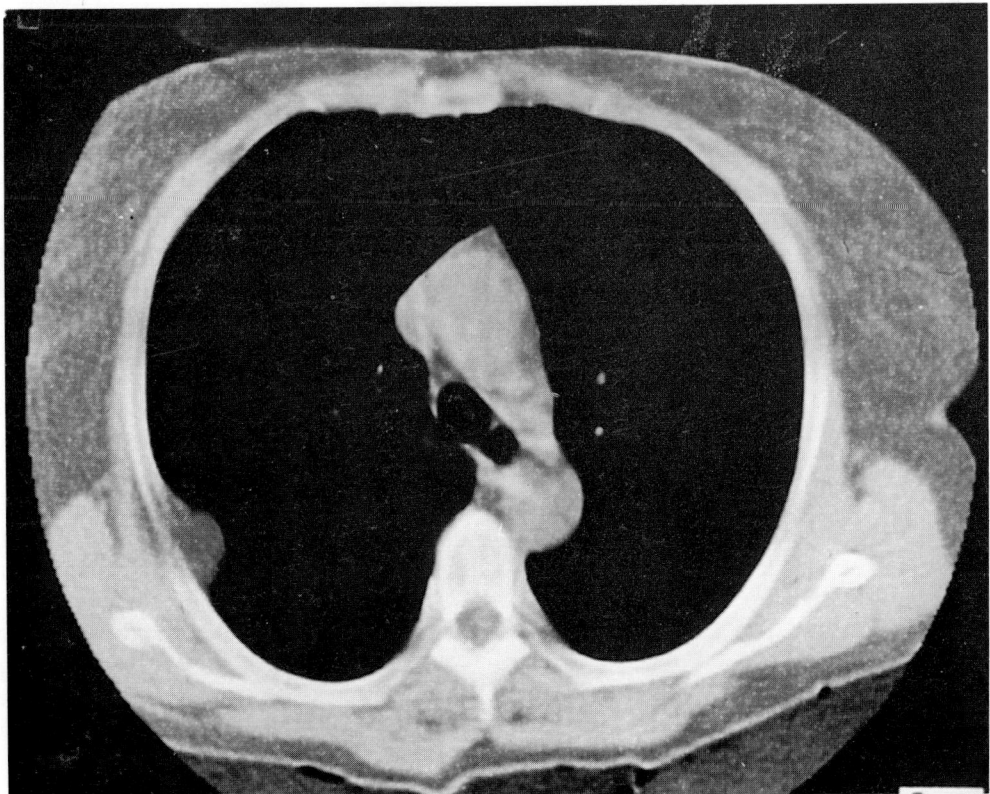

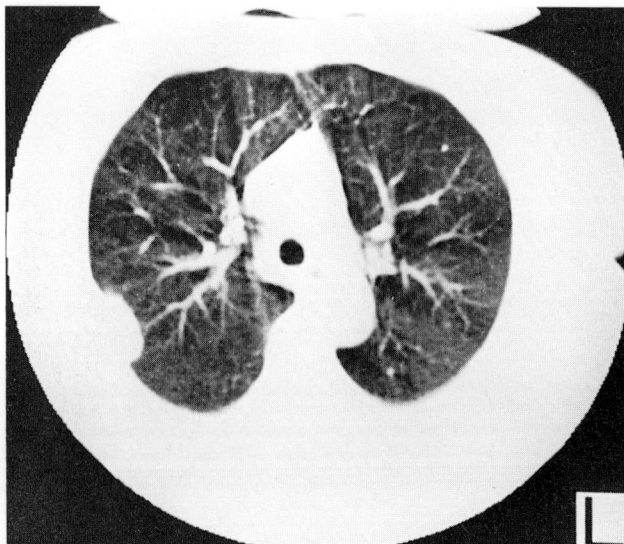

Figure 4c

Figure 4d

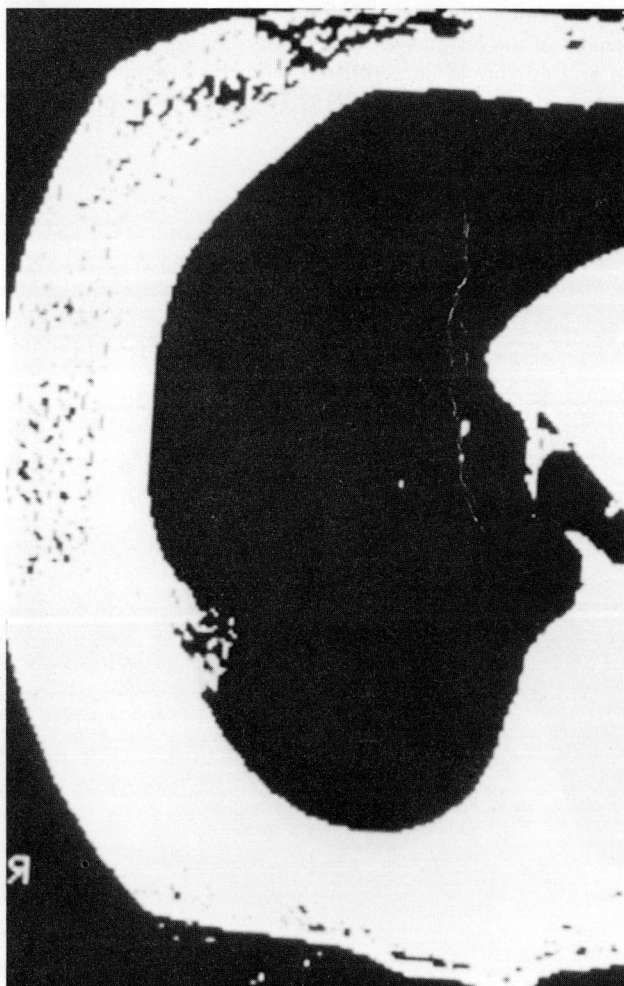

lipoma was made. The benign nature of the condition and ease of diagnosis by CT obviated the necessity of further investigation. Computed tomography thus enabled a biopsy to be avoided and the demonstration of the benign nature of the lesion removed the patient's anxiety.

Differentiation of benign from malignant disease by the presence of calcification shown by computed tomography

This is a controversial subject. Recent papers have detailed methods of analysing CT numbers of pulmonary nodules [11, 12]. It has been stated that if a nodule has a representative number higher than a certain figure it can be assumed to be calcified and therefore benign. There had been some delay in confirming these findings until a recent report [12]. The reasons for difficulty in the use of numbers in this way had been cited as variation between scanners in measurement of numbers and variations from scan to scan and patient to patient on the same scanner. Phantoms have been devised to overcome these problems.

However, it is clear that the value of such discrimination on the basis of calcification depends to a large extent on the local pattern of disease. The two papers supporting the use of CT in this way came from areas in which histoplasmosis is very common. The majority of patients in whom the representative number was high were suffering from histoplasmosis. In areas in which the condition is rare, calcified granulomata are much less common. It must also be remembered that several primary tumours are known to give rise to metastases that either ossify or calcify [13]. The most usual tumour to do this is osteosarcoma (see Case 11). The other problem is a malignant lesion arising at the site of, or immediately adjacent to, a previously calcified lesion (such as an old TB focus). Moreover, in the case of multiple pulmonary nodules it is important to consider that a patient may have calcified granulomata and also have malignant metastatic deposits. The presence of calcium in one nodule is meaningless in regard to evaluation of a second nodule.

It is only if there is complete calcification of a nodule that the appearances are virtually diagnostic of a granuloma. Thus, in an area in which histoplasmosis does not occur, high CT numbers do not necessarily imply that the lesion is benign.

Ultrasound

As described in the first chapter, the use of ultrasound in the chest is limited to lesions that have an 'acoustic window'. Ultrasound, in the frequencies used for imaging, will not pass through air thus, if a pulmonary mass is to be studied by ultrasound, it must either abut the chest wall, mediastinum or diaphragm. If the lesion can be visualized, ultrasound may be useful by demonstrating whether the mass is cystic, solid or of mixed echogenicity (for example, necrotic tumour or abscess). Moreover, it is possible, using real-time scanning and Doppler, to demonstrate pulsation and blood flow. The use of ultrasound in the chest is, however, fraught with difficulty due to the limited access, and it must always be borne in mind that occasionally lesions shown to be 'cystic' by ultrasound criteria will turn out to be solid but homogeneous tumour.

Case 5

John R., aged 50, presented with a history of lassitude and slight weight loss over 1 year that, on careful questioning, had stabilized over the last few months. Chest radiographs, PA and right lateral, were performed.

Figure 5a

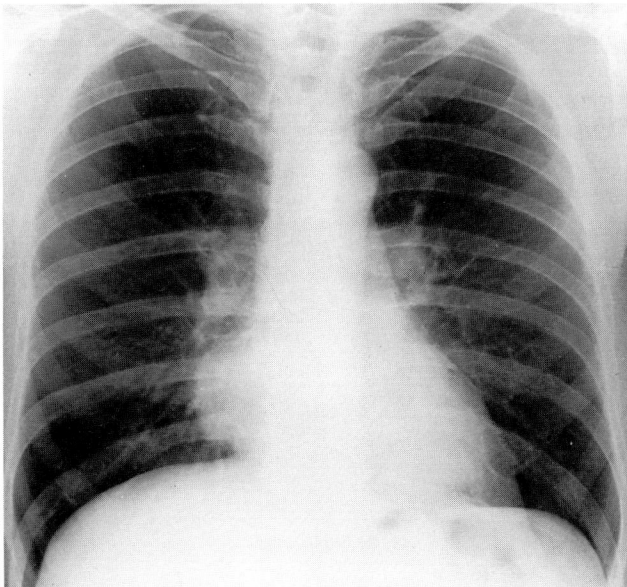

The PA chest film revealed an opacity obscuring the right heart border. The site was confirmed by the lateral film. On review of a chest radiograph of 1 year previously a small

Figure 5b

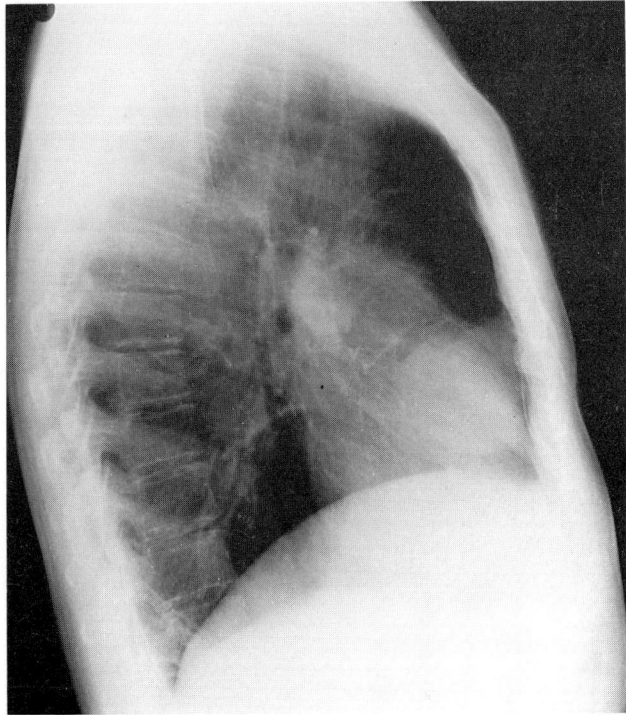

opacity was seen at the same site but there had been definite increase in size on the latest film. A diagnosis of bronchogenic carcinoma in the right middle lobe was considered. On further examination of the chest films it was, however, clear that the lesion could be mediastinal or cardiac in origin and ultrasound was thus undertaken prior to biopsy.

Real-time ultrasound (fig. 5c) showed the lesion to be immediately adjacent to the heart and transonic. Enhancement was present beyond the lesion. Doppler studies showed no flow in the lesion. It was thought initially that the opacity represented a pericardial or pleuropericardial cyst. Follow-up radiographs and ultrasound showed that the lesion was slowly growing and at surgery the opacity was found to be a haemangiopericytoma. *(Courtesy of Dr G Laszlo and Mr K Jeyasingham.)*

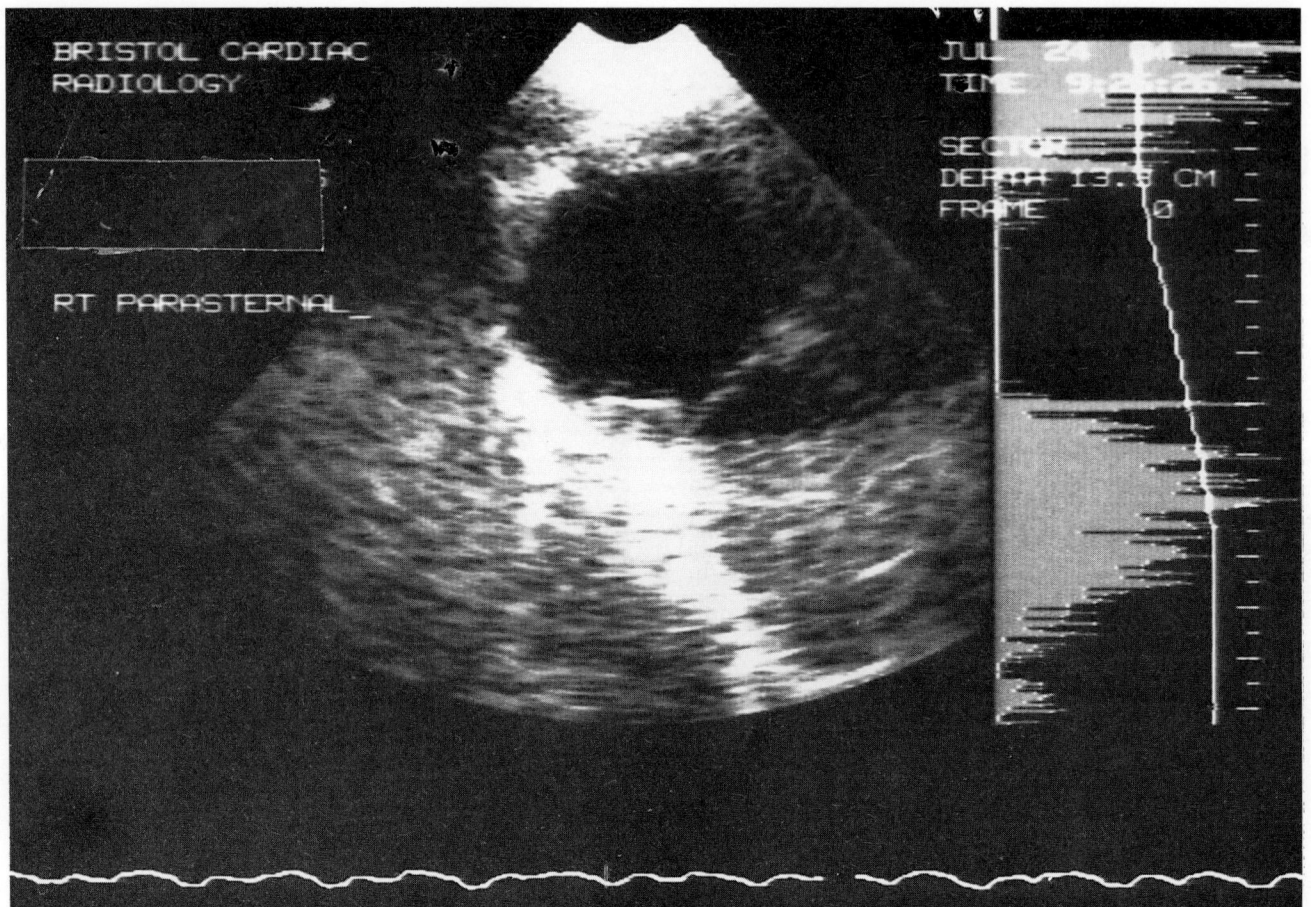

Figure 5c

Case 6

James B., aged 56, presented with a long history of mitral valve disease, and had the following chest radiographs (figs. 6a and 6b).

The heart is enlarged and has a straight left heart border due to left atrial enlargement. On the PA film a rounded opacity is seen in the right mid-zone and there is slight pleural reflection. On the lateral view the opacity is seen to be elliptical in shape and lies in the horizontal fissure.

Ultrasound of the pulmonary opacity showed it to be anechoic with distal enhancement. The pictures are not shown but were very similar to those seen in the last case.

A follow up chest x-ray was done after further diuretic therapy (fig. 6c).

The opacity is much smaller confirming the diagnosis of encysted effusion.

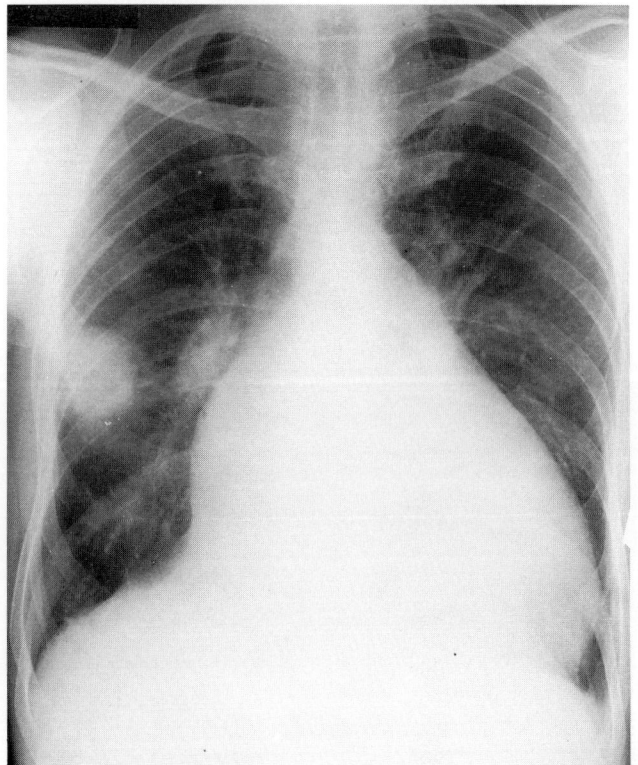

Figure 6a

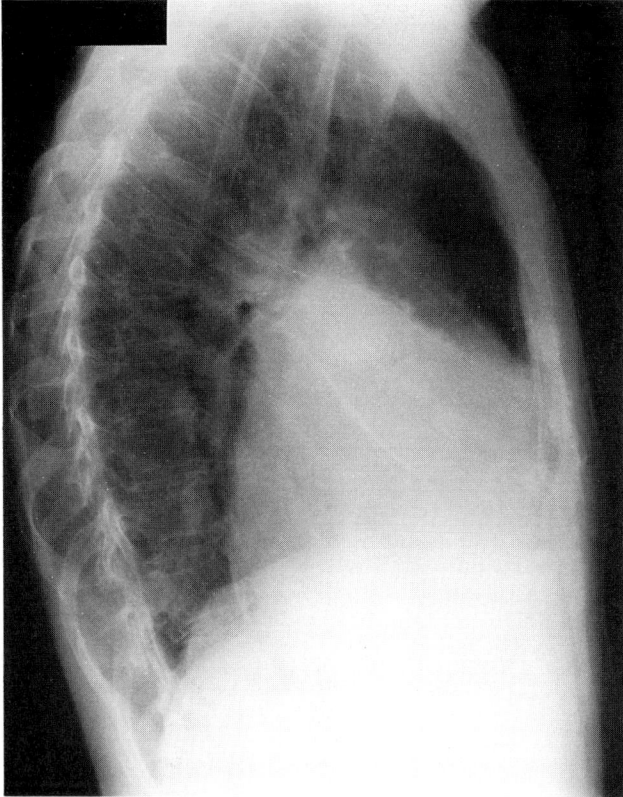

Figure 6b

Figure 6c

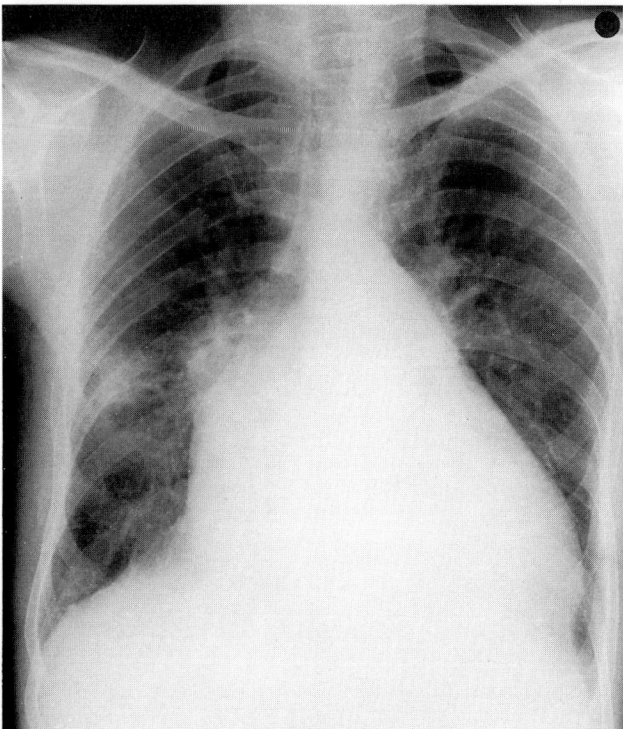

Angiography of pulmonary masses

If an arteriovenous malformation or other vascular lesion is suspected from chest radiography and tomography but some doubt remains, confirmation by pulmonary angiography can be helpful. Other methods of diagnosis include digital vascular imaging (DVI) and CT with contrast medium injection and rapid sequential scanning.

Case 7

Heather, a 13 year old girl, presented slightly short of breath and with recurrent bronchitis. A soft systolic murmur was noted.

Figure 7a

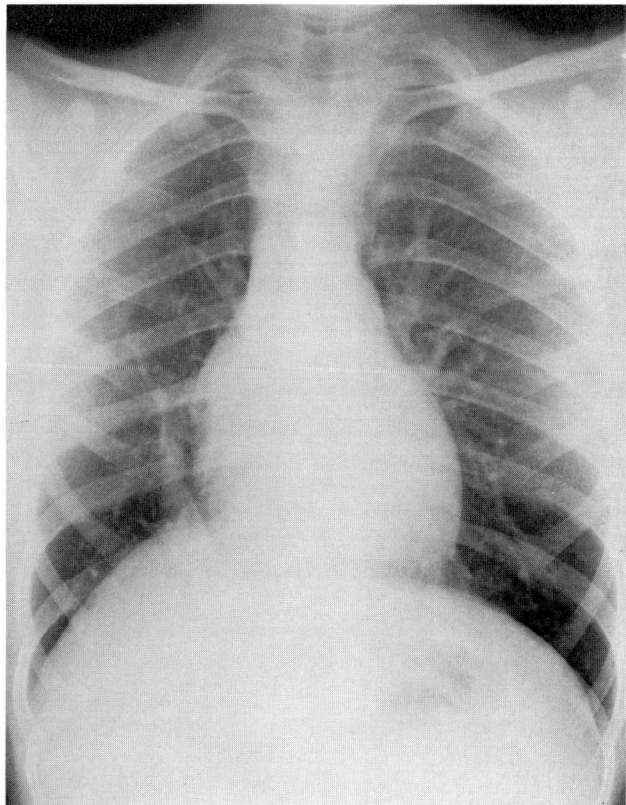

The chest x-ray showed a linear opacity in the right lower zone. The right hilar vessels were small. A pulmonary angiogram was done and a subtraction film of the venous phase is shown.

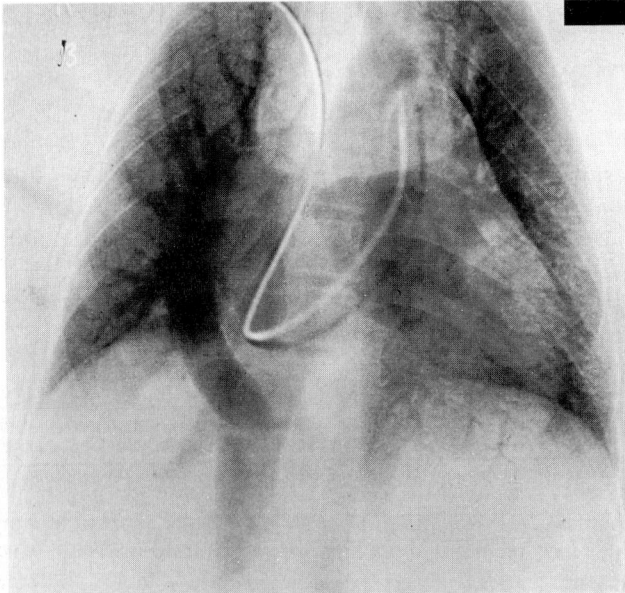

Figure 7b

This shows an anomalous vein draining the whole of the right lung into the inferior vena cava. This is an example of partial anomalous venous drainage and this particular configuration is known as the 'scimitar syndrome' [14].

Aortography (fig. 7c) shows a small aberrant vessel supplying the medial basal segment of the right lower lobe. This segment is sequestrated.

Figure 7c

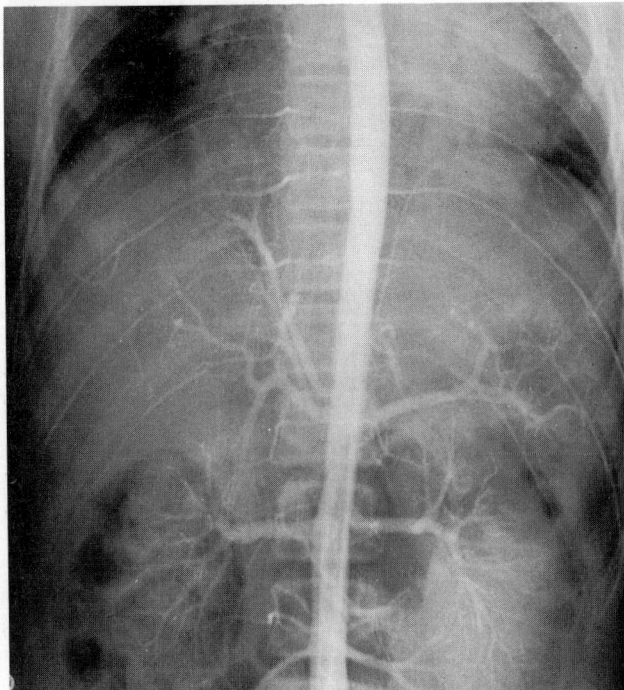

Case 8 (*Courtesy of Dr P Wilde*)

A woman with mitral valve disease was admitted for cardiac catheterization and angiography.

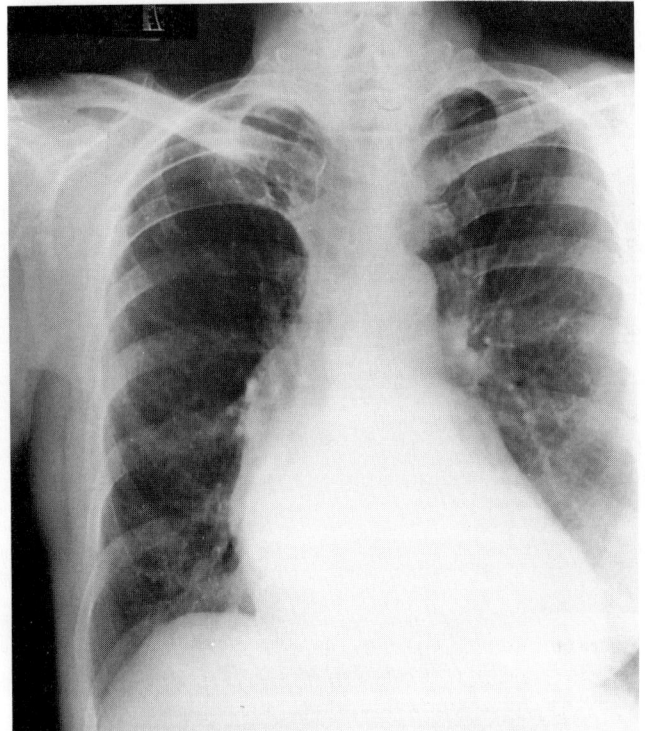

Figure 8a

Figure 8b

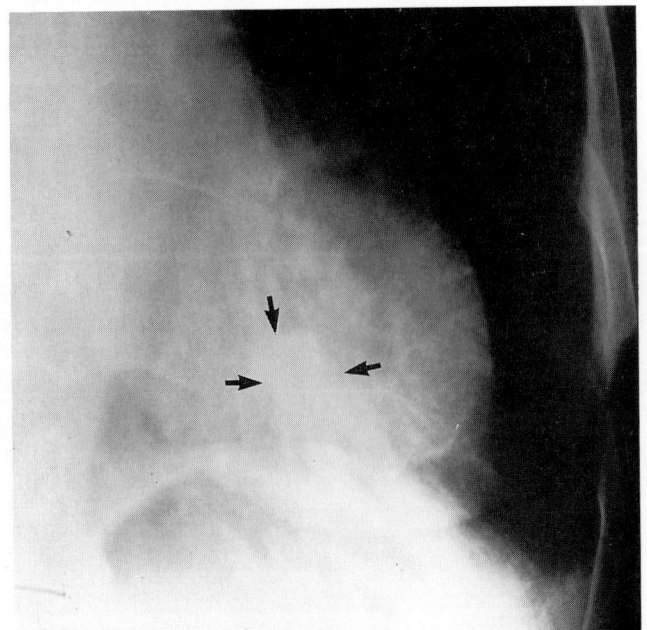

Bronchoscopy and mediastinoscopy

The development of the flexible bronchoscope has considerably extended the role of bronchoscopy. Segmental and subsegmental bronchi may be visualized. With the use of biopsy brush or forceps diagnostic material can usually be obtained from centrally placed lesions.

If enlarged mediastinal nodes are present in addition to a pulmonary mass, it may be sensible to sample the nodes first. If the pulmonary mass is biopsied first and a diagnosis of malignancy made, it will not be known whether the nodes are involved or the changes are reactive. This may be important in deciding upon management, e.g. involved nodes may render the patient inoperable. Performing mediastinoscopy first may give this information. If the results are negative, the lung lesion may still be biopsied.

If mediastinoscopy is contemplated, it is useful to detail the exact sites of abnormal lymph nodes in the mediastinum. This may be done by CT. On computed tomography, most normal mediastinal nodes are less than 1 cm in diameter. If a node is greater than 1.5 cm, it should be considered as abnormal [15]. In order to distinguish vascular structures from nodes, intravenous contrast medium is used. Most commonly a bolus technique is employed using an 18-gauge needle in the medial antecubital vein. Aberrant vessels in the mediastinum should be remembered and not confused with nodes, e.g. aberrant subclavian artery, persistent left SVC (see Case 110). Thus, it is important to follow any unusual structure on contiguous scans and to use IV contrast medium if in doubt. Transcervical mediastinoscopy obtains biopsy samples from the pretracheal nodes. If the abnormal nodes are shown to be anteriorly placed and hence away from the pretracheal region, mediastinotomy may be necessary. Conversely, reports would indicate that mediastinoscopy or mediastinotomy are unnecessary when the mediastinum appears tumour-free on CT [16, 17].

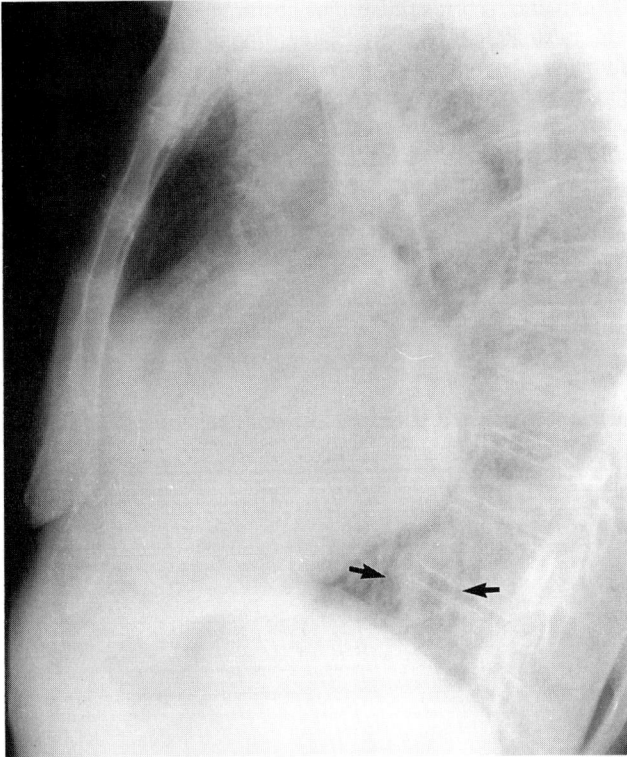

Figure 8c

The PA and lateral chest x-rays showed an enlarged heart with a prominent atrial appendage. They also revealed an opacity behind the heart (*arrowed*). The opacity was ill-defined and was situated in the left lower lobe.

At angiography an aberrant vessel was seen to supply the mass from the aorta (*open arrows*, fig. 8d)

The opacity was therefore diagnosed as a sequestrated segment. (See also Case 28.)

Figure 8d

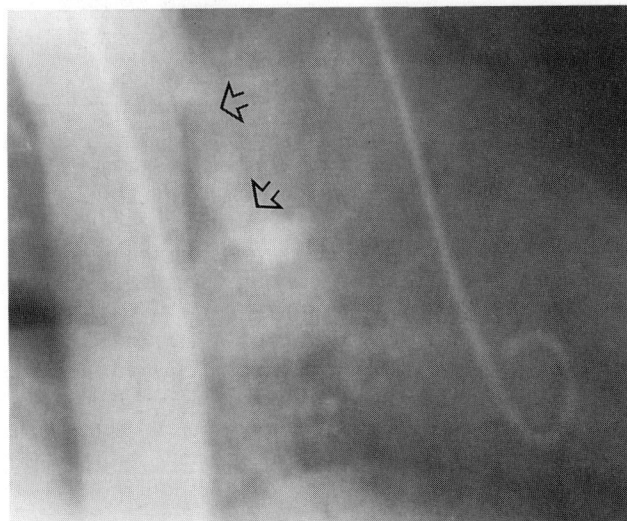

Case 9

Andrew D., 56 years of age, and previously a smoker, presented with a history of breathlessness. On auscultation there were fine mid and late inspiratory crepitations. Spirometry revealed a restrictive defect, decrease in lung volume and markedly impaired carbon monoxide transfer

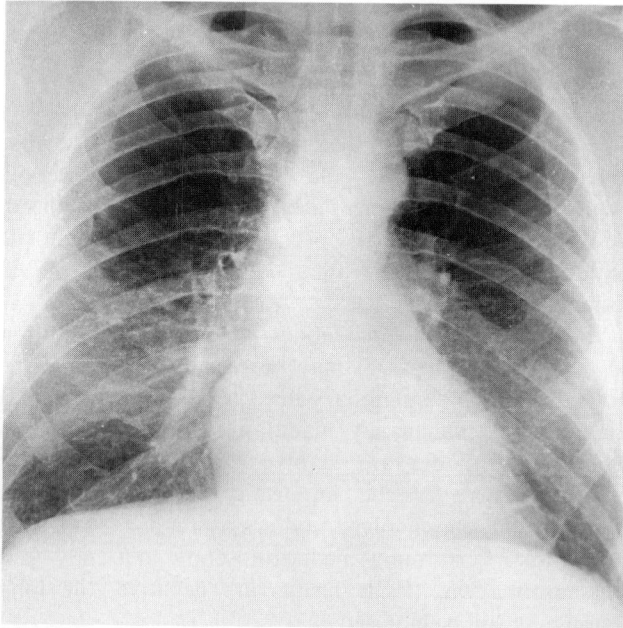

Figure 9a

factor. Routine biochemical and haematological tests were normal. The chest x-ray is shown (fig. 9a).

Chest x-ray showed reduced vascularity in upper zones and reticulonodular shadows in lower zones. The history and investigations were considered consistent with cryptogenic fibrosing alveolitis.

Two years later the patient presented with haemoptysis and worsening of his breathlessness. A further radiograph was performed (fig. 9b).

Figure 9b

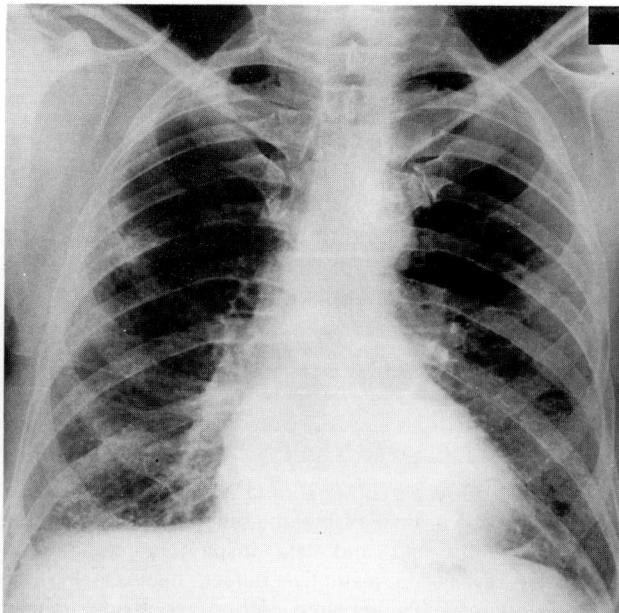

Ventilation/perfusion studies at the time showed matched and mismatched defects. Such findings are common in fibrosing alveolitis and probably account for the decreased carbon monoxide transfer factor and the hypoxia. The chest x-ray was unchanged apart from further opacification in the right mid to upper zone.

CT was performed in view of the possibility of carcinoma.

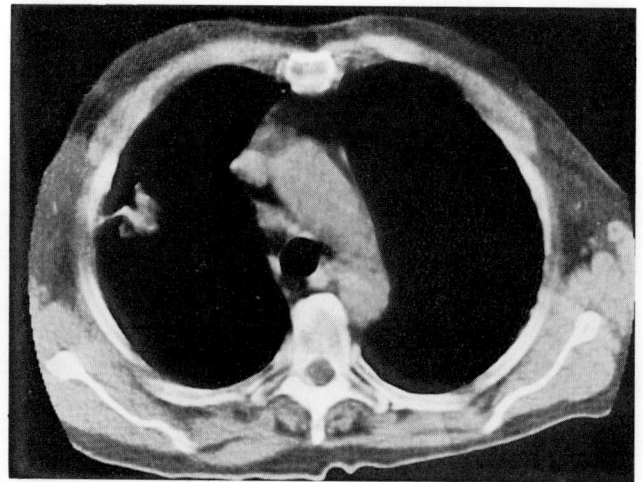

Figure 9c
Figure 9d

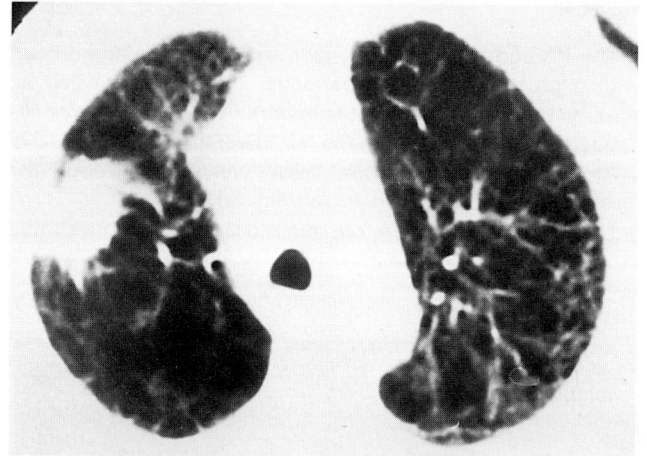

CT shows a large mass in the right lung field, containing slight calcification. In the area in front of the trachea and between the SVC and aorta, there is an enlarged lymph node (nodes in this site should not be more than 1.5 cm in diameter) and enlarged nodes are also present on the immediately inferior scans.

In the upper zones there is emphysema and in the lower zones there is, bilaterally, a 'honeycomb' pattern of cystic holes due to fibrosing alveolitis. Carcinoma of the bronchus is more common in fibrosing lung conditions. In this case the nodes were biopsied by mediastinoscopy and found to invade the wall of the trachea. Histology showed adenocarcinoma.

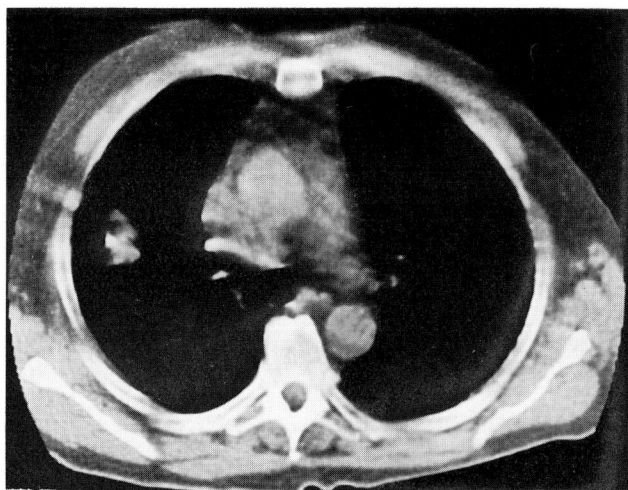

Figure 9e

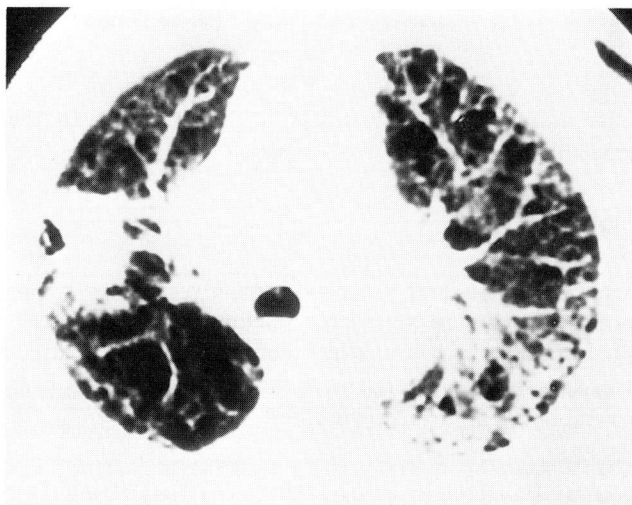

Figure 9f

Figure 9g

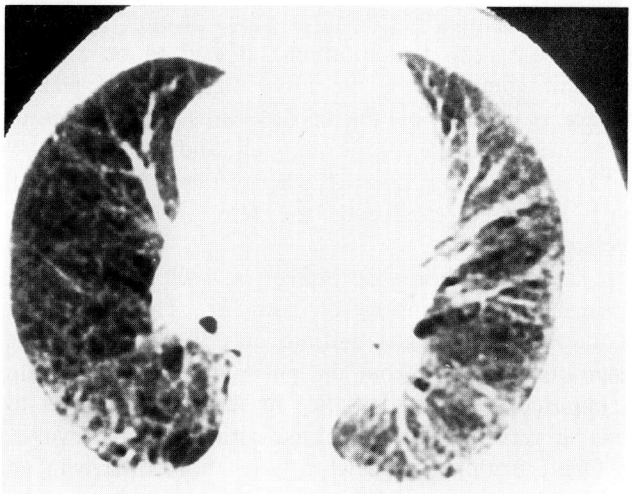

Needle biopsy

The main indication for performing needle biopsy is an undiagnosed pulmonary mass or nodule. Needle biopsy is easiest when the lesion is peripherally positioned. If there is consolidation present, this may be distal to a lesion and it may thus be difficult to decide upon the best biopsy site. Centrally placed lesions are often best biopsied using the flexible bronchoscope.

A chest radiograph should always be performed within the 24 hours before the procedure since the mass may well have changed. It may even have disappeared! As discussed at the beginning of this chapter, it is mandatory to find any previous chest films for comparison.

The procedure may be performed on an out-patient basis but always with the proviso that a bed must be available if admission is necessary due to complications. A simple check on the respiratory function is useful. The simplest method is to enquire whether the patient can climb stairs. If respiratory function is significantly impaired, then full respiratory function studies should be performed and overnight hospital care arranged prospectively.

Contraindications

Contraindications to lung biopsy include uncorrectable bleeding tendency, a possible vascular lesion or an echinococcal cyst, uncontrollable cough or inability of the patient to cooperate for some other reason. In patients with severe bullous emphysema, with widespread fibrosis, or on mechanical ventilation the risk of pneumothorax is greater. Lung biopsy is contraindicated if the patient has respiratory functional impairment such that a pneumothorax could not be tolerated [17]. Cavitating lung lesions can be more difficult to biopsy satisfactorily than solid masses.

Apparatus

The biopsy apparatus available must include the biopsy needle, syringe, local anaesthetic, glass slides, formal saline and specimen pots. Full resuscitation equipment is essential and should include chest drains. The Heimlich valve and narrow gauge tubing were commonly used in the USA.

There are many different needles including the Greene needle, the Franseen needle and the Nordenstrom needle. One particular warning regarding the selection of needles· is that, if the biopsy site is likely to be near vascular structures, one should avoid using a core-type needle (i.e. a needle that removes a core of tissue). Bleeding from a puncture in a pulmonary vessel is not usually a problem when a narrow gauge needle has been used but, if a core of tissue had been taken from the vessel wall, the haemorrhage could be catastrophic [18]. The needle used should theoretically be the smallest, most flexible needle that will do the job. It is best to select one favourite needle and learn to use it well.

Technique

Biplane or C-arm screening is first used to check the position of the mass and to mark the skin. Local anaesthetic is infiltrated into the subcutaneous tissues and intercostal muscles at the site for insertion of the biopsy needle. It is important that the injection of local anaesthetic should be sufficiently deep that the biopsy is painless but also that penetration through the pleura should be avoided if possible since this will increase the risk of pneumothorax. The position for insertion of the biopsy needle should again be checked by screening. If the position of the mass for biopsy appears to be considerably different despite the patient not having moved, this could be due to a pneumothorax resulting from the local anaesthetic injection. If the position is accurate, a scalpel blade is used to pierce the skin. The biopsy needle is held in position using forceps and screened to check that it is directly over the lesion. The needle is advanced using biplane screening until correctly sited in the lesion. The stilette is removed and a finger put over the end because of the theoretical risk of air embolus into a pulmonary blood vessel. A connecting tube may now be connected with a 20-ml syringe, or alternatively the syringe may be connected directly to the needle. Hard suction is applied whilst moving the needle up and down in a jogging motion. The needle is withdrawn with the suction released. Slides are then made of the aspirate and any tissue put into saline. Another two passes may be performed.

Modification of technique

Percutaneous needle biopsy is usually performed under fluoroscopic control. In certain circumstances computed tomography (CT) can be useful. CT can either be used to assist in planning biopsies that will be performed under fluoroscopic control, or it can be used instead of fluoroscopy as the method of guidance of the needle. Professor Gamsu considers CT-guided aspiration biopsy

of the thorax to be helpful when the type, size or position of the lesion makes fluoroscopic guidance of the needle unreliable [19]. The lesions thus biopsied are usually not amenable to biplane fluoroscopy, for example, lesions in or adjacent to the mediastinum or hila, peripheral lesions, and small or ill-defined lesions such as cavitating masses.

Cytology

The slides are taken straight to the cytopathologist. The biopsy should be repeated if the results are not conclusive. The immediate access to cytology is essential in order that the patient does not have to return to the department. There will be considerable inconvenience to the patient if asked to return, and loss of confidence. There is often impatience on the part of the clinicians if the result is negative and must be repeated. This impatience may well lead to too many open biopsies being performed. Therefore it is necessary to obtain as much information as possible at the first visit to the department.

Follow-up

A chest x-ray is performed immediately after the needle biopsy in order to look for a pneumothorax. A further film is done 4 hours after the biopsy. The delay is necessary since a pneumothorax may develop even several hours after the procedure.

Complications and their management

The most common complication is pneumothorax, occurring between 10 and 50 per cent in different series with most centres reporting a rate of around 25 to 35 per cent [20–22]. Pneumothorax is said to be a more common complication the more frequently a pleural surface is crossed by the needle. Thus the number of passes should be kept to a minimum and one should try to avoid crossing fissures whenever practicable [18]. With increased experience the rate of complications decreases [23].

If a pneumothorax is present, it will need a chest drain in only a minority of cases [22]. The practice in many centres is to use a drain only if the patient has respiratory distress from the pneumothorax. If a drain is required, it is the practice in the United States to insert a very narrow tube fitted with a Heimlich valve. In Great Britain a somewhat larger bore tube with an underwater seal would be more commonly used.

If a pneumothorax occurs whilst the biopsy is being performed, it is not necessarily a reason to abandon the investigation. In fact it is probably in the patient's best interests to proceed with further passes of the needle until diagnostic material is obtained, since the most common complication has already taken place.

The other important complication is haemorrhage. It is a sensible precaution when planning the biopsy to aim such that large pulmonary vessels are avoided. When the lesion is centrally positioned it is advisable to use only an aspiration technique. Central lesions should, as discussed above, be preferentially biopsied by bronchoscopy.

Summary: the pulmonary mass or nodule

There are many causes of a solitary pulmonary mass. Having discovered an opacity on a chest radiograph, if there are previous films, they should be examined to determine whether or not the lesion is significant. A lateral chest x-ray is required to show the site of the mass. There may be clinical pointers to the cause of the mass and laboratory investigations should be considered, including serology for various precipitating antibodies and sputum for cytology and culture.

Computed tomography, if available, is useful for analysis of the characteristics of the lesion with regard to the site, size, shape, density and vascularity. CT may also show further unsuspected pulmonary nodules or enlarged mediastinal nodes.

If there is a single central lesion, bronchoscopy and transbronchial biopsy may be indicated but, if the lesion is peripheral, percutaneous needle biopsy may provide the answer. Thoracotomy may be necessary if the aforementioned investigations do not provide the diagnosis or if at any stage the investigations indicate that surgical removal of the opacity would be the best treatment.

3 | Multiple coin lesions

Many of the causes of a solitary, well defined mass (listed in Table 2) can also result in multiple opacities. However, some conditions more commonly give rise to multiple lesions than others. The list of differential diagnoses is given in Table 3.

Table 3 Multiple pulmonary 'coin' lesions

Common
1 Metastatic deposits
2 Abscesses
3 Rheumatoid nodules
4 Granulomata—histoplasmosis is a common cause of nodules in the USA

Less common
1 Infarcts
2 Sarcoidosis
3 Haematomata
4 Lymphoma
5 Tuberculosis

Rare
1 Multiple arteriovenous malformations
2 Hydatid (common in some countries)
3 Amyloidosis
4 Wegener's granulomatosis

Metastatic deposits are by far the most common cause of multiple pulmonary nodules in patients in Great Britain but this is not the case everywhere. As mentioned in Chapter 2, histoplasmosis is endemic in some parts of the United States of America and multiple lesions due to this condition may be more common than those due to malignancy.

In certain circumstances the likelihood of nodules being malignant may be so high that no further diagnostic investigation may be required. In Great Britain, for example, if a patient has a known malignancy with a predilection for metastasizing to the lungs and presents with multiple pulmonary nodules greater than 1 cm in size, they will almost certainly be secondary deposits.

If, however, any doubt remains, it is important to investigate the patient carefully so that a diagnosis of terminal disease is not wrongly given to a patient with a potentially curable condition.

The flow chart for the diagnosis of a single pulmonary mass should again be examined (page 7). Many of the investigations and comments pertain when dealing with multiple 'coin' lesions although the emphasis is different. Access to previous films may prove invaluable since lesions that are unchanged over many years are unlikely to be malignant. Laboratory investigations may be helpful, including blood culture in case the lesions are abscesses, and serology should be undertaken for rheumatoid factor and to look for antibodies to histoplasmosis and to hydatid. In some cases it may be necessary to do the Kveim test for sarcoidosis and Heaf test for tuberculosis.

At some stage it may be useful to examine the liver using one of the imaging techniques, ultrasound, CT or scintigraphy, whichever is best performed in the particular hospital. If the liver is found to be packed with metastatic deposits, there will be little point in proceeding further! In the final analysis, if the diagnosis has not been made, a biopsy may be required. Percutaneous needle biopsy may be a sensible examination in order to obtain a tissue diagnosis.

If the lesions are found by biopsy to be malignant but there is no known primary, a search for the primary may be undertaken. It must be stated at this point that this is frequently a futile exercise, and once histological proof of malignancy is obtained from the pulmonary opacities (by one of the methods described in the previous chapter) then it may be wise to treat symptomatically. If histology or cytology is obtained, it may give a pointer to the site of the primary. Very often, however, the findings are vague as to the origin of the malignancy. A cytology or histology report of 'poorly differentiated malignant cells of uncertain origin' is not uncommon. Routine clinical tests should be performed, including urine testing for blood and palpation of the thyroid and abdomen. Almost all malignant neoplasms may metastasize to the lungs especially if the terminal phase is included. Some malignancies more commonly give rise to pulmonary metastases and this may occur before metastases are apparent in other sites such as bone or liver. This list would include:

Primary neoplasia with predilection for pulmonary metastastases

1 Renal cell carcinoma

2 Thyroid carcinoma

3 Teratoma/seminoma

4 Chorion epithelioma

5 Osteosarcoma

6 Nephroblastoma (Wilms' tumour).

7 Carcinoma of the breast

8 Carcinoma of the bronchus

Carcinoma of the breast and of the bronchus have been included because, although lymph node and bone metastases usually occur before pulmonary metastases, they are such common tumours that pulmonary deposits from these tumours will frequently be seen.

Computed tomography is often used as a staging procedure for a variety of malignancies including testicular tumours, osteosarcoma and bronchogenic carcinoma. Smaller nodules can be detected using CT than using either plain radiography or whole lung tomography (see Chapter 2 page 8). As discussed above the discovery of multiple lesions raises considerably the likelihood that the lesions are secondary deposits.

Scintigraphy is sometimes useful in malignant disease by demonstrating specific uptake in pulmonary nodules. Thus osteosarcoma metastases, being bone-forming, may take up bone-scanning radiopharmaceuticals containing phosphate. Radioactive iodine is avidly sequestered by some pulmonary metastatic deposits from thyroid carcinoma. There is uptake of gallium in a large number of inflammatory and neoplastic conditions but uptake occurs particularly in abscesses, lymphoma and sarcoidosis.

New scintigraphic methods for showing malignant disease are being developed. Monoclonal antibodies have been raised against antigens that are found on tumours ranging from ovarian carcinoma and seminoma to oat cell carcinoma and neuroblastoma.

Case 10

A girl with an osteosarcoma in the left tibia was treated by excision and prosthesis. A follow-up chest x-ray was done (fig. 10a) and a radioisotope bone scan (figs. 10b and 10c).

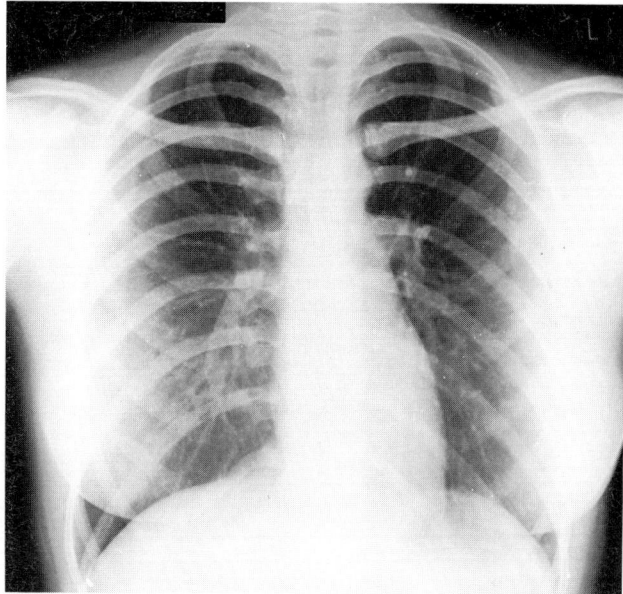

Figure 10a

The chest x-ray was reported as normal. The bone scans (fig. 10b, anterior, fig. 10c, posterior) showed uptake over the posterior end of a right rib and in the right sacroiliac region. Plain films and computed tomography showed recurrence of osteosarcoma in the right sacroiliac region. Computed tomography of the chest showed three small nodules. Emission computed tomography of the bone scan was performed to determine the site of the right chest lesion since a pulmonary metastatic deposit had not been identified at that site.

The emission CT of the bone scan showed uptake of MDP just lateral and to the right of the vertebral body. A repeat CT scan was performed (fig. 10e) and overlay of the emission CT image on the computed tomograms showed the lesion to be a large intrapulmonary deposit previously mistaken for a blood vessel (fig. 10f). There is also a small nodule anteriorly in the left lung (fig. 10e) which is a metastatic deposit.

This is an example of computed tomography showing several metastatic deposits that were not visible on the chest x-ray and the value of the bone scan in both showing the recurrence of the osteosarcoma and in demonstrating an intrapulmonary deposit.

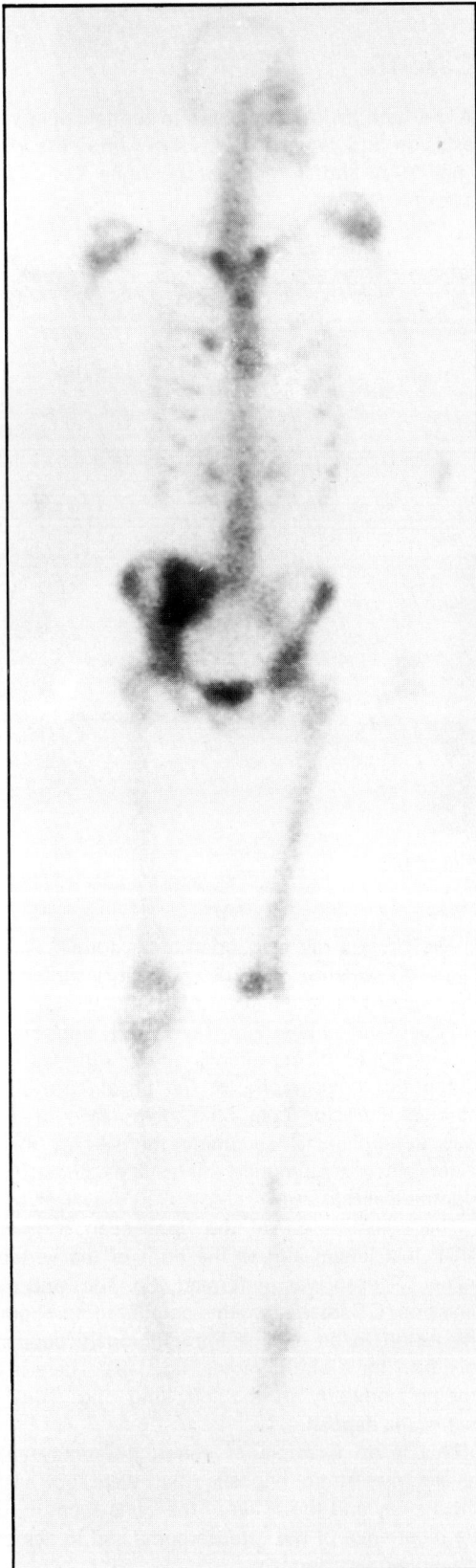

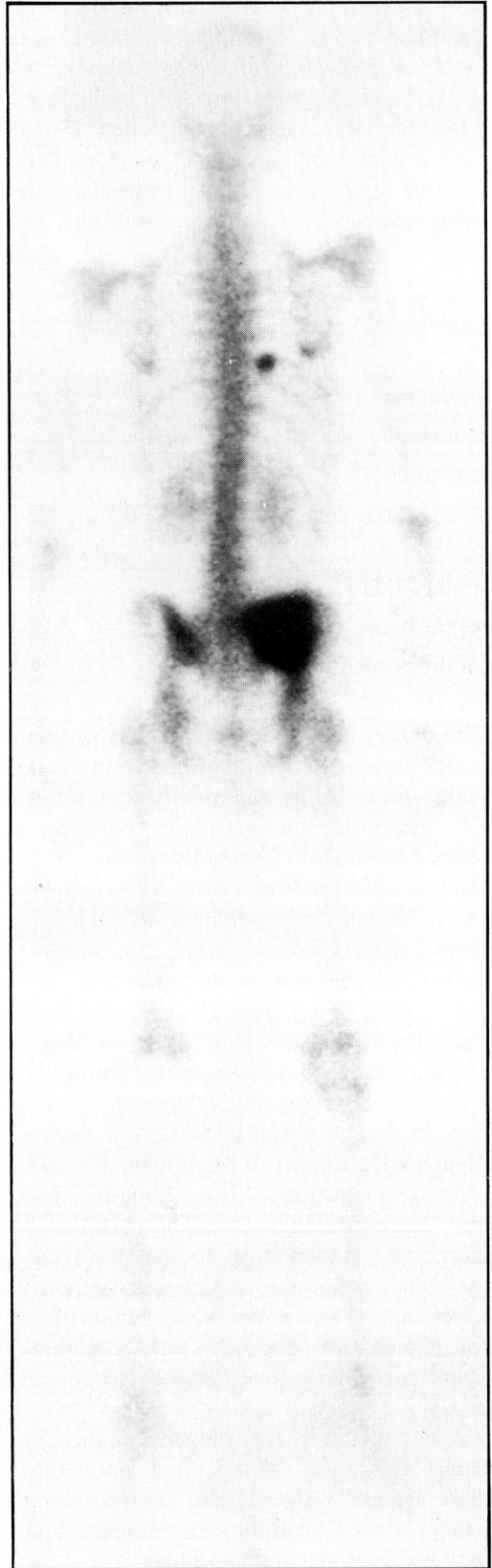

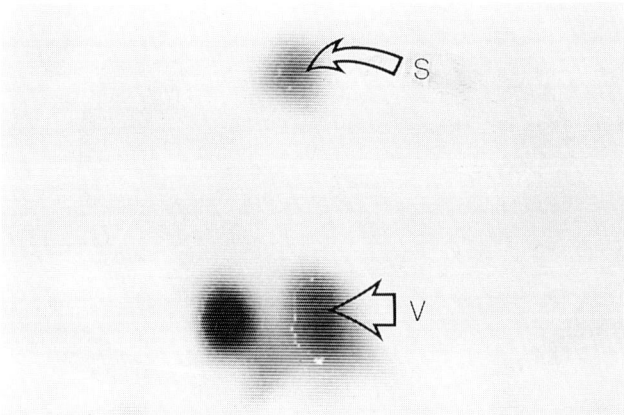

Figure 10d (S = sternum, V = vertebral body)

Figure 10e

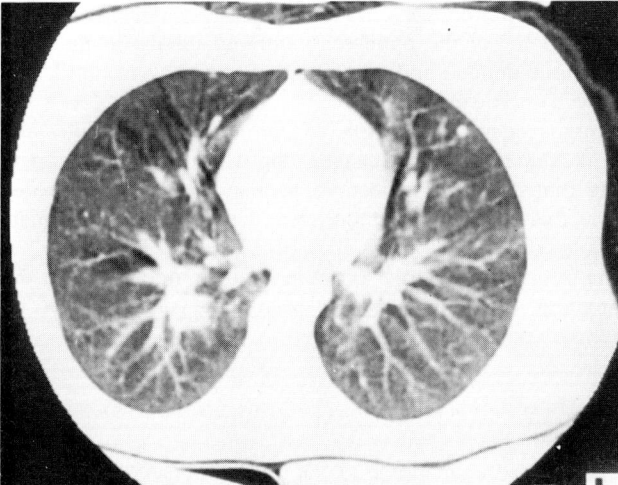

Figure 10f

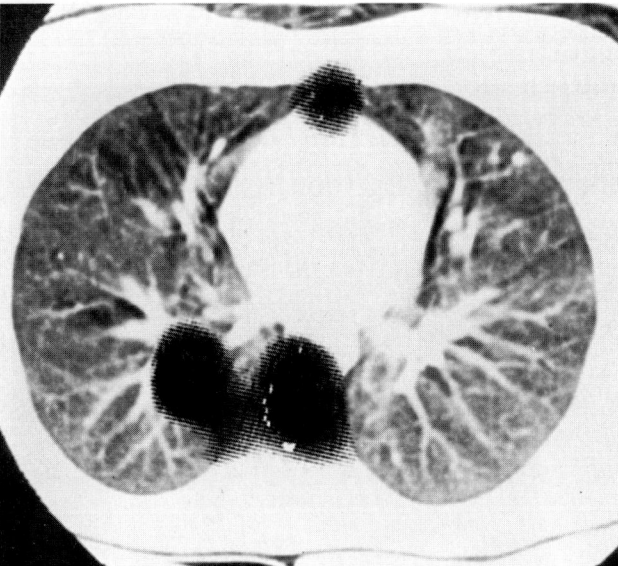

Case 11

This is a similar case to the last one. A girl with osteosarcoma of the left femur had been treated with excision of the affected bone and prosthesis. Chest x-rays, PA and lateral, were done.

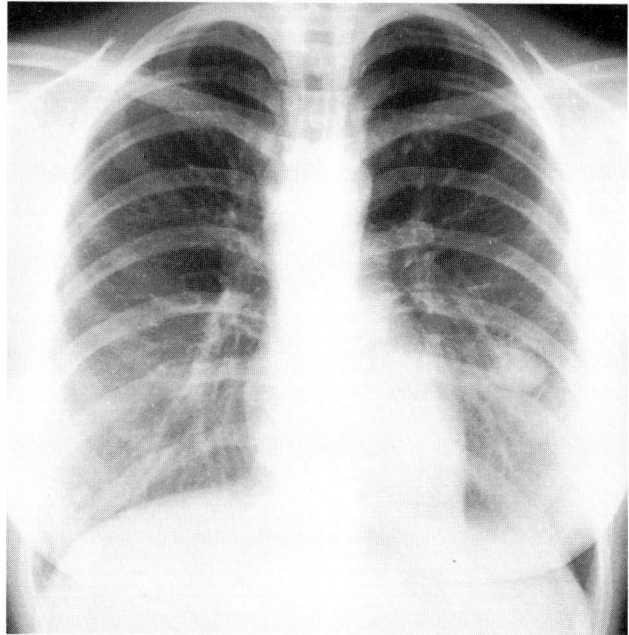

Figure 11a

Figure 11b

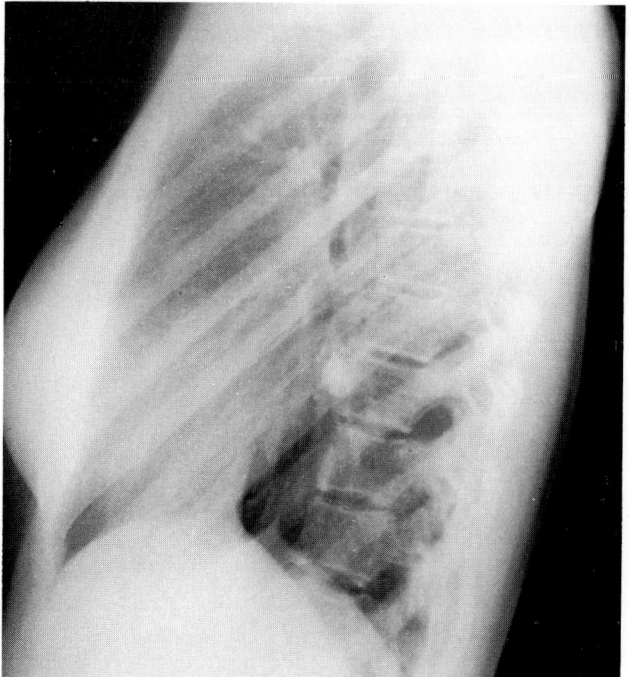

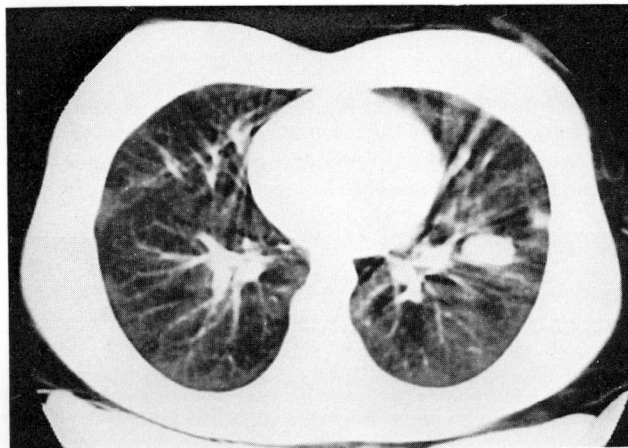

Figure 11c

Figure 11d

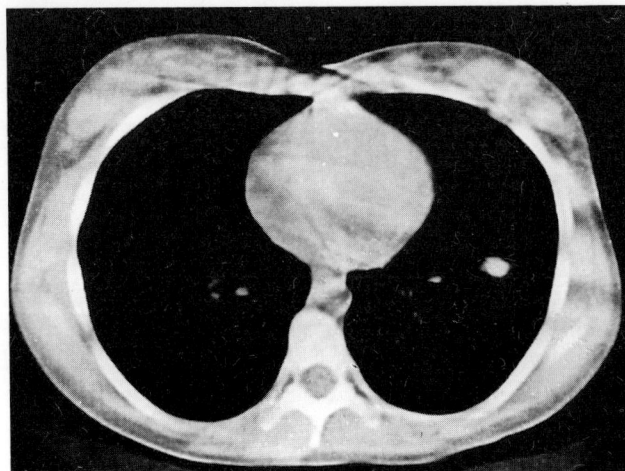

Figure 11e

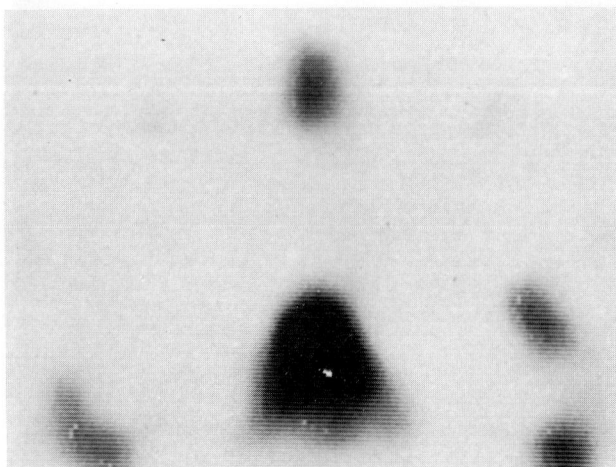

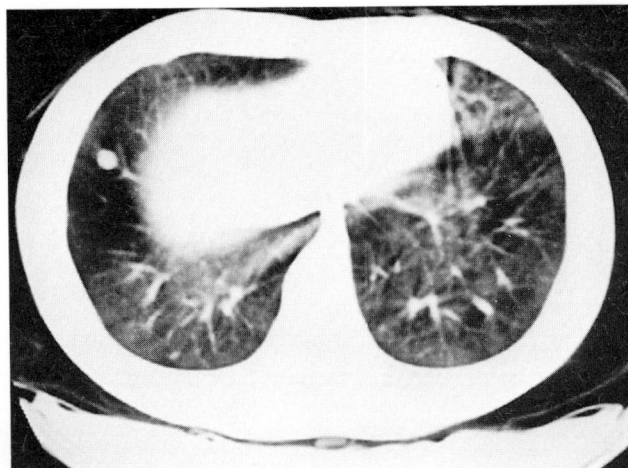

Figure 11f

One large dense opacity was seen in the left lung fields. CT was performed and showed several metastases. Emission CT of the bone scan showed uptake in the large metastatic deposit and computed tomography of that lesion showed it to be ossified.

This is again an example of computed tomography and bone scan showing metastatic deposits. It is interesting to note that the large metastatic deposit was heavily ossified since this is a demonstration that calcium in a pulmonary nodule does not prove that the lesion is benign. A discussion of the role of computed tomography in the detection of calcification in pulmonary nodules can be found on page 14 in Chapter 2.

Case 12

A patient with carcinoma of the thyroid presented with pain in the left hip.

A radiograph of the pelvis (fig. 12a) revealed a large lytic lesion destroying the left ilium. CT showed the lesion and

Figure 12a

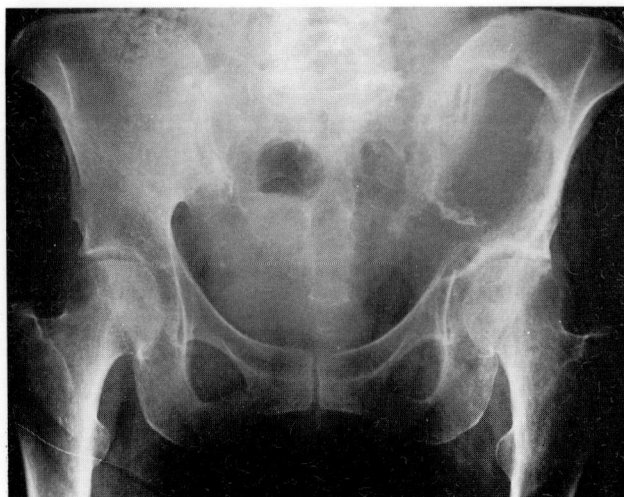

its associated large soft tissue component. The appearances were typical of a slow growing metastatic deposit (fig. 12b).

Figure 12b

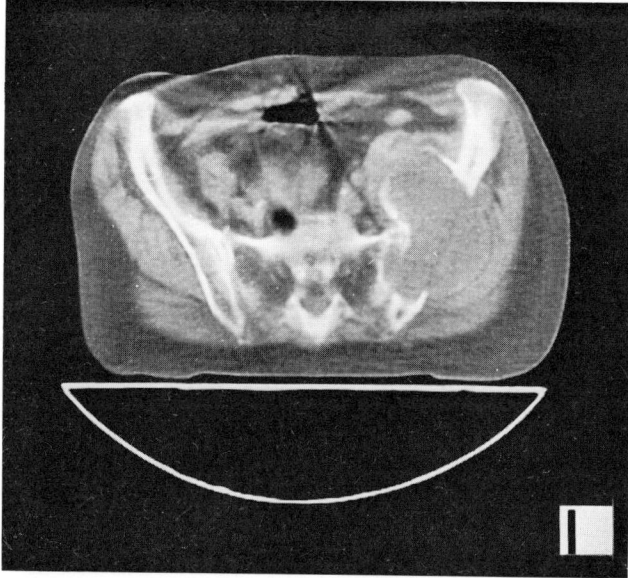

Chest x-ray (fig. 12c) showed several pulmonary nodules and radioisotope scan (fig. 12d) confirmed that these were metastatic deposits from thyroid carcinoma.

Figure 12c

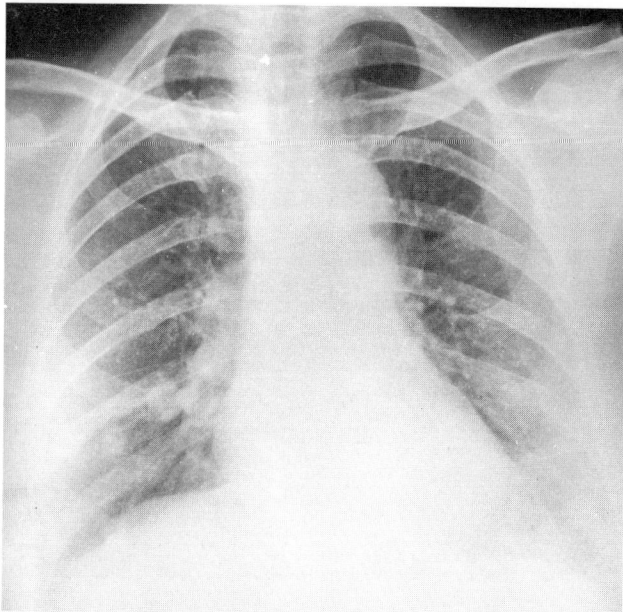

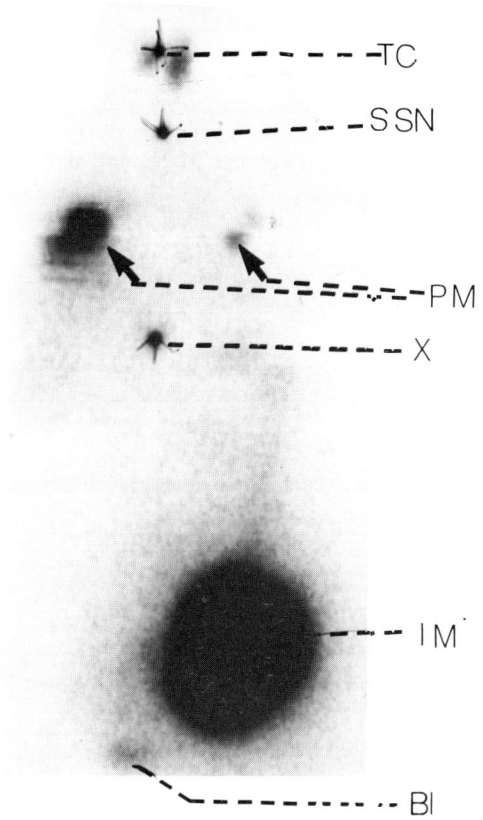

Figure 12d Key: TC: marker on thyroid cartilage, SSN: marker on suprasternal notch, PM: pulmonary metastatic deposits, X: xiphisternum marker, IM: iliac metastatic deposit, BL: bladder

Case 13

A man was found to have multiple opacities on computed tomography whilst being investigated for suspected malignancy. The opacities were subsequently shown to be

Figure 13a

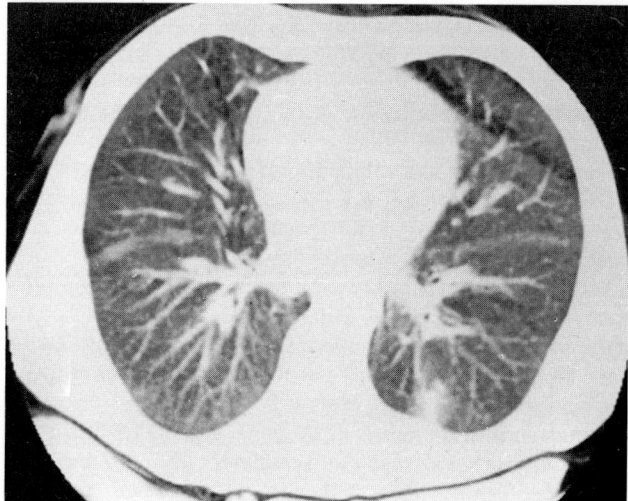

due to pulmonary infarcts due to emboli from deep vein thromboses. Note that the opacities are all peripherally positioned and rather ill defined. These appearances should be compared with cases 10 and 11 in which the metastatic deposits are better defined. It is, however, possible to have metastatic deposits that look almost exactly like the infarcts shown in this case.

Figure 13b

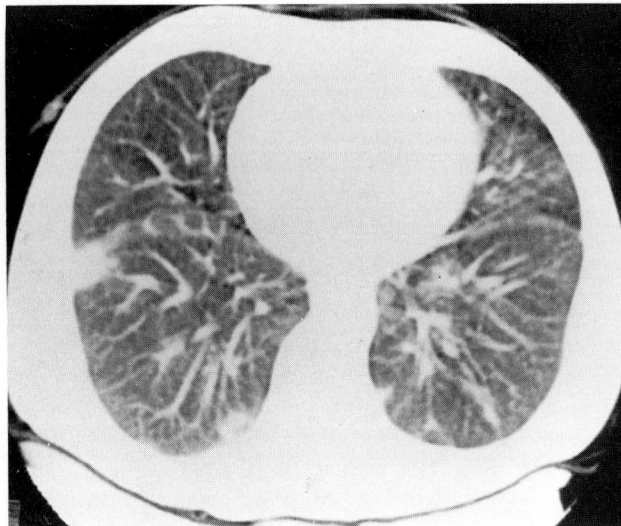

Figure 14a

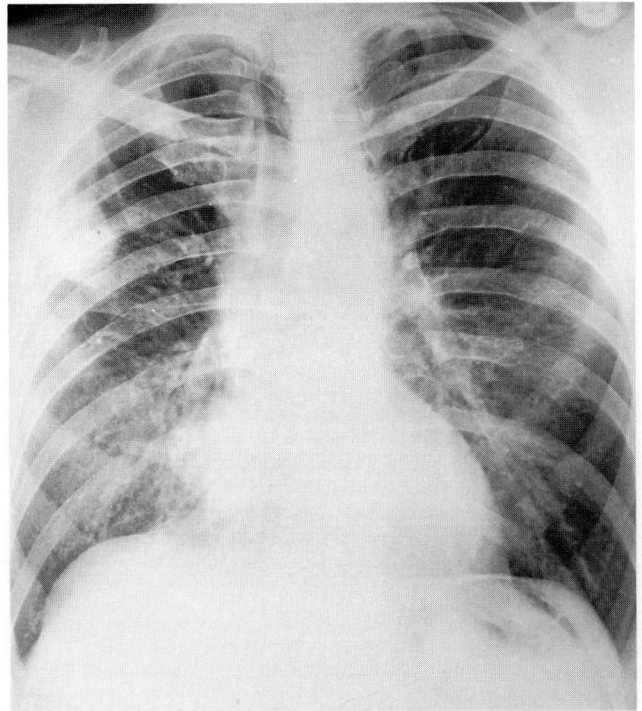

Figure 14b

Case 14 (*Courtesy of Dr G Laszlo*)

Frank, aged 63, presented with diplopia, and orbital swelling. On examination there was marked proptosis of the right eye and mucosal swelling in the nasal cavity. He had also recently developed chest pain. His chest x-ray and CT of the orbits are shown in figures 14a and 14b.

The chest radiograph shows an opacity in the right mid to upper zone and a further lesion immediately adjacent to the right heart border.

The CT scan of the orbits shows a normal left orbit but on the right side the eyeball is considerably displaced forwards by a mass of soft tissue density. There is also swelling of the surrounding soft tissues.

Thoracotomy was performed and the right mid-zone lung lesion was removed. Biopsy showed this to be granulomatous tissue. The right orbit and the turbinates were biopsied several times but the histology only showed non-specific inflammatory tissue.

A presumptive diagnosis of Wegener's granulomatosis (or a close variant) was made and treatment with steroids and cyclophosphamide was instigated. The orbital swelling disappeared and the second pulmonary mass also resolved.

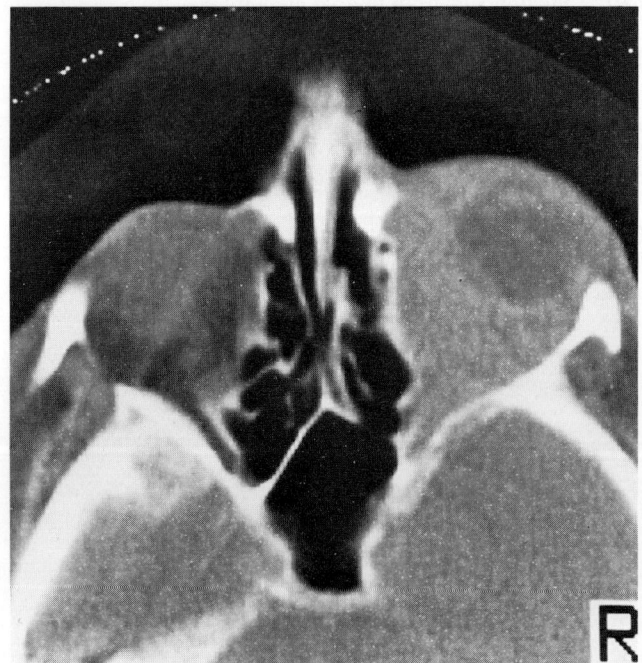

A repeat chest radiograph some months later (fig. 14c) shows signs of the right thoracotomy with a segment of rib missing and scarring in the right mid to upper zone. The right lower zone lesion has disappeared and there is also slight fibrosis in the left mid to upper zone laterally.

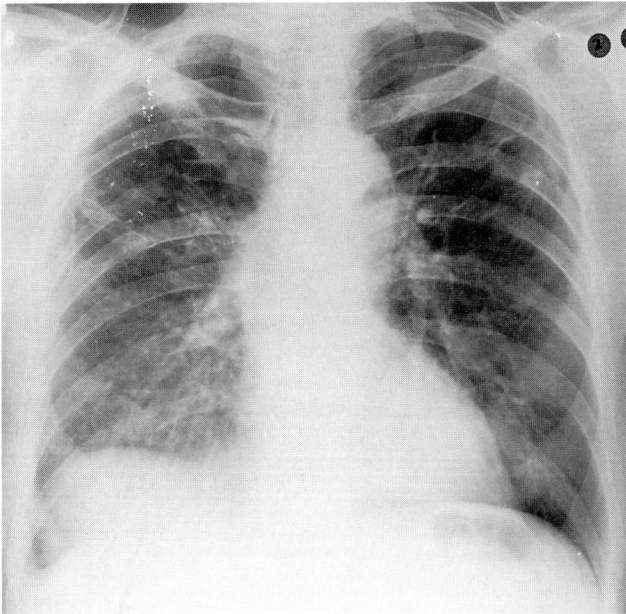

Figure 14c

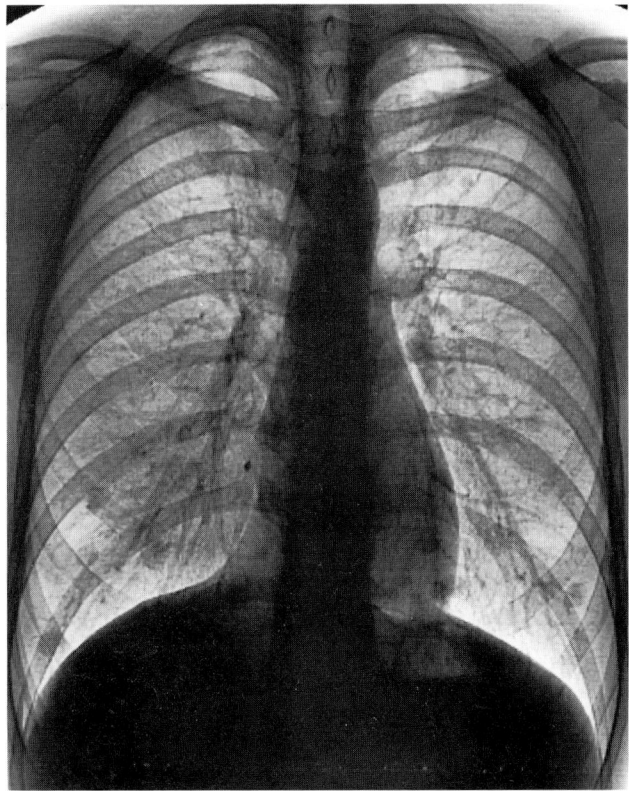

Figure 15a

Figure 15b

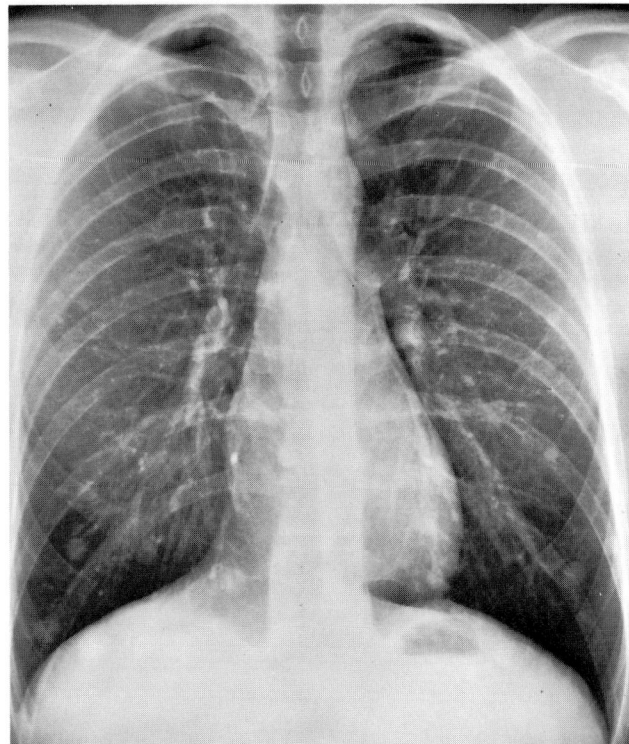

Digital chest radiography

Digital chest radiography was discussed in Chapter 1, page 5. The Picker machine appears to be particularly good at demonstrating pulmonary nodules and the use of edge enhancement or reversal of the image permits demonstration of nodules that are otherwise hidden by the heart and mediastinum [8]. If the completely digital department of the future is developed, it will be essential to have some form of digital chest radiography.

Various different forms of filmless radiography are being developed by manufacturers such as Digi-rad and Fuji. Another method of improving the chest radiograph is Raster scanning [24–26].

Case 15 (*Courtesy of Professor R Fraser*)

A patient with metastatic seminoma of the testis had the following digital chest radiographs. In figure 15a the image is in the positive (reversal) phase and in figure 15b it is in the negative (traditional) phase.

There are multiple small opacities visible in both lung fields. Note also how the blood vessels are clearly seen.

Case 16 (*Courtesy of Professor R Fraser*)

This is a similar case to the last one. In this case the primary tumour was a teratoma of the testis.

Both of the digital chest images are in the positive phase but the window settings differ slightly. Multiple coin lesions are clearly seen.

Figure 16a

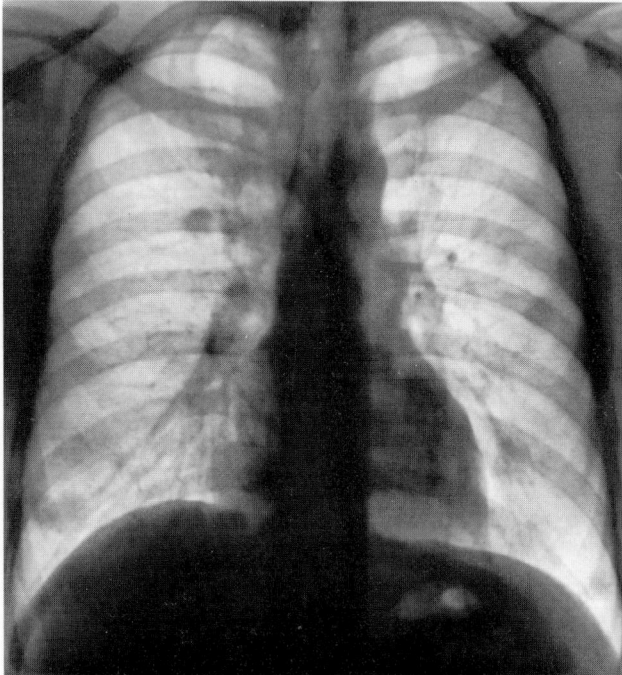

Figure 16b

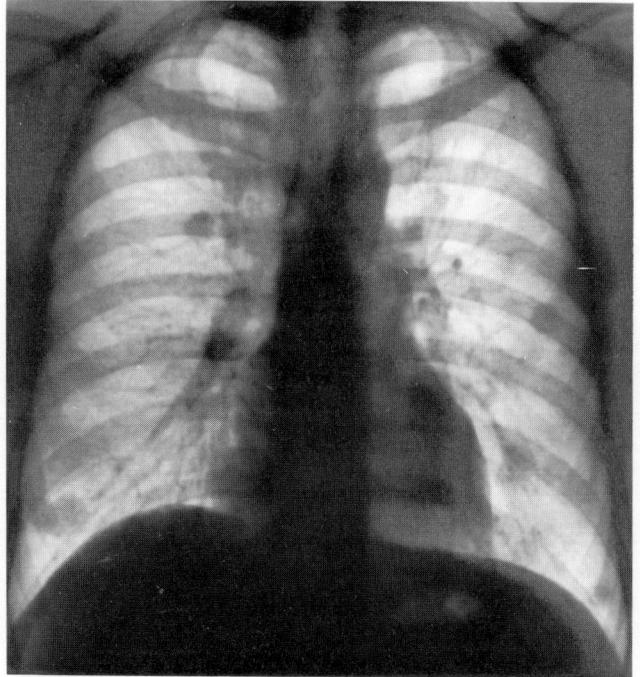

Summary: multiple coin lesions

In Great Britain metastatic deposits are by far the most common cause of multiple coin lesions. However, before ascribing a diagnosis of terminal disease to a patient it is important to consider the other possibilities. Multiple abscesses, rheumatoid nodules and infarcts are the next most likely diagnoses and it may well be necessary to undertake investigations with these conditions in mind. In the United States of America granulomatous conditions such as histoplasmosis are so common in some areas that they may be more frequent than metastatic deposits, even in patients with known malignant disease!

Computed tomography and various scintigraphic examinations may be helpful and newer techniques, such as digital chest radiography, are being developed to assist in the detection of nodules. Needle biopsy under fluoroscopic control will usually provide sufficient material to tell whether or not the lesions are malignant but the nature of the primary often remains obscure. A search for the primary malignant lesion may be undertaken but too exhaustive a search can prove to be a futile exercise.

4 | Miliary nodularity and pulmonary fibrosis

Miliary nodularity

Miliary nodularity is a term referring to multiple small nodules detected on a plain chest radiograph. The term is usually used to describe nodules that are so multiple that they cannot be counted and are less than 5 mm in diameter. The most important cause is miliary tuberculosis, not because it is the most common cause but because it is eminently treatable, but if untreated is a rapidly progressive and potentially fatal condition.

The causes of miliary nodularity are numerous because a similar appearance can be produced both by a combination of linear or reticular opacities (as in pulmonary fibrosis) and by true nodules (as, for example, in tuberculosis).

It is only by careful clinical history and close examination of the plain films that differentiation between the different causes can be made. Particularly important features are:

1 The age of the patient
2 Whether the patient is symptomatic or not
3 History of occupation and hobbies
4 The distribution and shape of the nodules

Table 4 shows the different diagnoses that may be of importance at different age groups. If the patient is completely asymptomatic and miliary nodularity is picked up on a routine chest radiograph, the most common cause by far is sarcoidosis. Another cause of miliary nodularity without symptoms is an uncomplicated pneumoconiosis particularly of a rather inactive form (for example, china clay worker's lung or uncomplicated coal-miner's pneumoconiosis). On the contrary, if the patient is excessively ill, two conditions that must be considered are miliary tuberculosis and carcinomatosis. If the condition is slowly progressive and the patient presents with clubbing of the fingers, cryptogenic fibrosing alveolitis must be considered. If

Table 4 Diffuse miliary nodules

Adulthood
Important causes
   Miliary tuberculosis
   Miliary carcinomatosis
   Sarcoidosis
   Pneumoconiosis
   Fibrosing alveolitis: cryptogenic fibrosing alveolitis,
                       rheumatoid arthritis,
                       scleroderma
   Allergic alveolitis
   Cystic fibrosis (child or young adult)
   (pulmonary oedema)
   (Pneumocystis carinii pneumonia)

Other causes are numerous but include
   Histiocytosis
   Amyloidosis
   Histoplasmosis, coccidioidomycosis (USA) and many more

Childhood
   Respiratory distress syndrome (newborn)
   'Wet lung' (newborn)
   Cardiac failure and pulmonary oedema
   Cystic fibrosis
   Histiocytosis X
   Viral pneumonia
   Allergic alveolitis.

Other causes in childhood
   Gaucher's disease
   Tuberose sclerosis

there is any history of exposure to allergens (for example, pigeon breeding), then one must consider allergic alveolitis. Occupational history is very important indeed because of the possibility of inhalation of inorganic dusts, as in a pneumoconiosis, or organic dust, as in an extrinisic allergic alveolitis. On examination of the nodules, if the nodules vary in size considerably, this may point towards carcinomatosis. If the nodules are widespread, tuberculosis, sarcoidosis or carcinomatosis may well be the cause. Classically in miliary tuberculosis the nodules are said to be all the same size and so well defined that they look 'as if you could pick them out with tweezers'.

Case 17

Mrs Margaret J., aged 60, presented with the following chest x-ray (fig. 17a). Figure 17b is a close up of the left mid-zone.

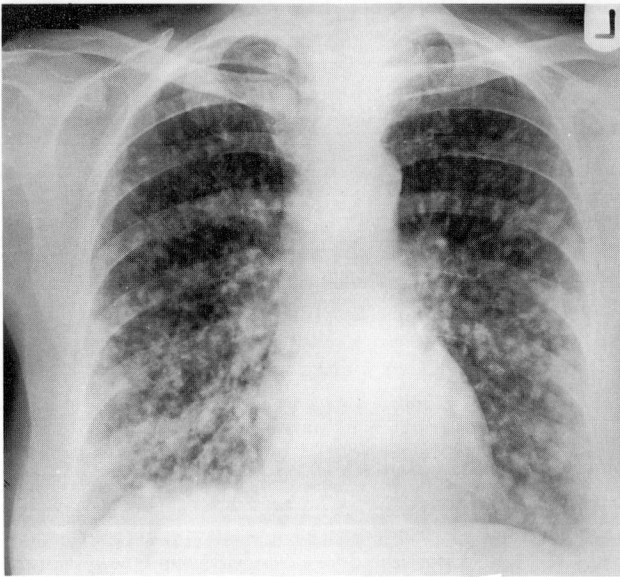

Figure 17a

Figure 17b

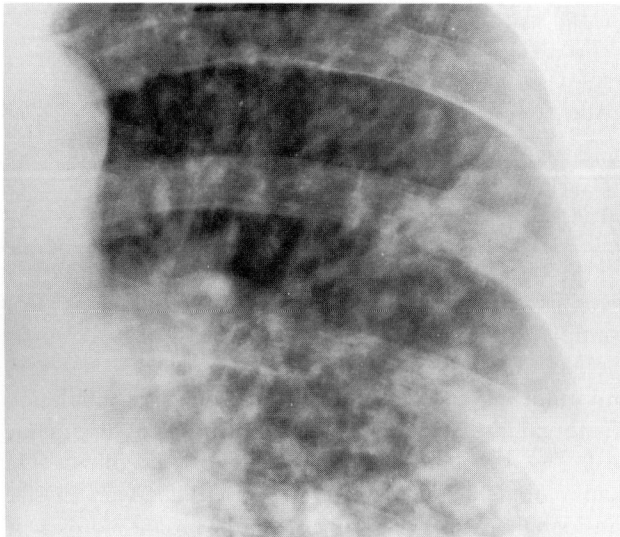

Nodules are seen throughout both lung fields. The nodules vary considerably in size. These are the features of metastatic carcinoma. In this case the primary was carcinoma of the thyroid and the trachea can be seen deviated to the right by a large thyroid mass.

There is often confusion in terminology between metastatic carcinoma and lymphangitis carcinomatosa. In the latter there is obstruction of the lymphatic channels due to neoplasia, resulting in interstitial oedema and infiltration. On the radiographs septal lines are usually evident in lymphangitis cartinomatosa and nodularity, if present, is ill-defined (see Case 82).

A number of clinical investigations may be of assistance in a patient with miliary nodules. These include, Heaf testing, a Kveim test and pulmonary function studies. If carcinomatosis is suspected, a search for the primary may be undertaken although it is often a futile exercise (see Chapter 3, page 30).

Other radiological studies to assist in direct visualization or assessment of the miliary nodules are rather limited. Gallium scanning may show active inflammation in a large number of diseases including sarcoidosis. Computed tomography may give further information about the opacities. In particular it may show whether or not there are cystic holes associated with the nodules as would be the case in conditions such as fibrosing alveolitis or histiocytosis X (see Case 9). The distinction between nodules and fibrosis may be more easily made by CT and associated abnormalities, such as pleural thickening, may give diagnostic information.

Case 18

A 36 year old lady with known sarcoidosis had been followed up for years with little alteration of the appearances on her chest radiograph. She now presented with worsening shortness of breath and the following chest x-ray and gallium scan (figs. 18a and 18b).

The plain chest radiograph shows reticulonodular shadowing in both lungs but most marked in the right mid and lower zones. As stated above, there was little change compared with previous films. The gallium scan shows uptake in the right mid and upper zones indicative of active inflammation. The role of gallium scanning in sarcoidosis is discussed on page 130 in Chapter 12.

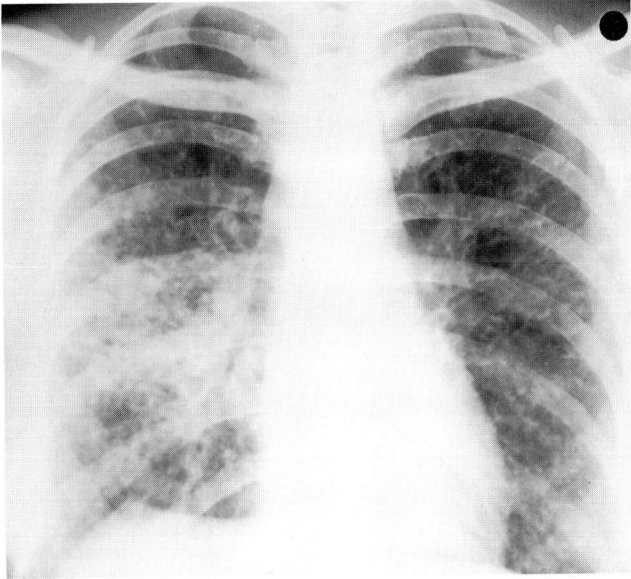

Figure 18a

Figure 18b

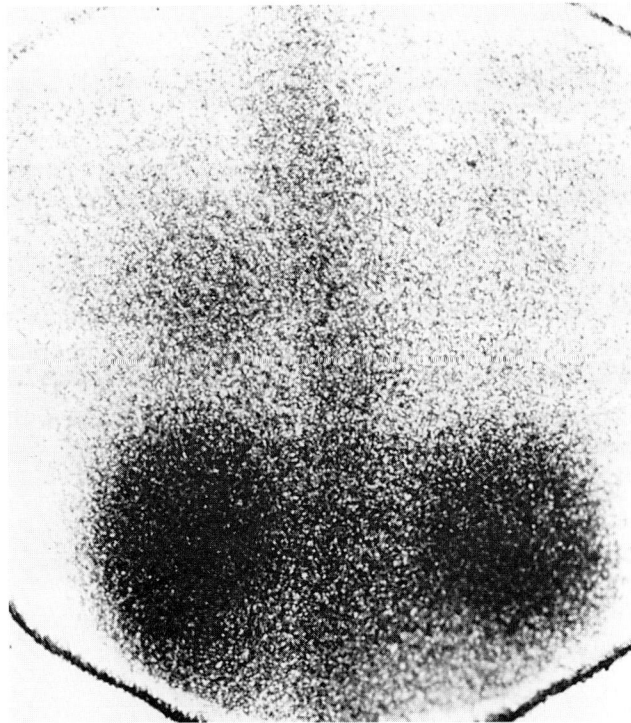

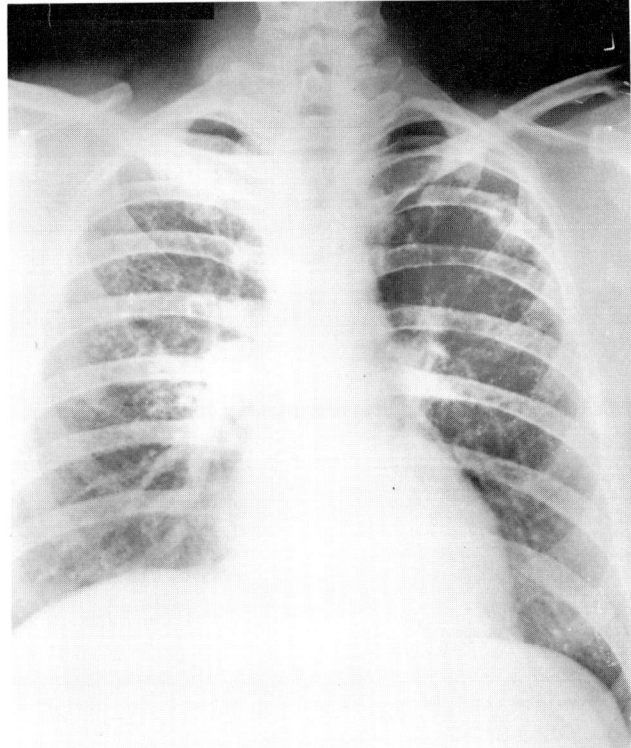

Figure 19a

The appearances are those of diffuse nodularity and fibrosis with gross disorganization of the lung architecture and multiple small cystic spaces containing air. The patient was suffering from histiocytosis X which is the generic name for a group of diseases now generally regarded as an inflammatory histiocytosis. Proliferation of reticuloendothelial cells occurs in bone marrow, spleen, liver, lymphatic glands and lungs. The final result in the lungs is widespread pulmonary fibrosis and air-filled cysts with an appearance known as 'honeycomb lung'. Computed tomography shows

Figure 19b

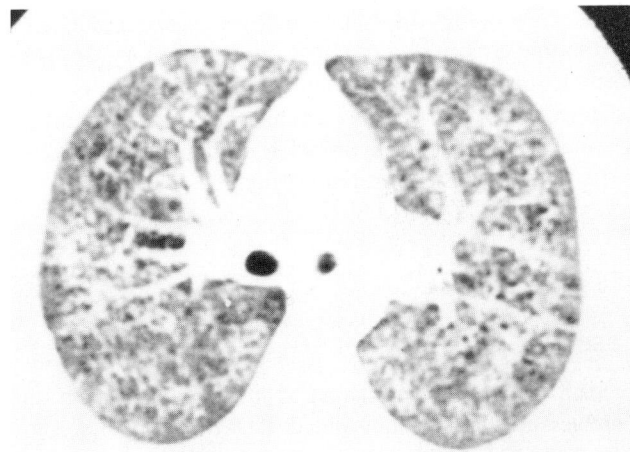

Case 19

A young man with a history of chronic pulmonary nodular shadowing and multiple lytic lesions of the skeleton had the following chest x-ray and CT scans of his chest (figs. 19a, b and c).

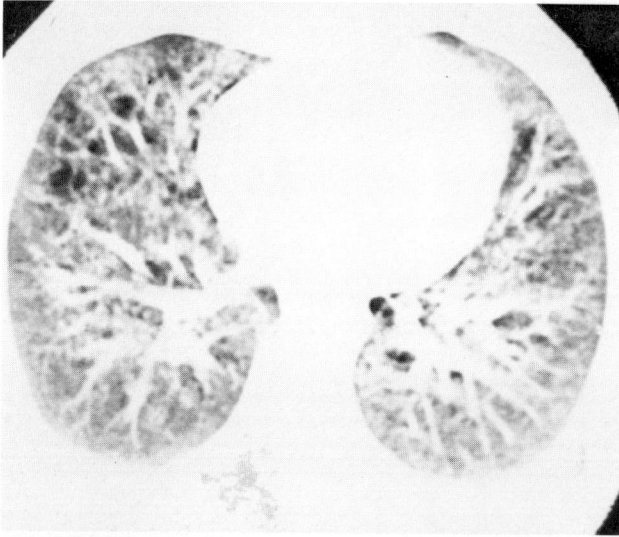

Figure 19c

the nodular opacification, the fibrosis and the cysts to be more regularly distributed when compared with sarcoidosis or fibrosing alveolitis. Note also, on the chest x-ray a pathological fracture can be seen through a lytic lesion in the left 4th rib.

Pulmonary fibrosis

If the nodules are associated with ring or line shadowing, it is likely that the appearance is due to a fibrosing lung condition. Again the history is very important since pulmonary fibrosis is a predominant feature of conditions such as silicosis and asbestosis and is also a major factor in long-standing allergic alveolitis. Connective tissue disorders such as scleroderma and rheumatoid arthritis may also cause pulmonary fibrosis. Positive rheumatoid factor and antinuclear factors may indicate the diagnosis. Joint changes are predominant in rheumatoid arthritis and in scleroderma changes occur in the skin and gastrointestinal system.

Case 20

A man aged 53 presented with gradual onset of breathlessness and the following chest x-ray.

He also had a long history of joint problems.

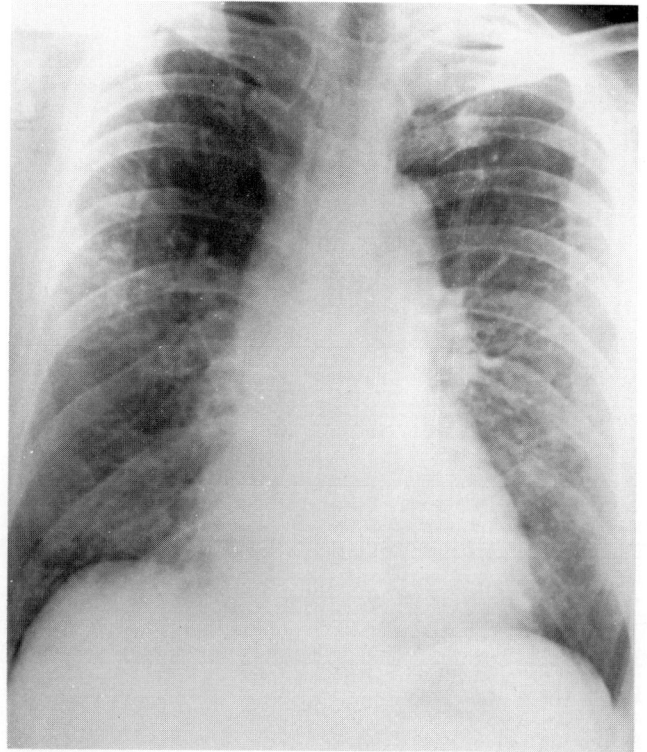

Figure 20a

The chest radiograph showed interstitial opacification in both lungs with nodules and line shadows.

The x-rays of his wrists and hands showed a bilaterally symmetrical erosive arthritis (fig. 20b) with particularly nodular joint swelling. The patient had a very high rheumatoid factor.

Pulmonary fibrosis is uncommon in relation to the population of patients with rheumatoid arthritis (about 1 in 70) but rheumatoid arthritis is relatively common among patients with pulmonary fibrosis, accounting perhaps for 1 in every 6 patients [27].

Pulmonary changes that can occur in association with rheumatoid arthritis include:

1 Pleurisy with or without effusion
2 Nodules
3 Caplan's syndrome
4 Pulmonary fibrosis
5 Respiratory infections
6 (Sjögren's syndrome)
7 (Cricoarytenoid arthritis)

There is a less certain link with:

1 Empyema
2 Bronchiectasis
3 Obliterative bronchiolitis
4 Selective IGA deficiency

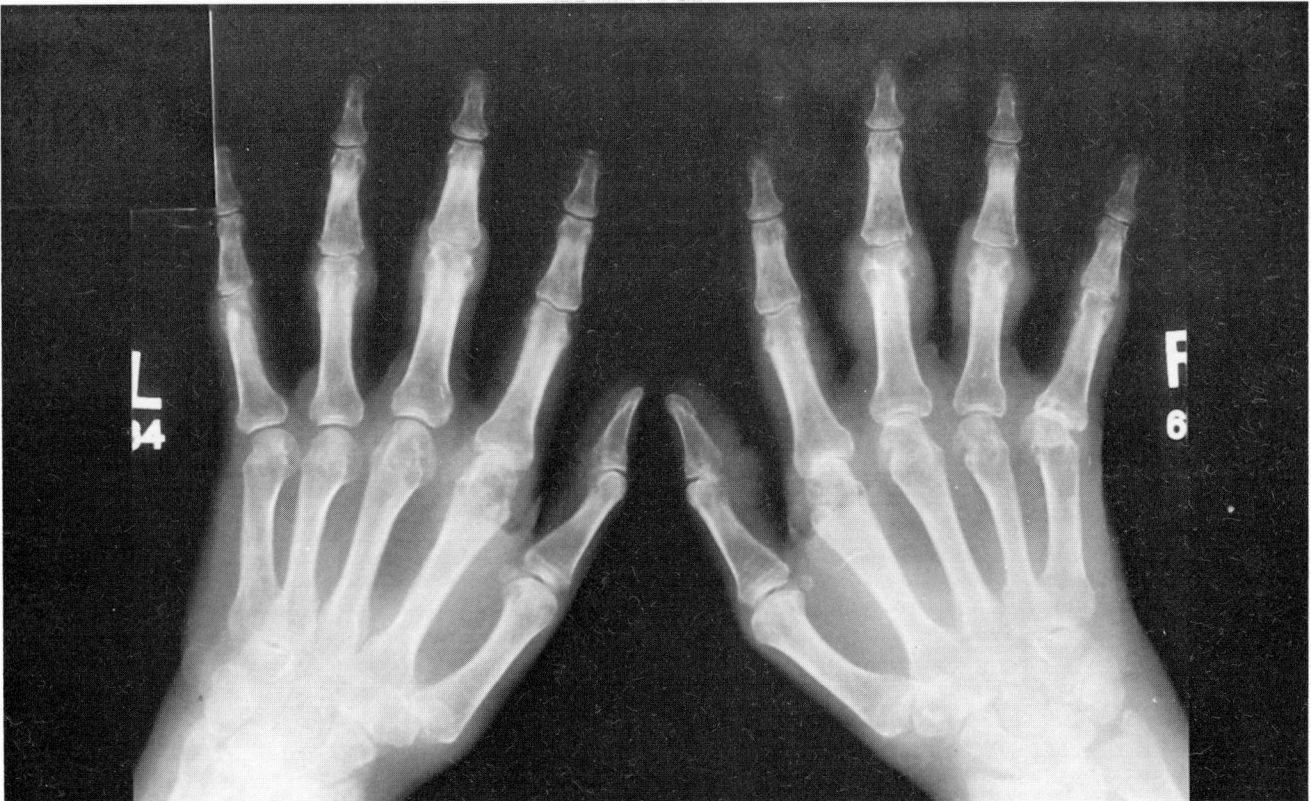

Figure 20b

Case 21

Mildred, aged 64, had a history of pulmonary fibrosis and skin abnormalities. She presented on this occasion with heartburn. A barium swallow examination was carried out and the results are shown in figure 21a. Due to the patient's history and physical examination x-rays of the hand and forearm were taken (figs. 21b, 21c and 21d). The findings on the hand and forearm radiographs were related to the results of the barium swallow.

The patient is suffering from diffuse systemic sclerosis (scleroderma). The oesophagus is the most easily recognized and probably the most common part of the gut to be involved in this condition. The barium swallow (fig. 21a) shows a widely dilated oesophagus. On screening there was no peristalsis. The cardia is widely patent permitting gastro-oesophageal reflux which leads to oesophagitis.

The patient suffered from atrophic changes in the skin, most marked in the digits. Figures 21b and 21c show multiple small opacities in the soft tissues of the digits which represent deposits of calcium. There is also absorption of the tufts of the terminal phalanges. Figure 21d shows marked deposition of calcium in the soft tissue of the forearm.

Systemic sclerosis is a rare chronic disease the main features of which are intimal thickening of small arteries, patchy loss of specialized tissue and replacement fibrosis. In addition to skin lesions, the gastrointestinal tract, heart, skeletal muscles, kidneys and lungs are most often affected. Clinical features include dysphagia and oesophagitis and other disturbances of the gastrointestinal tract. Respiratory insufficiency may result from progressive pulmonary fibrosis. Calcium deposits occur in degenerated collagen and are seen on x-ray as in this case.

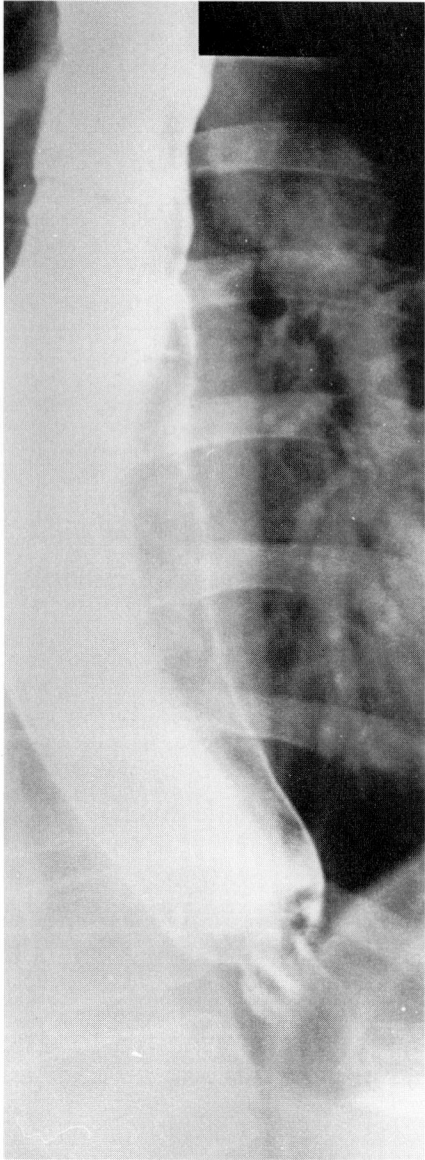

Figure 21a

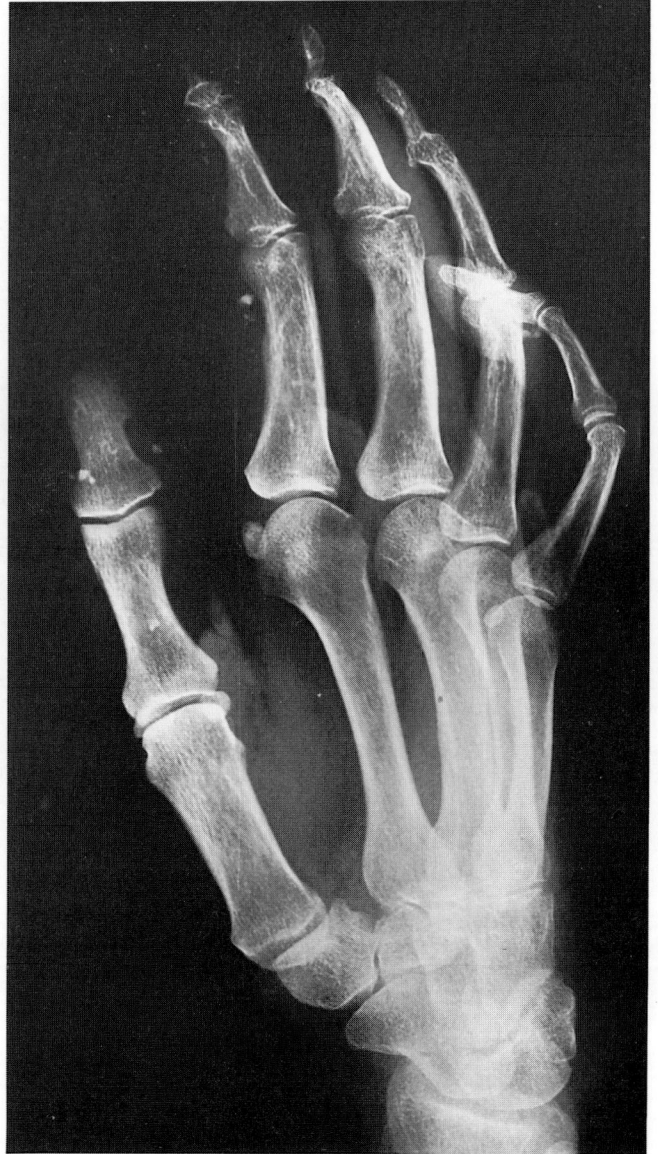

Figure 21b

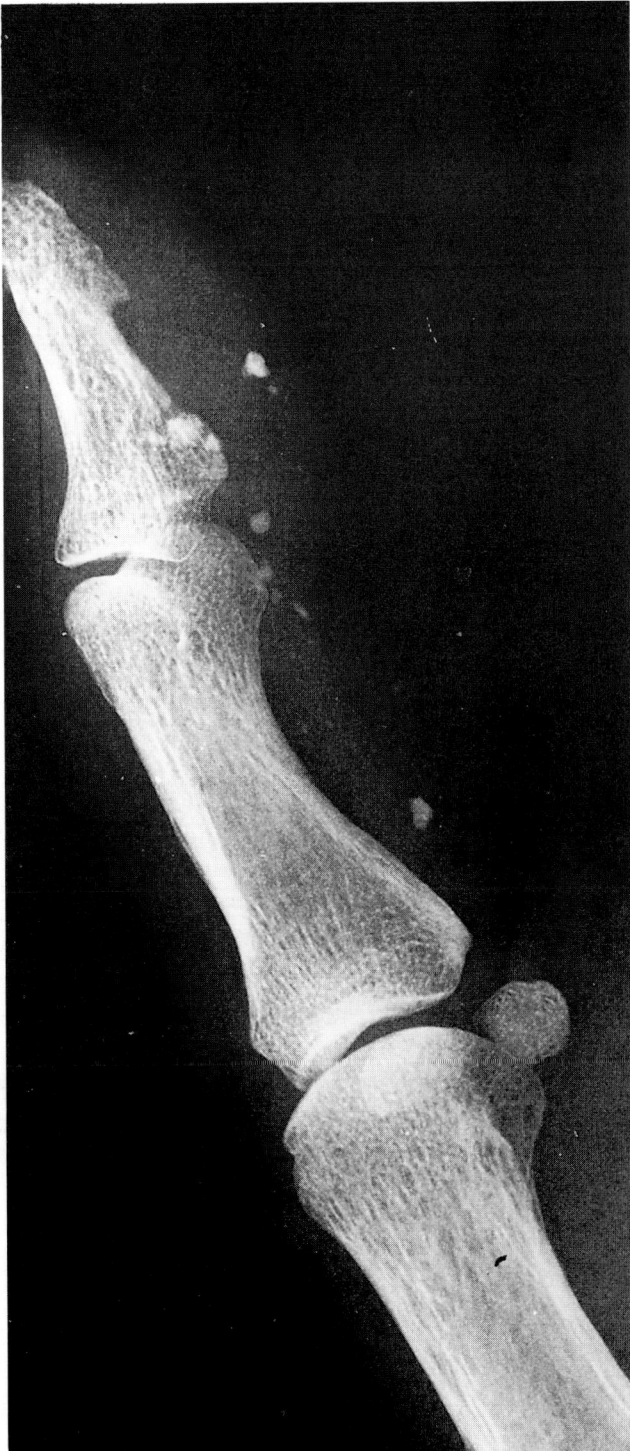

Figure 21d

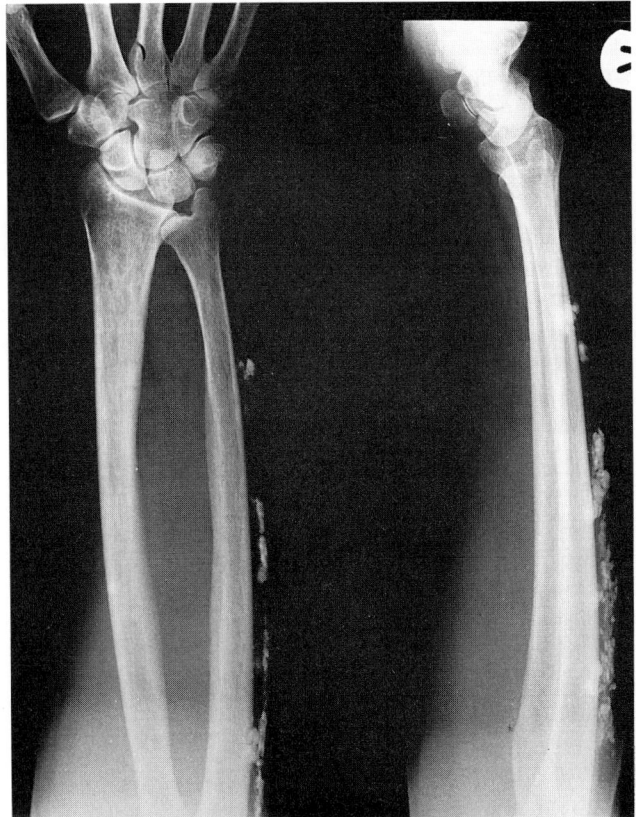

Figure 21c

The aetiology of systemic sclerosis is unknown. Antinuclear autoantibodies may be present in the serum. Patients with systemic sclerosis occasionally show the features of a variety of other connective tissue or autoimmune conditions. These associated diseases include dermatomyositis, systemic lupus erythematosus, polyarteritis nodosa, Sjögren's syndrome and ulcerative colitis. An association with silicosis has been reported.

Treatment of systemic sclerosis is, unfortunately, unsatisfactory and corticosteroids are of little value.

If no cause is found for the pulmonary fibrosis, the diagnosis of exclusion is cryptogenic fibrosing alveolitis. If the diagnosis cannot be made by serological or other tests, and is in doubt on clinical grounds, it may be necessary to proceed to biopsy. Transbronchial biopsy using fibreoptic bronchoscopy may provide a specimen that is sufficient for the diagnosis of sarcoidosis but is not usually diagnostic in the other causes of miliary nodularity or pulmonary fibrosis. Further information can be obtained by bronchoalveolar lavage.

Bronchoalveolar lavage (BAL) is a technique that can be performed as an adjunct to fibreoptic bronchoscopy. Bronchoalveolar lavage has diagnostic value in the investigation of diffuse pulmonary opacification if the cell profile is considered in conjunction with other information. It provides a representative sample of the inflammatory cells within diseased alveoli and the lavage fluid cell population has been characterized in a number of conditions [28]. The cell counts are useful in assessing inflammatory activity in sarcoidosis and cryptogenic fibrosing alveolitis. The results are not, however, pathognomonic except where infective organisms can be identified by culture or by microscopy.

Increased lymphocyte percentages in the BAL differential cell count usually indicate sarcoidosis or tuberculosis while increases in other inflammatory cells without increased lymphocytes usually indicate cryptogenic fibrosing alveolitis, pneumoconiosis or infection. A very high neutrophil count usually indicates infection.

While the results are often not specific they can provide useful supporting evidence for a particular diagnosis. In cryptogenic fibrosing alveolitis, transbronchial biopsies often show non-specific features and an open lung biopsy may still be necessary for a definitive diagnosis. If the patient is not fit for thoracotomy, a characteristic BAL profile may be very useful. In suspected tuberculosis bronchoscopy is already often preferred to laryngeal swabs and gastric washings in the investigation of sputum negative disease. If microscopy for acid fast bacilli and transbronchial biopsy are negative, a characteristic BAL cell profile may help support the diagnosis whilst culture is awaited.

It is quite often the case that the techniques discussed above do not result in a definite diagnosis. In such patients a limited thoracotomy may be necessary in order to obtain sufficient biopsy material to provide a histological diagnosis.

Alveolitis and pulmonary fibrosis

Many of the conditions discussed in this chapter initially cause an alveolitis which then progresses to pulmonary fibrosis. In the early stages there may be widespread, ill-defined pulmonary opacification—this is discussed along with other causes of such appearances in Chapter 6. Diseases causing alveolitis and pulmonary fibrosis are listed in Table 5.

Table 5 Alveolitis and pulmonary fibrosis

Disease or condition	Agent
Cryptogenic fibrosing alveolitis	Cause unknown
Mineral dust inhalation	Asbestos, silica
Extrinsic allergic alveolitis	Avian proteins (bird fancier's lung)
	M. faeni (farmer's lung)
Drug reaction	Nitrofurantoin
	Busulphan
	Bleomycin
Chemical inhalation	Beryllium
	Mercury
Poison	Paraquat
Radiation fibrosis	Ionizing radiation
Sarcoidosis	Unknown
Mitral valve disease	Chronic elevation of left atrial pressure
Uraemia	Renal failure
Adult respiratory distress syndrome	Acute severe illness, often septicaemia

Many of these conditions are also discussed in Chapter 6.

In some of the conditions, such as adult respiratory distress syndrome and bleomycin lung, there is rapid progression of the lung changes. In others, e.g. radiation pneumonopathy, the progression is moderate and in some, such as asbestosis, the disease process is fairly slow.

Some of the conditions in the later stages will particularly cause fibrosis in the lower zones. This occurs in cryptogenic fibrosing alveolitis, rheumatoid lung and scleroderma. Fibrosis in the lower zones is also a predominant feature of asbestosis. Fibrosis in the upper zones occurs as the result of tuberculosis, extrinsic allergic alveolitis, bronchopulmonary aspergillosis, sarcoidosis and radiation fibrosis. It also occurs in association with ankylosing spondylitis and progressive massive fibrosis in pneumoconiosis.

Case 22

A 40 year old lagger presented with slight shortness of breath. His respiratory function studies showed low vital capacity and decreased gas transfer. The chest x-ray is shown.

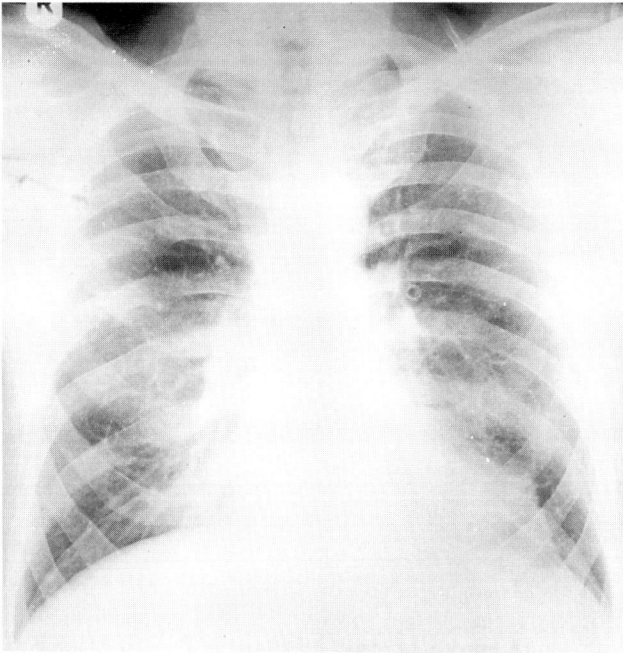

Figure 22a

There is slight haziness adjacent to the heart borders but no other definite abnormality can be seen.

Figure 22b

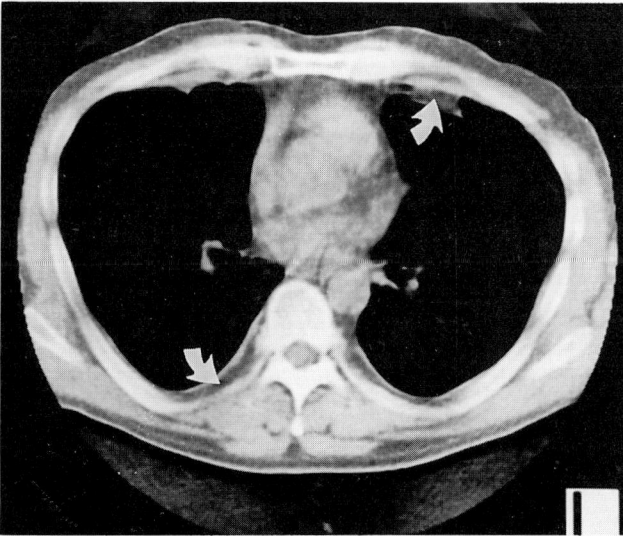

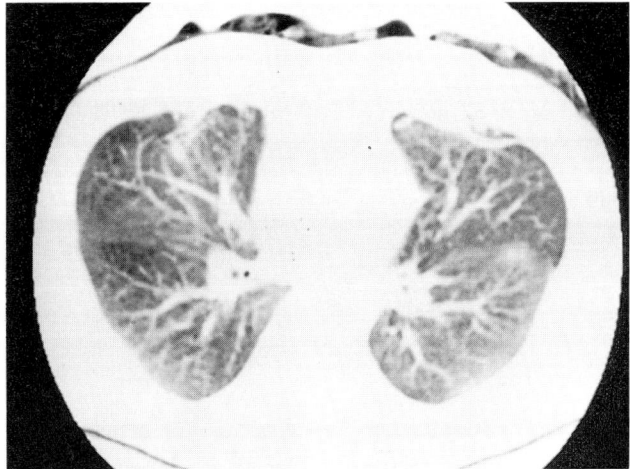

Figure 22c

Figure 22d

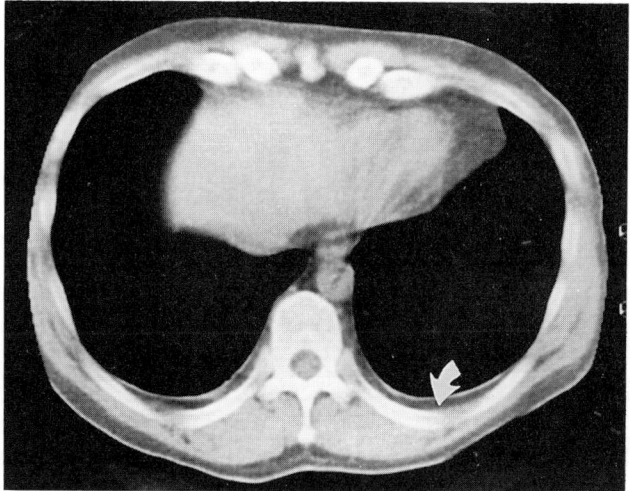

Figure 22e

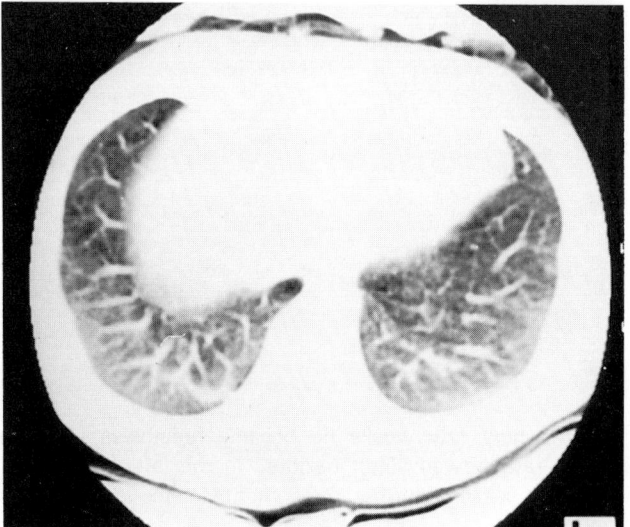

Computed tomography (figs. 22b–e) shows that there is marked pleural thickening bilaterally, particularly posteriorly. There is fat under the pleural thickening both anteriorly and posteriorly (*arrowed*) indicating that it has been present for some considerable time and is almost certainly 'benign'. There is patchy increased density of the lungs due to fibrosis. The appearances are those of asbestosis with pulmonary fibrosis and pleural plaques. The subject of pleural lesions and asbestos disease is also covered in Chapter 11.

Case 23

A man aged 37 presented with an enlarged testis and the chest x-ray below.

Figure 23a

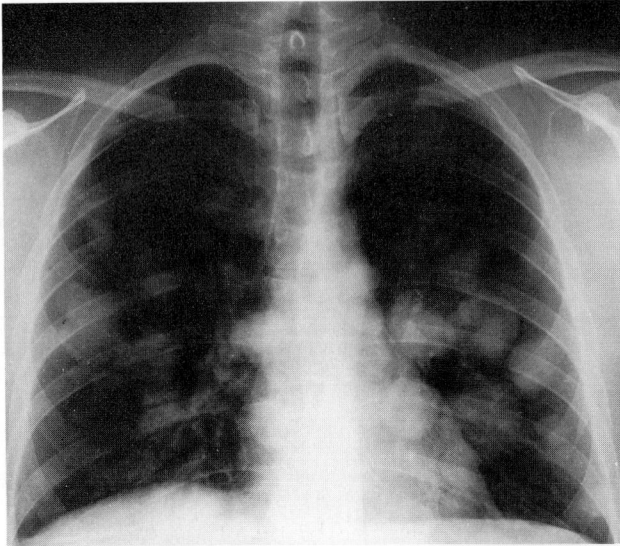

The large rounded opacities of varying size were secondaries from teratoma. Chemotherapy including bleomycin resulted in considerable reduction in size of the metastatic deposits. The chest x-ray below (fig. 23b) was taken two months later.

Figure 23b

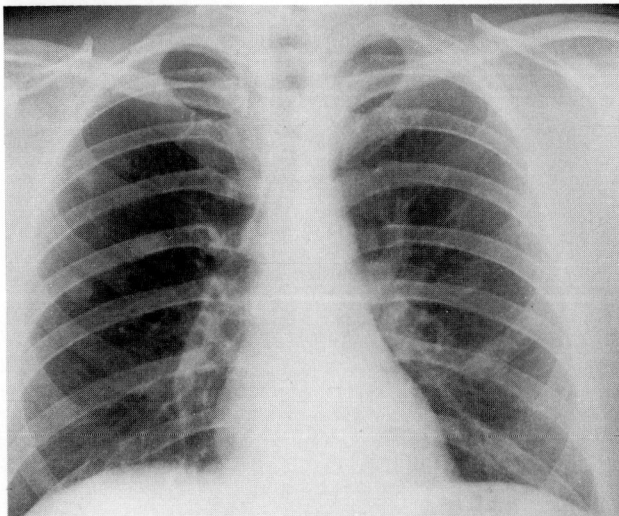

In the next few weeks he became breathless and the chest x-ray showed slight haziness in the left lower zone. The chest x-ray a further three months later is shown in figure 23c.

Figure 23c

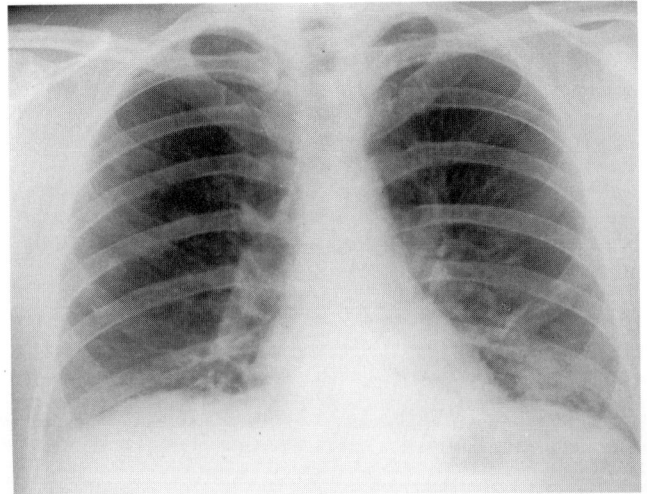

CT had been performed on several occasions for staging and follow-up. These showed increased opacification in both lungs due to fibrosis, presumably due to bleomycin. Figure 23d shows the appearances of the chest CT at the time of the second radiograph and figure 23e shows CT at the time of the last radiograph shown in figure 23c.

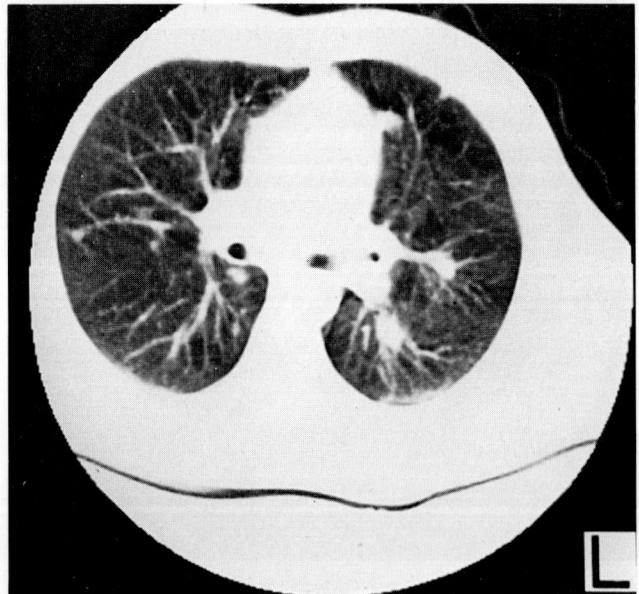

Figure 23d

The CT scan in figure 23d shows a few small nodules which represent the considerably shrunken metastatic deposits. There is also a small line of subpleural fibrosis in the left lung field posteriorly. In figure 23e the fibrosis has progressed considerably and it is interesting to note that it is still mainly subpleural but is extending into the lung. On the left side it is almost solely affecting the lower lobe and

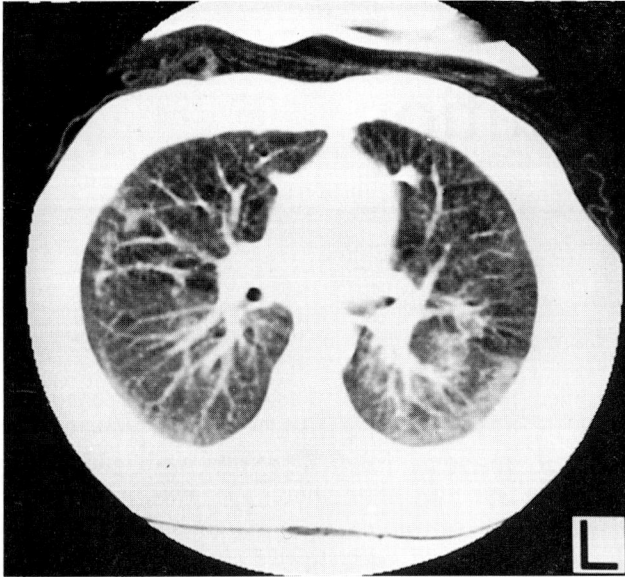

Figure 23e

the upper lobe anteriorly is unaffected. These appearances are rather similar to those seen in the last case in which the cause of the pulmonary fibrosis was completely different.

CT is often used in follow-up of patients with teratoma and seminoma. Bleomycin toxicity can be detected by computed tomography before definite changes are seen on the chest x-rays and at a time when the patient is not symptomatic. The characteristic changes seen on CT include small linear opacities in the lower zones progressing

to widespread pulmonary opacification due to fibrosis. The fibrosis initially affects the subpleural lung but progresses to involve the more central pulmonary areas. Although characteristic of bleomycin toxicity the appearances in other fibrosing lung conditions can be very similar. If the series of CT scans is examined, it is possible to be specific with regard to the cause of pulmonary opacification in the case of bleomycin toxicity.

Summary: miliary nodularity and pulmonary fibrosis

An enormous number of conditions can cause miliary nodular opacification. This is because the chest radiographic appearances can result either from a combination of fibrotic lines and ring shadows or from true nodules. Pulmonary fibrosis of some form or another is the end result of most chronic lung diseases, hence the vast differential (137 at the last count!).

Imaging techniques such as gallium scanning and CT can give information with regard to the activity of the disease and whether or not there is fibrosis. However, more important are the clinical details, the occupation and the hobbies.

In the final analysis, if no diagnosis is forthcoming, open biopsy may be necessary.

5 Pulmonary cavitation

The discerning reader, having perused the preceding chapters may have noticed that many of the same conditions appear on all the lists. The lungs, like other tissues, have only a limited number of responses to all stimuli. Most pulmonary conditions can present with a variety of radiological abnormalities. The lists have been compiled in the order of likelihood of the condition being the cause of that particular sign on a chest film. Thus, if an adult patient presents with pulmonary cavitation on the chest film, the two most likely diagnoses are carcinoma or infection and appropriate clinical tests should be instigated. In children infection is a much more common cause of cavitation than milignancy. In all age groups it is important to consider tuberculosis since it is treatable, unlike many of the other conditions that cause cavitation. The clinical history and examination are, as always, of vital importance.

The pattern of diagnostic investigation is very similar to that outlined in Chapter 2 for a solitary pulmonary mass. A few important differences will be discussed in this chapter.

Table 6 Causes of pulmonary cavitation

Common

1 Carcinoma of the bronchus
2 Infections particularly:
    (i) pyogenic abscess, pneumatocele, cavitation in consolidation
    (ii) tuberculosis (histoplasmosis and coccidioidomycosis in USA)
3 Haematoma, laceration, contusion (including post-surgery)

Less common

1 Other malignancies
    (i) cavitating metastases
    (ii) lymphoma
2 Infarction
3 Other infections including *Klebsiella, Aspergillus, E. coli* and *Pseudomonas*
4 Sarcoidosis
5 Pneumoconiosis with cavitation of progressive massive fibrosis
6 Rheumatoid nodule
7 Cystic fibrosis (child and young adult)
8 Bronchiectasis
9 Infected bulla (see also Chapter 9)
10 Mycetoma*
* mass within a cavity

Rare

1 Rare infestations or infection, histoplasmosis (common in USA), coccidioidomycosis, hydatid
2 Congenital lesions—sequestrated segment, bronchogenic cyst (cystic adenomatous malformation [infant])
3 Wegener's granulomatosis

Case 24

Matthew, aged 11, presented in the A and E department coughing blood. He gave no past history of chest problem or other symptoms, but on questioning admitted that he had been knocked off his bicycle by a car some two hours previously. Although he had been hit on the chest he did not complain of chest pain. At the time of presentation he was slightly febrile.

The chest x-rays (figs. 24a and 24b) show cavitation within an area of hazy consolidation in the right lung field. No rib fractures can be seen. The appearances could be due to a variety of conditions. These include infective causes such as pyogenic pulmonary abscess, post-inflammatory pneumatocele and pulmonary tuberculosis. However, in view of the history, pulmonary laceration due to trauma appeared to be a likely cause in this case. Sorting between the different differential diagnoses of these cavitating lesions is usually possible if the patient's history and clinical course are kept in mind. The history of trauma usually within two hours, as in this case, and the absence of previous symptomatology are typical of pulmonary

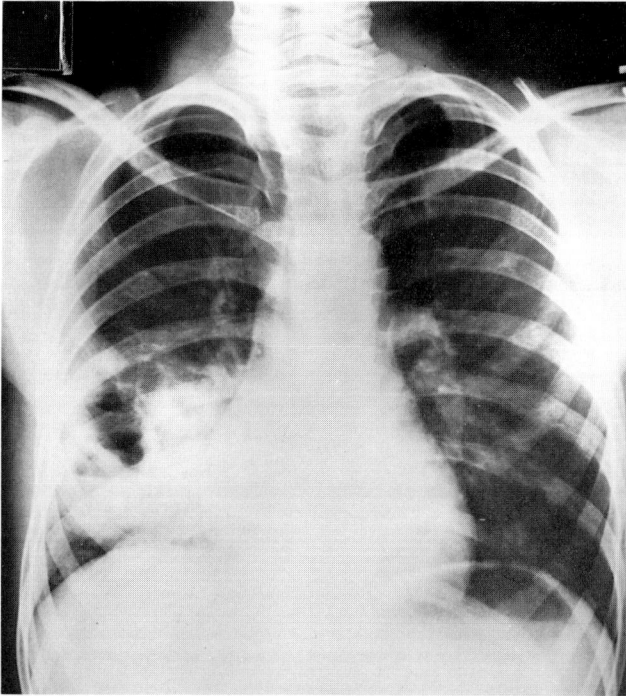

Figure 24a

Figure 24b

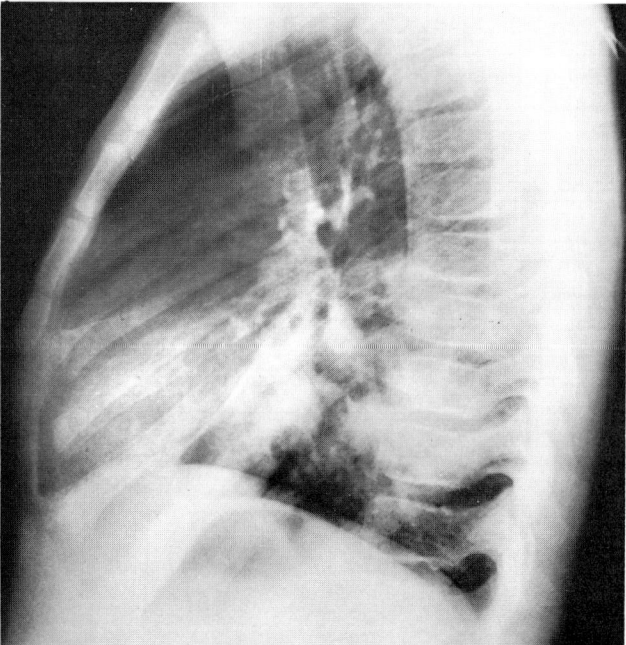

laceration. Haemoptysis is the most constant clinical finding and other symptoms include minimal cough, chest pain and dyspnoea which usually occur only on the first day. Mild temperature elevation and leucocytosis are recognized features.

It is very important to consider the possibility of infection having been present before the trauma—hence the importance of the exact timing of the symptoms. If there is any cause for doubt, a Heaf test should be performed and sputum sent for microscopy and culture.

Most authorities feel that prophylactic antibiotics are not indicated in patients with pulmonary laceration and that the condition should be followed by serial chest radiographs. Superimposed pneumonia is a rare occurrence but, if it should develop, it is recognizable by the presence of purulent sputum and worsening of the consolidation. Traumatic pulmonary changes can be divided into three main groups:

1 Pulmonary contusion: this is the most common lesion with areas of homogeneous infiltrate representing peribronchial and perivascular haemorrhage. These changes clear within a few days.

2 Pulmonary laceration: this is a cavitating lesion often containing an air-fluid level and surrounded by a variable amount of consolidation.

3 Intrapulmonary haematoma: a rounded solid density arising within an area of pulmonary contusion or laceration and taking many weeks or months to resolve.

Injury to the underlying pulmonary parenchyma occurs commonly in major non-penetrating chest trauma. In children the elasticity of the ribs results in pulmonary contusion being more common than rib fractures [29].

This case is an example of the importance of taking a good history. Although the radiographic changes could have been due to a variety of causes, the typical history and awareness of the condition resulted in the correct diagnosis being made.

Much is said about differentiation between benign and malignant disease by the thickness of the wall of the cavity. Whilst it is true that malignant lesions tend to have thick walls, on occasions the walls are relatively thin. Conversely an abscess can have apparently thick walls due to surrounding consolidation. It is only when the walls are extremely thin (1–2 mm) that the sign is helpful in indicating that the lesion is likely to be benign —in children such a lesion would be almost pathognomonic of a pneumatocele due to staphylococcal infection.

The main radiological investigations of value in patients with pulmonary cavitation have been described in detail in the chapter on the pulmonary mass or coin lesion (Chapter 2). A few modifications or additions can be made.

Linear or computed tomography may prove of value particularly in confirming the presence of cavitation, showing masses within cavities (mycetoma) and showing whether there is hilar or mediastinal gland enlargement (see also Cases 9, 63).

Computed tomography can be used to diagnose bronchiectasis (pages 51, 52, 63) and bullous emphysema (page 85).

Case 25

A man aged 48 presented with weight loss and night sweats. The chest x-ray is shown (fig. 25a).

Figure 25a

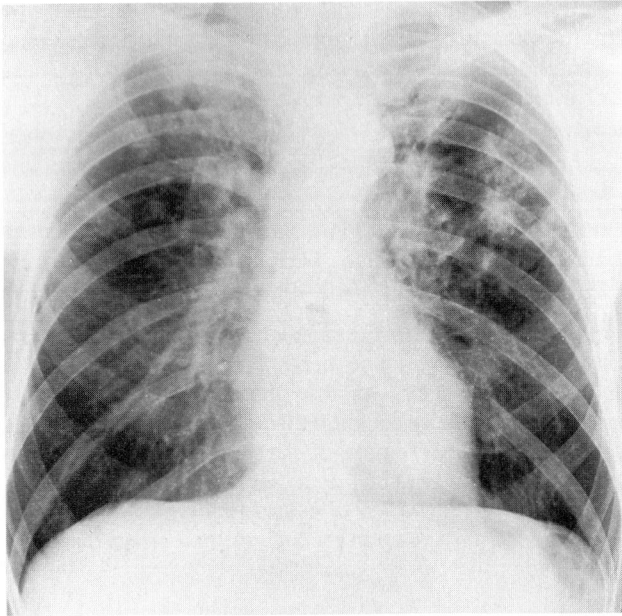

Figure 25b

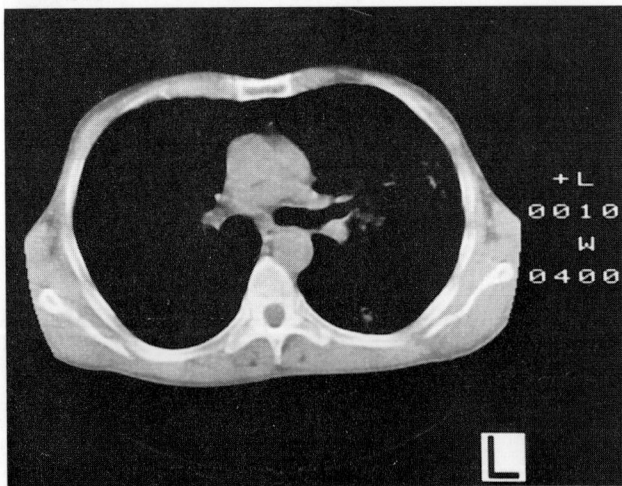

Figure 25c

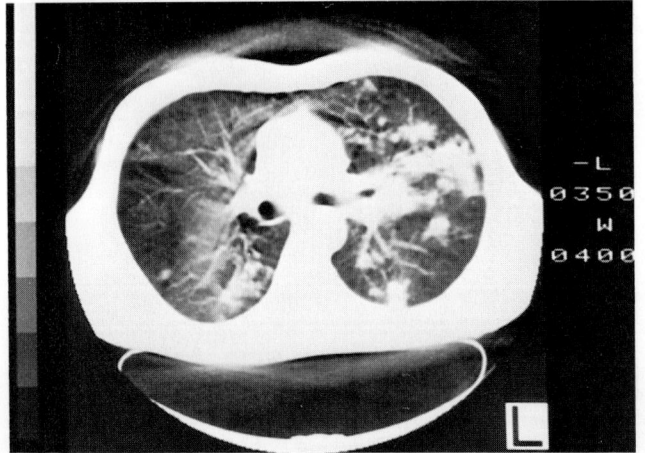

Figure 25d

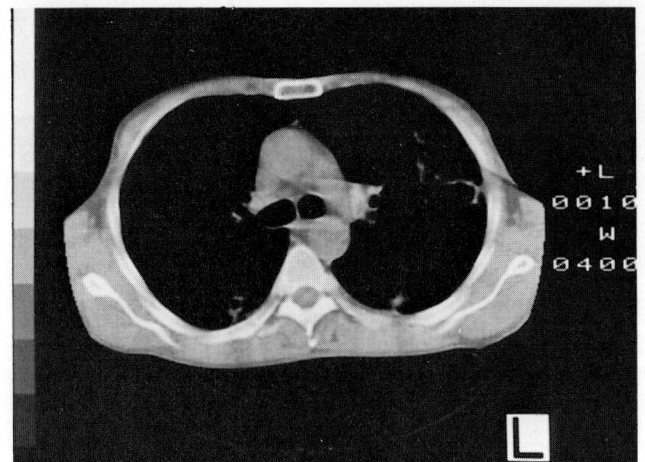

Figure 25e

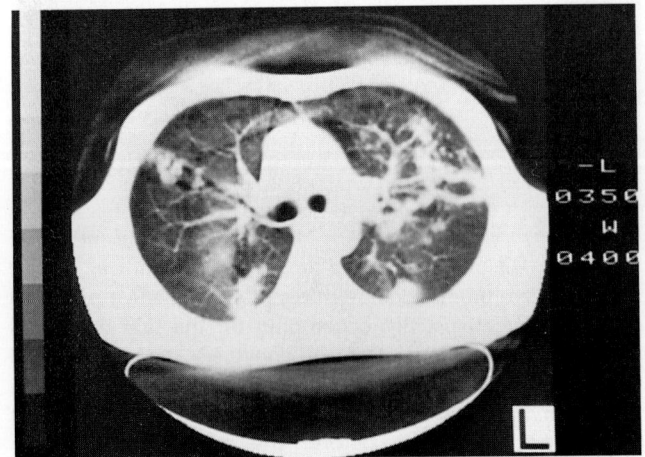

The chest x-ray shows ill-defined opacification in both upper zones. CT was undertaken.

CT confirmed the presence of a cavitating pneumonia in both upper zones and enlargement of left hilar nodes. The Heaf test was positive and acid fast bacilli were detected. Diagnosis: tuberculosis.

Case 26

A patient with a long history of pulmonary cavitation due to sarcoidosis had the following chest x-ray.

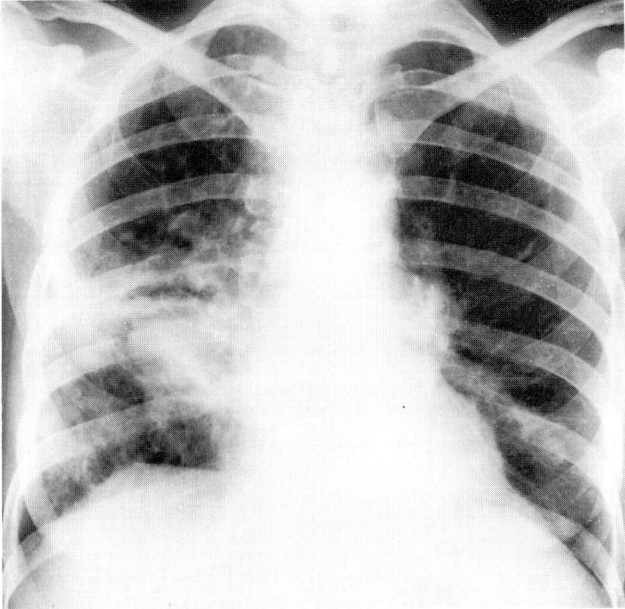

Figure 26a
Figure 26b

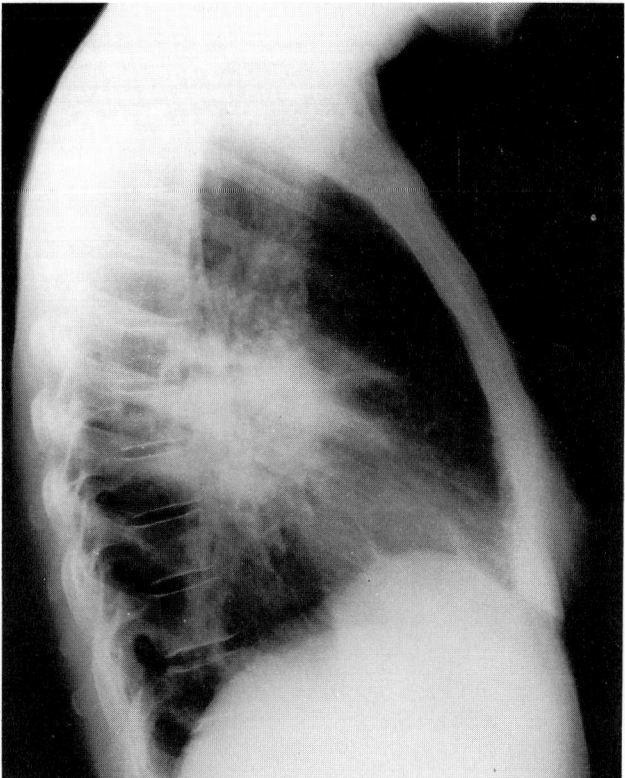

Linear tomography was undertaken.
This confirmed the presence of an intracavitary mass. Diagnosis: mycetoma (aspergilloma).

Figure 26c

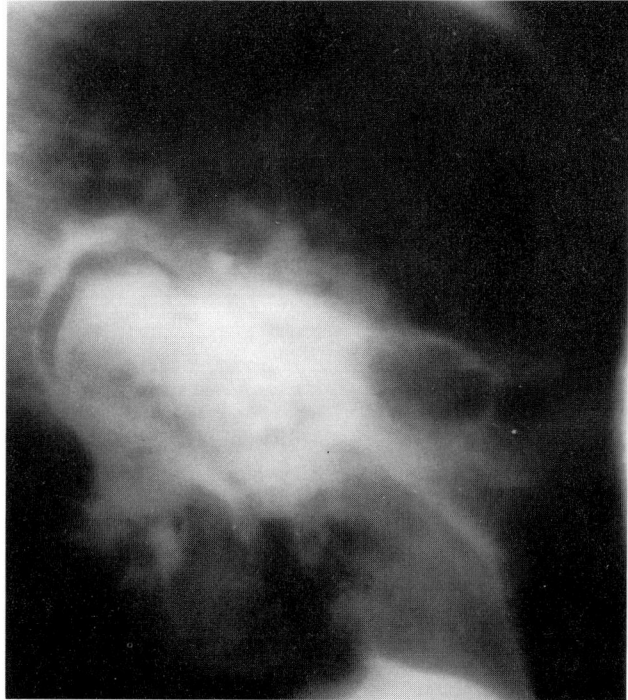

The next case demonstrates the wide variety of tests that are available in patients in whom the cause of pulmonary abnormality is not readily discernible. Most cases are thankfully not as complex as this one but it does demonstrate the large number of diagnostic tools available to study intrathoracic problems.

Case 27

A 39 year old woman was admitted to hospital with increasing breathlessness and cough productive of green sputum over three months. An oesophageal carcinoma had been resected three years previously and she had received prophylactic radiotherapy to the thorax postoperatively.

On admission the patient was thin, febrile and breathless. She had a regular tachycardia of 120/minute. Inspiratory crackles were heard over the right upper lobe. The remainder of the examination was normal.

The chest radiograph showed an enlarged heart shadow and opacification in the right lung field, particularly in the right upper zone. Computed tomography was undertaken.

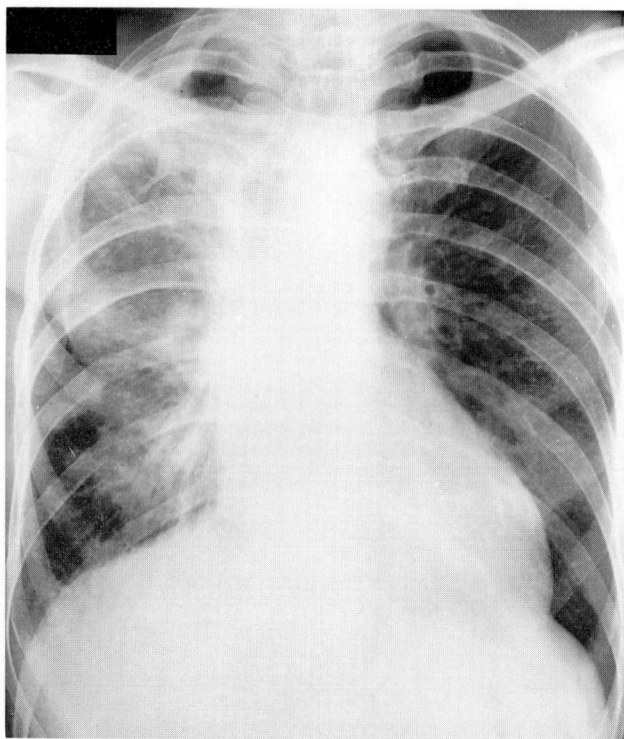

Figure 27a

Figure 27b

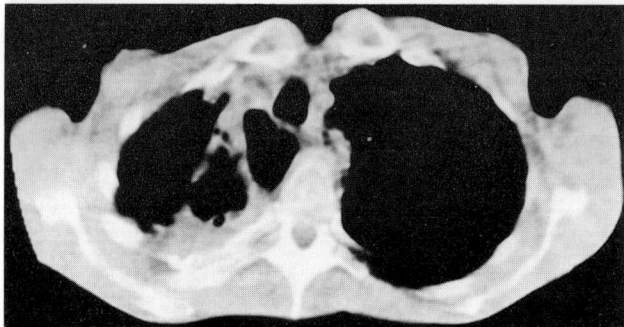

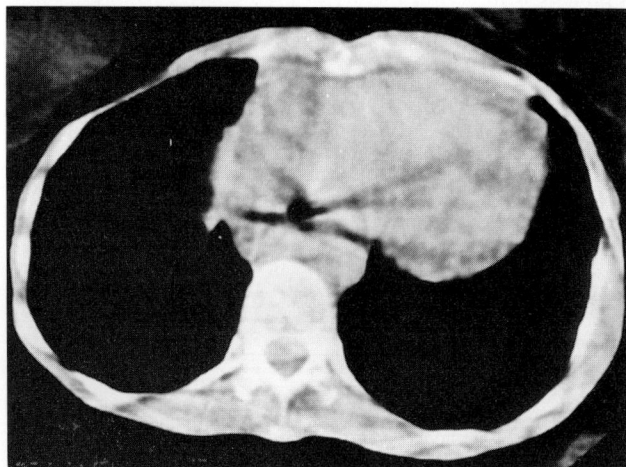

Figure 27c

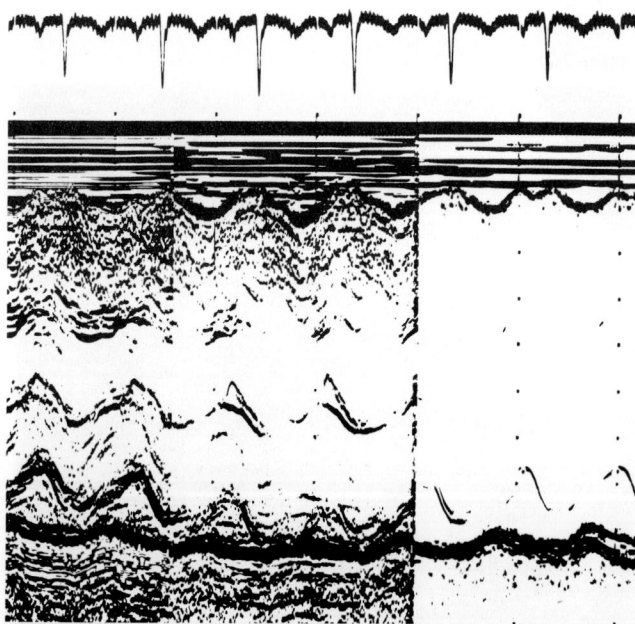

Figure 27d M-mode echocardiography

This showed a large cavitating lesion in the apex of the right lung with pleural thickening. There was patchy opacification within the right upper and middle lobes. The appearances were due to destructive pneumonia in an area of radiation fibrosis. Subsequent review of the chest radiographs showed that the pulmonary changes had developed slowly, but the cavitation had been masked by dense pleural thickening. Cavitation was readily visible on the cross-sectional image. In figure 27c the heart is shown with a surrounding rim of lowered attenuation.

The heart was further studied using echocardiography.

M-mode echocardiography confirmed that the apparent cardiomegaly was due to a pericardial effusion.

Diagnostic possibilities included tumour recurrence, tuberculosis, pyogenic infection or opportunistic infection such as aspergillosis. Initial sputum culture yielded no

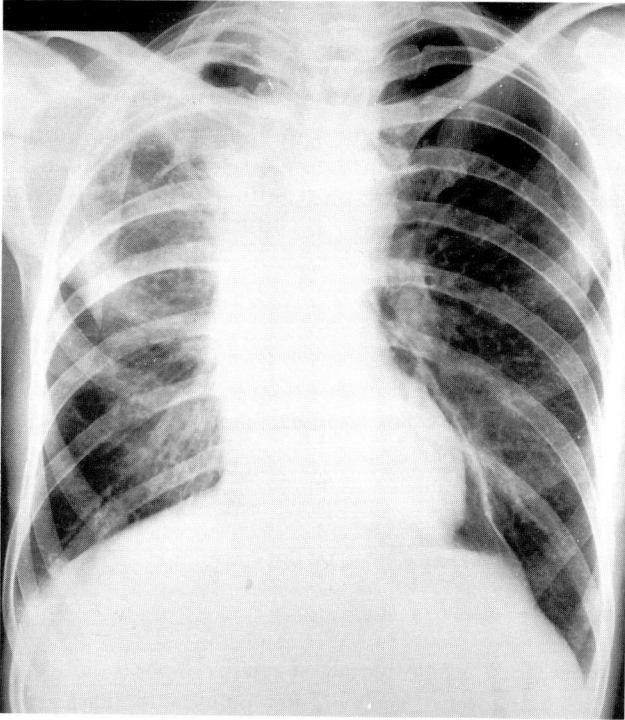

Figure 27e Post-aspiration pneumopericardium

Figure 27f

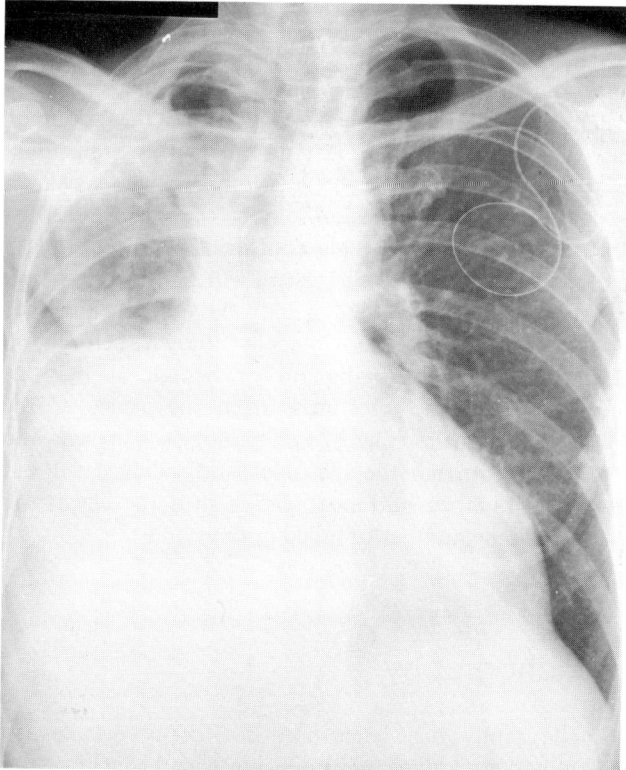

pathogenic organisms and previous treatment with oral amoxycillin had been ineffective. Additional antibiotic treatment with oral cotrimoxazole was initiated and subsequently intravenous cefuroxime and oral metronidazole were given, without clinical improvement. Acid-fast bacilli were not found in the sputum and a tuberculin test was negative. Extensive investigation, including sputum cytology, upper gastrointestinal endoscopy and biopsy and pericardial aspiration, failed to demonstrate evidence of malignancy.

Thin barium swallow showed no evidence of tracheo-oesophageal fistula or other cause for aspiration into the lung. *Aspergillus* pneumonia was supported by the finding on the blood film of a modest eosinophilia and confirmed by high titres of circulating precipitins to *Aspergillus* (1/32, rising to 1/64 and 1/128). *Aspergillus fumigatus* was subsequently isolated from the sputum.

Treatment was commenced with daily intravenous infusions of 40 mg amphotericin after an initial test dose of 10 mg. The fever persisted and serial radiographs showed increasing opacification in the upper and mid zones of the right lung. Fibreoptic bronchoscopy showed no evidence of bronchial obstruction. Corticosteroid therapy was introduced with marked clearing of pulmonary opacification and resolution of fever. Erythromycin was given to cover the remote possibility of additional opportunist infection such as *Legionella* (serology was negative). After a brief improvement she became more breathless. Chest radiograph showed extensive opacification of the right mid and lower zones (fig. 27f).

Ultrasound was done to see whether or not a pleural effusion was present (figs. 27g, h, i).

Figure 27g

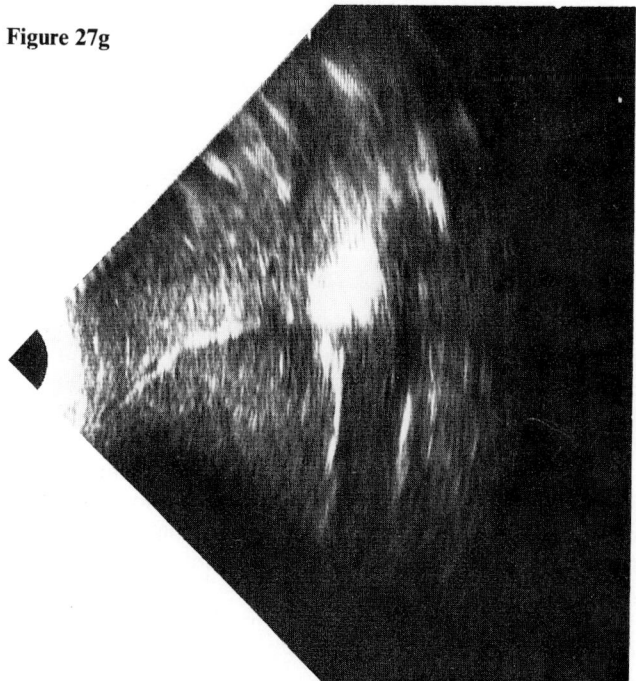

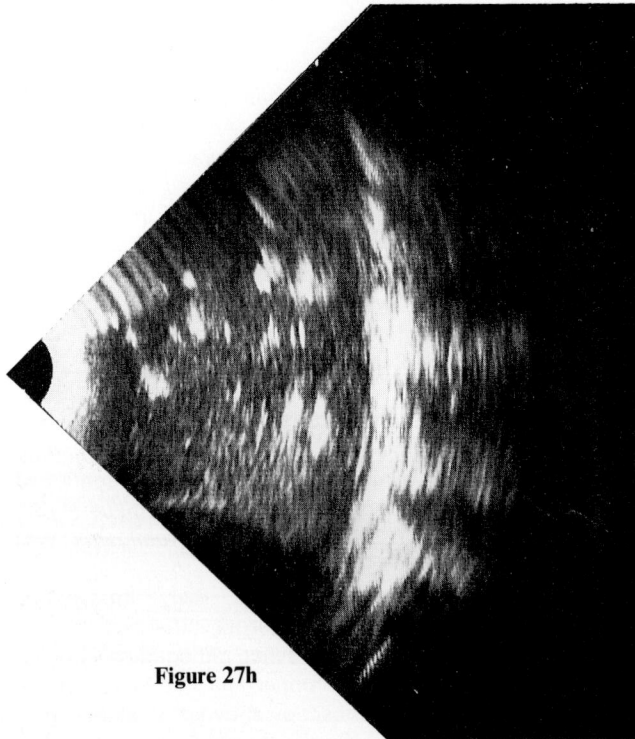

Figure 27h

Figure 27i

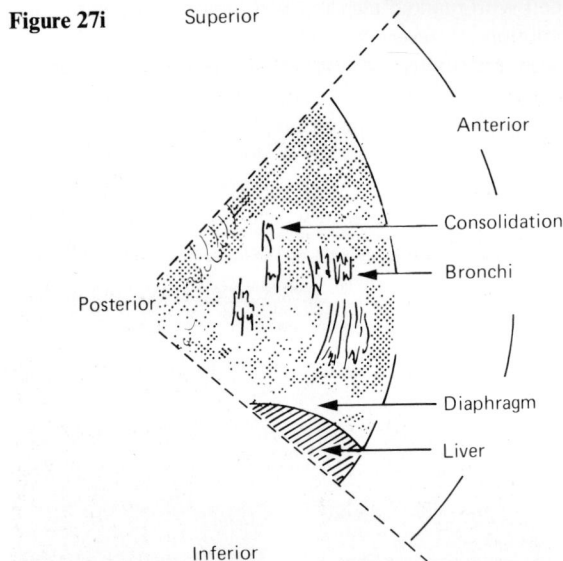

The patient was scanned from behind in the erect position. The scans have been reproduced with the line drawing for comparison. Ultrasound examination of the lung showed pulmonary consolidation but no intrapleural fluid.

Despite continued treatment the patient deteriorated further and died two months after admission. Autopsy confirmed a destructive pneumonia in the right lung and a fibrinous pericarditis. There was no evidence of recurrent or metastatic carcinoma.

This case has been published in the *Bristol Medico-Chirurgical Journal* [30] and has been reproduced with the permission of the editor.

Fungal pneumonia

Fungal pneumonias are rare and usually occur as opportunistic infections in immunocompromised patients. *Aspergillus* pneumonia is well recognized in this context [31, 32]. Despite antifungal therapy there is a high mortality from *Aspergillus* pneumonia [31]. Nevertheless, successful treatment of this infection in some patients [33, 34] underlines the importance of early diagnosis and treatment.

Diagnosis may be difficult and should not depend on the isolation of the fungus which may take some days. As in the last case eosinophilia may be a valuable clue and high titres of circulating *Aspergillus* precipitins are the best hope of an early diagnosis.

Needle biopsy

Percutaneous needle biopsy is relatively contraindicated in the diagnosis of a cavitating pulmonary mass. It is only when all other relevant tests have proved negative (including bronchoscopy) that needle biopsy should be contemplated. There is a greater incidence of complications such as pneumothorax and empyema following biopsy of a cavity compared with biopsy of a solid mass.

Specimens from biopsy require both cytology and culture. It is important to have the cytologist readily available in the x-ray department since the specimen may macroscopically appear useful but contain only necrotic debris. If the lesion is an abscess, the specimen from the centre of the lesion may be the most useful for culture of organisms. The contrary is the case with malignant lesions since the centre will be necrotic—thus the specimen from the edge may be more helpful for cytology. Since it is not usually known beforehand whether a lesion is malignant or benign, it may be necessary to obtain specimens from the centre of the lesion and from the edge. If the cytologist is present and able to confirm that the specimen is of value, it will cut down the number of repeat passes into the chest and also reduce the number of failed examinations.

Bronchography

Bronchography has been used for many decades to show whether cavities communicate with bronchi or are indeed dilated bronchi (bronchiectasis: see Cases 37 and 42).

The investigation has become less common, partly due to a lessened frequency of bronchiectasis and partly because of the advent of fibreoptic bronchoscopy. Computed tomography is also able to show bronchiectasis (Case 36) and as it becomes more generally available CT is further reducing the need to resort to bronchography. Bronchography is a rather unpleasant examination for the patient and rigorous physiotherapy is required after the examination in order to keep morbidity to a minimum.

Biopsy

If the diagnosis is not forthcoming despite diagnostic imaging, bronchoscopy and transbronchial biopsy, sputum culture and microscopy and other clinical tests, the diagnosis may only be made by open biopsy. If at an early stage in the proceedings it is decided that surgical intervention will be necessary whatever the outcome of the tests, then there is little point in performing all of the investigations except as staging procedures. The staging of carcinoma of the bronchus is discussed in Chapter 2.

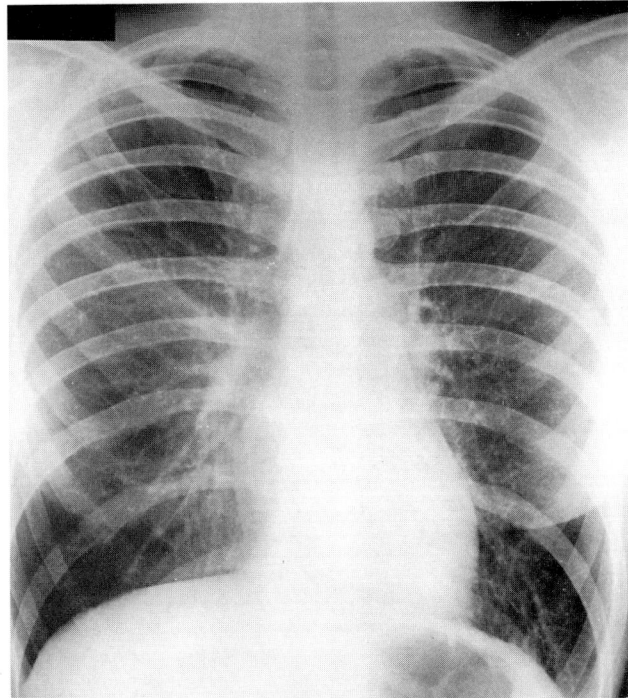

Figure 28a

Figure 28b

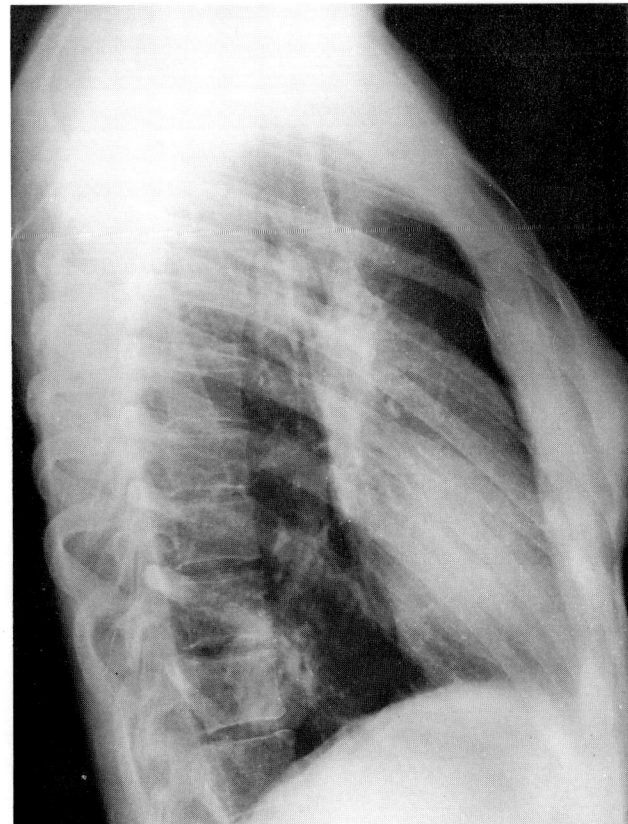

Case 28

Jill, aged 23, had suffered from intermittent chest infections for some years. Chest x-ray showed a lesion about the size of a Victoria plum in the left lower lobe.

Bronchoscopy was normal but the bronchogram is shown below.

The bronchogram shows cyst-like spaces in the posterior basal segment of the left lower lobe. Computed tomography was also performed.

The computed tomography shows a rounded density in the posterior basal segment of the left lower lobe. Anterior and slightly lateral to it is a cystic area containing air and traversed by septa. The opacity is seen to communicate with the aorta by a band of tissue. This is the vascular pedicle of the mass and the lesion represents a sequestrated segment.

Sequestrated lung segments arise as a congenital anomaly [35]. They are usually asymptomatic unless they become infected. There are two forms, intralobar and extralobar. The intralobar segments arise through failure of development of the normal arterial supply to an area of lung tissue and derive their arterial supply from systemic vessels,

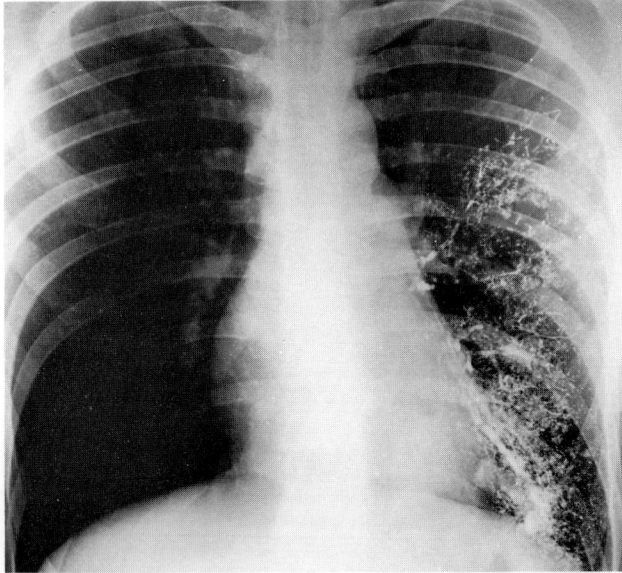

Figure 28c
Figure 28d

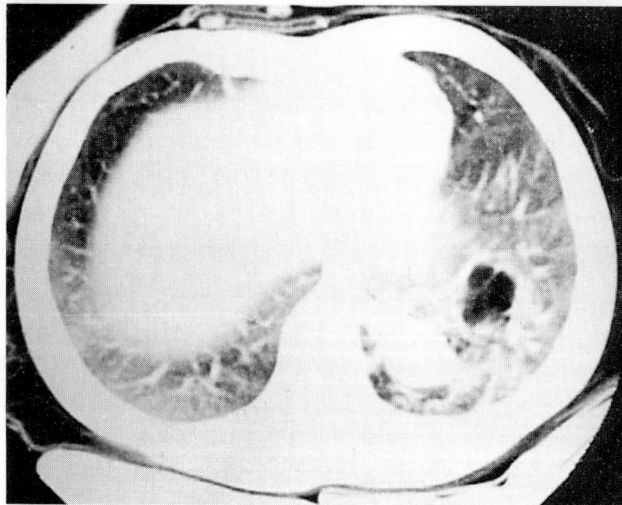

Figure 28e

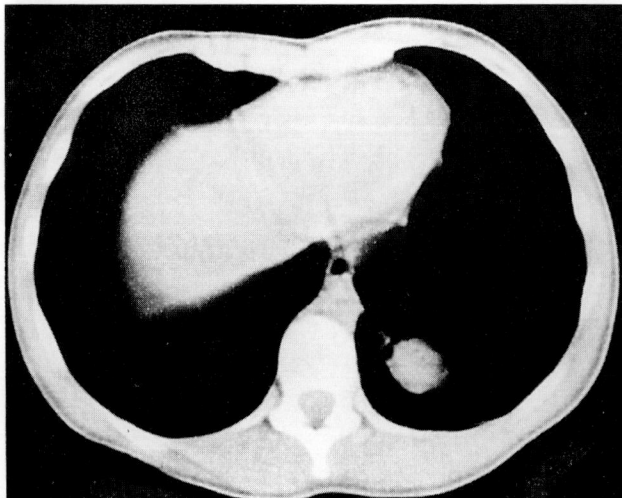

usually the thoracic aorta. Their venous drainage, however, is always via the pulmonary veins and they may therefore cause a left to right shunt. If they become infected, the surrounding lung is often also involved and the nature of the sequestrated segment will only become apparent with resolution of the pneumonia.

The extralobar sequestrated segments have a different embryological origin, arising from abnormal budding of the tracheobronchial tree. They have their own pleural sac which makes them far less likely to become infected. Their arterial supply is usually from the aorta, often the abdominal aorta, but their venous drainage is always via the systemic veins. They usually occur related to the left hemidiaphragm and may be either intrathoracic or intra-abdominal.

The diagnosis of sequestration may be suspected on plain radiography and confirmed by demonstration of the arterial supply arising from the aorta either by aortic contrast medium injection (see Case 8), by digital vascular imaging with intravenous injection, or by CT as in this case.

Summary: pulmonary cavitation

The two most likely diagnoses, in an adult patient presenting with pulmonary cavitation, are carcinoma or infection. Tuberculosis must, as always, be remembered and appropriate tests considered. Rare conditions, such as sequestrated segment may be encountered because the aphorism of Professor Charles Dent remains true: 'Any one rare disease is, of course, rare. Rare diseases are, however, common.' This is the case because there are innumerable different rare diseases!

The pattern of diagnostic investigation in a patient with pulmonary cavitation is similar to that outlined in Chapter 2 for a solitary mass. CT may prove of value by confirming the presence of cavitation and the exact size, site and shape of the adjacent or surrounding mass. Bronchoscopy and CT are replacing bronchography in determining whether bronchiectasis is present.

Biopsy can be performed transbronchially, percutaneously or by thoracotomy. It is more difficult to obtain a useful result from percutaneous needle biopsy of a cavitating mass than from a solid mass and the risks are greater. Conversely it is more likely that positive results will be obtained from the culture and microscopy (including cytology) of the sputum in a patient with a cavitating mass. The least invasive test should be performed first, especially if there is a good chance of a useful yield.

6 Widespread alveolar opacification

Widespread ill-defined pulmonary opacification ('alveolar opacification')

Widespread ill-defined pulmonary opacification can be due to any condition that opacifies the alveoli. The pattern is most commonly seen in *pulmonary oedema* due to transudation. However, the appearances may be due to any cause of fluid in the alveoli, in particular *exudation, transudation* and *inhalation*. Moreover a similar appearance can result from *infiltrating masses* invading the parenchyma. In Table 7 the causes of 'alveolar opacification' are outlined. The conditions that cause alveolar opacification may also cause consolidation. The distribution is the main distinguishing factor between 'alveolar' opacification and consolidation, with the former being more widespread and consisting of multiple ill-defined fluffy opacities. If the opacification is more localized and confluent, it is usually described as consolidation—in such cases exudation is a more common cause than transudation (see Chapter 7).

Sometimes it is difficult to distinguish between a pattern of rather ill-defined miliary nodular shadowing and widespread alveolar opacification. In such cases it may be necessary to follow the investigative procedures discussed in the first part of Chapter 4.

Careful examination of the chest radiograph, coupled with the clinical details, may reveal the cause of the opacification. If the opacification is due to pulmonary oedema, this is often the result of raised pulmonary venous pressure secondary to heart failure or mitral value disease. In such cases there is often upper zone diversion of blood and interstitial oedema. The former is shown by enlargement of upper zones vessels and the latter is indicated by septal (Kerley B) lines and bronchial wall thickening. The upper lobe anterior segment bronchi and arteries can show these features

Table 7 Widespread ill-defined pulmonary opacification (alveolar shadowing)

Alveolar opacification	Cause

Transudation (Pulmonary oedema)	Heart failure*
	 Mitral valve disease*
	 Overtransfusion*
	 Renal failure*
	 Hepatic failure*
	 Hypo-albuminaemia*
	   (Raised intra-cranial pressure
	   Morphine overdosage)*

Exudation	Infection
	   bronchopneumonia
	   atypical and viral pneumonias*
	   *Pneumocystis carinii**
	   (Tuberculosis)
	 Adult respiratory distress syndrome
	 Alveolar proteinosis
	 Pulmonary eosinophilia
	 Contusion
	 Fat emboli

Inhalation	Gastric contents
	 'Near-drowning'
	 Toxic fumes
	   (Paraquat)
	 Oxygen toxicity
	   (Oxygen lack—altitude sickness)

Infiltration	Lymphoma Alveolar cell carcinoma Lymphangitis carcinomatosa* and widespread carcinomatosis

The conditions marked with asterisks can also be associated with *septal lines* (Kerley B lines). Other conditions that result in septal lines include veno-occlusive disease, haemosiderosis and pneumoconiosis. Bullous emphysema can result in lines that mimic septal lines.

elegantly. Although the heart is usually enlarged in cardiac failure, it may be normal or near normal immediately following acute myocardial infarction. The heart may also be nearly normal in size in pure mitral stenosis without regurgitation. Further investigation of the cardiovascular system is to be covered in another book in this series, but includes imaging techniques such as radionuclide ventriculography, real-time ultrasound and Doppler (echocardiography), and cardiac catheterization and angiography.

Case 29

A lady with a history of heavy smoking and triple cardiac valve disease was well when chest x-ray (fig. 29a) was taken but was suffering from shortness of breath and paroxysmal nocturnal dyspnoea when figure 29b was taken.

In figure 29a there is enlargement of the heart and slight bulging of the left heart border due to an enlarged left atrial appendage. No lung lesion is seen. In figure 29b there is slight increase in opacification throughout the lung fields, there is enlargement of the upper zone vessels and interstitial oedema. The features are those of cardiac failure.

When figure 29c was taken some 18 months later she was still suffering from shortness of breath but also had a chronic cough productive of mucopurulent sputum. At this

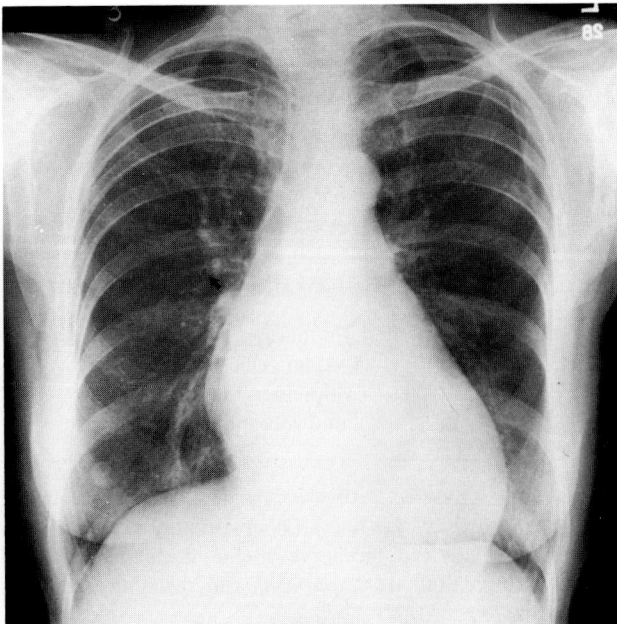

Figure 29b

stage she was suffering from chronic bronchitis but the cardiac problems were well controlled.

The changes in fortune can be followed by close examination of the bronchi and pulmonary vessels. Knowledge of the distribution, shape and size of the pulmonary vessels is basic to the understanding of pulmonary parenchymal changes on chest radiographs.

Figure 29a

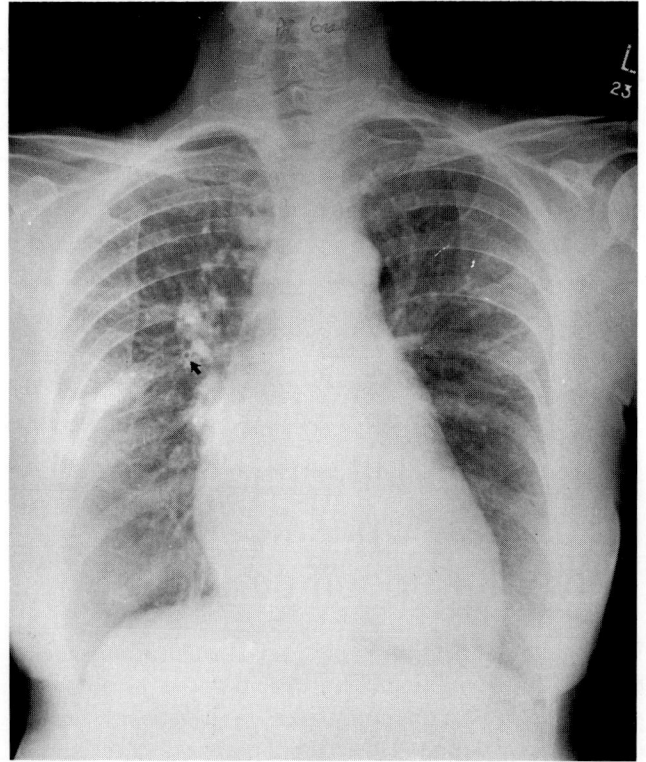

Figure 29c

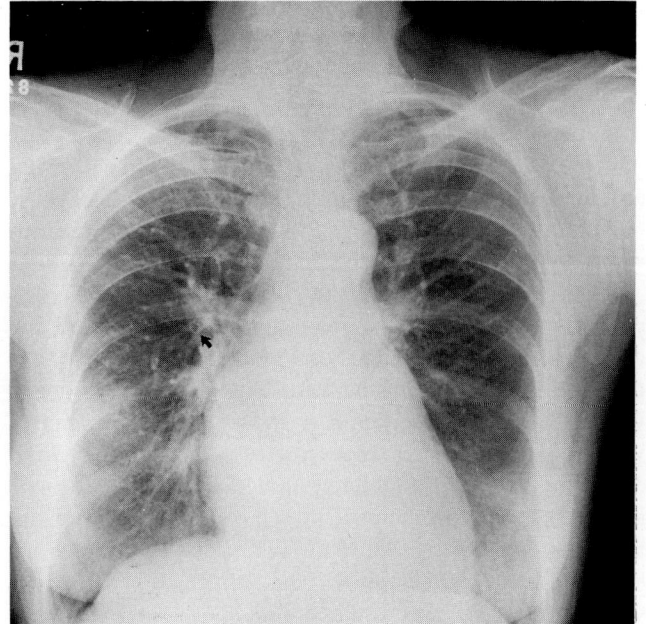

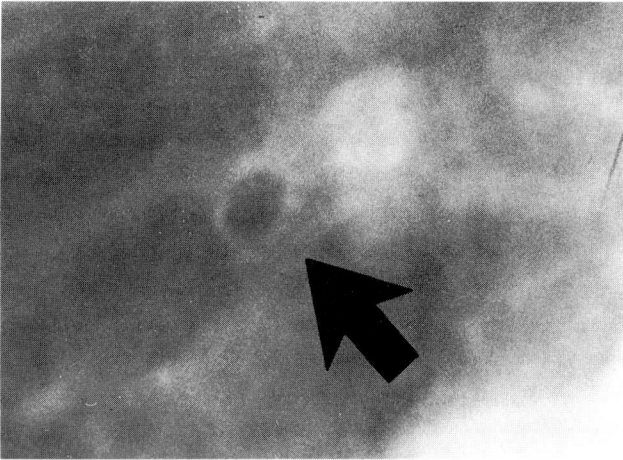

Figure 29d

Figure 29e

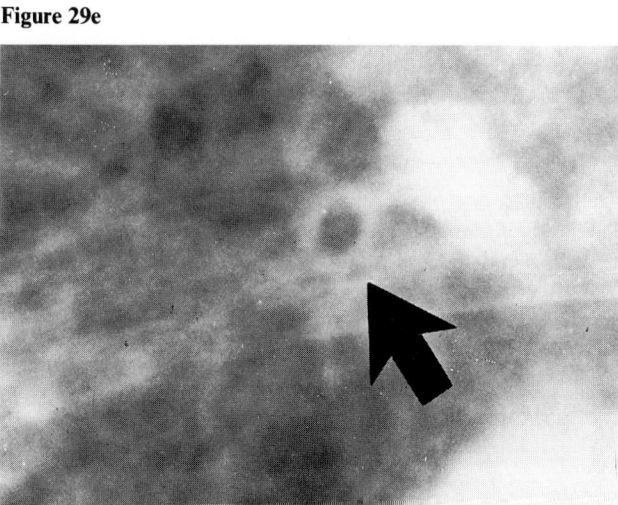

Figure 29f

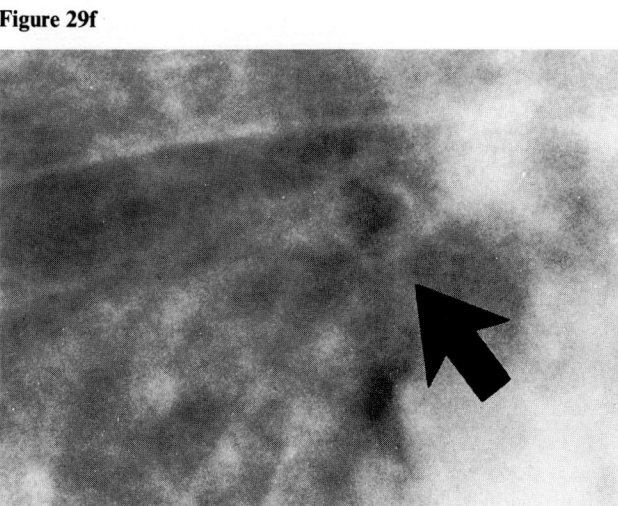

The right upper lobe anterior segment bronchus and artery are shown in detail in figures 29d, 29e and 29f and relate to the chest radiographs 29a, 29b and 29c, respectively.

In figure 29d the artery and bronchus are of comparable size and the patient was well.

In figure 29e the bronchial wall is markedly thickened, the septum between the bronchus and artery is also thickened (Milne's dumbbell sign) and the patient is in cardiac failure.

In figure 29f the bronchus is irregular in shape, the bronchial wall is irregularly thickened and the artery is about the same size as the bronchus. At this time the patient was suffering from chronic bronchitis.

The clinical features will usually indicate if the patient is suffering from infection and further laboratory investigations that may be of value include sputum culture and microscopy (including culture for tuberculosis) and blood should be taken for haemoglobin and white cell count, blood culture and search for viral antibodies.

Pulmonary eosinophilia is usually associated with a high or normal total white blood cell count and an absolute eosinophilia. The sputum may contain eosinophils. In tropical pulmonary eosinophilia the stool may contain parasites [36].

A multitude of diverse severe insults to the lung can result in alveolar opacification. If this fails to clear with antibiotics or diuretics the possibility of adult respiratory distress syndrome should be considered.

Case 30

A lady of 73 was in a car that plunged off the motorway into a flooded ditch. Her chest x-ray on admission is shown.

There is widespread 'alveolar' opacification. Over the next few days the chest x-ray did not clear.

The opacification became more confluent. A diagnosis was made of adult respiratory distress syndrome due to near-drowning. Note also that the ET tube is positioned too low: one of the values of ITU films is in showing the position of tubes (endotracheal tube, nasogastric tube, central venous pressure line etc).

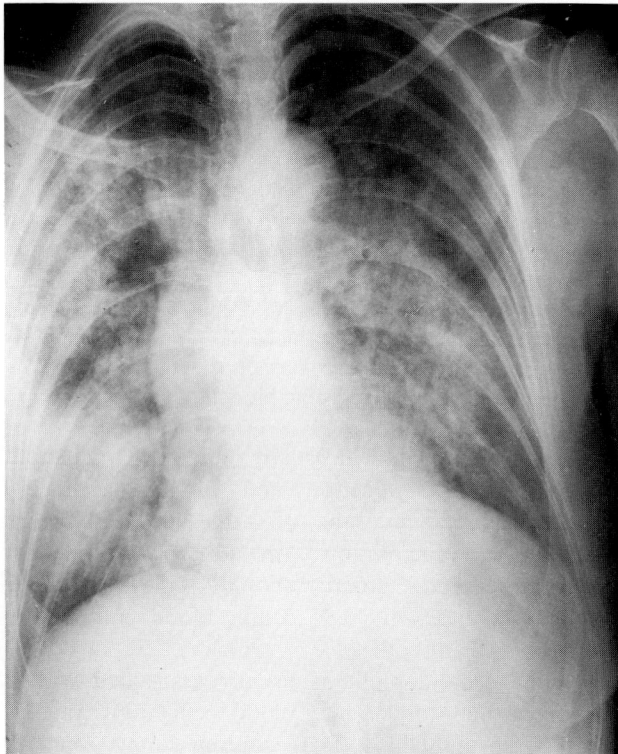

Figure 30a

Figure 30b

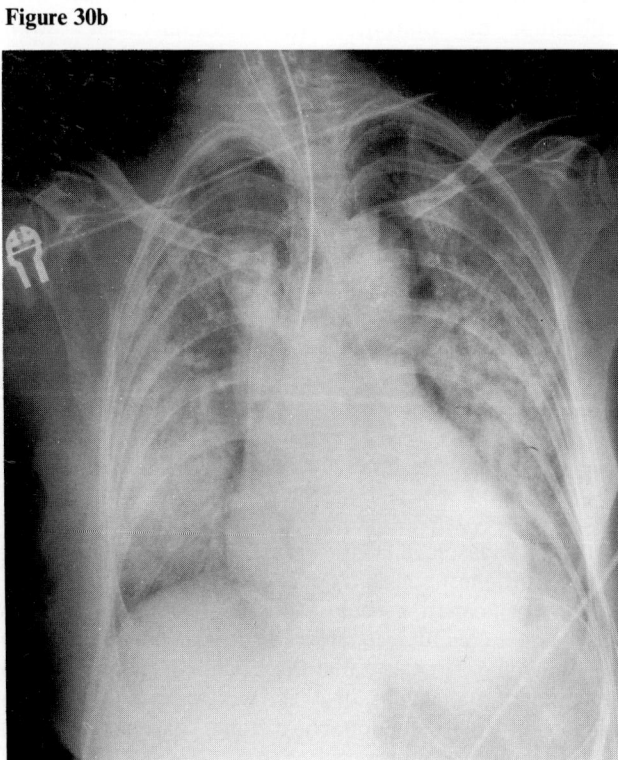

Many of the causes of alveolar opacification can result in adult respiratory distress syndrome (ARDS). This condition, also known as shock lung, is the final expression of a multitude of diverse insults to the lung. Its characteristic features are diffuse pulmonary opacification, refractory hypoxaemia and respiratory distress [37]. The various conditions which can result in shock lung are listed in Table 8.

Table 8   Adult respiratory distress syndrome

Conditions that may result in 'shock lung'

1   Sepsis
2   Aspiration of gastric contents or near drowning
3   Lung contusion
4   Burns
5   Multiple blood transfusions
6   Disseminated intravascular coagulopathy (DIC)
7   Long bone or pelvic fractures
8   Atypical pneumonia
9   Prolonged hypotension
10   Pancreatitis

If more than one of the above conditions occur together, the likelihood of developing adult respiratory distress syndrome rises considerably.

The pulmonary response to acute injury and subsequent repair is similar whether the insult is delivered by inhalation or mediated via the blood stream. Whatever the cause it progresses through exudative, proliferative and fibrotic phases. In the exudative phase of ARDS a 'hyaline membrane' forms in areas of severe epithelial damage and in this way it is similar to the respiratory distress syndrome that occurs in the neonatal period.

In adult respiratory distress syndrome, there is increased vascular permeability and fluid passes across the capillary wall into the interstitium and into the alveoli. This fluid has a higher protein concentration than that in transudation due to heart failure. Lung vascular permeability can be monitored by the use of radiolabelling of proteins. Basran, Burn and Hardy (1983) [38] showed increased vascular permeability in adult respiratory distress syndrome using a non-invasive technique. This involved the radiolabelling of protein transferrin with indium-113 metastable and labelling red blood cells with technetium. The radioactivity over the lung field and the cardiac blood pool were measured using a portable scintillation probe. An index of protein accumulation was calculated and it was found that vascular permeability was increased in severe pneumonia, but was far higher in adult respiratory distress syndrome. In one of their patients with ARDS the permeability index returned to normal following methyl prednisolone and the patient made a full recovery.

An alternative method of providing a measure that relates to permeability is for the patient to inhale a radioactive substance that is cleared from the alveoli via the blood stream. This may be done by inhalation of technetium-labelled DTPA.

In adult respiratory distress syndrome the hypoxaemia is caused by shunting. In some areas there is perfusion of unventilated lung, and in others relative mismatch. The normal mechanism of regional vasoconstriction in response to hypoxia appears to be damaged in adult respiratory distress syndrome, resulting in the mismatch of perfusion and ventilation [37].

Summary; widespread alveolar opacification

Generalized opacification of the alveoli can occur due to transudation, exudation, inhalation or infiltration. If it is widespread in both lung fields, the most common causes are pulmonary oedema or infection. Careful examination of the radiographs and assessment of the pulmonary vasculature, bronchi and parenchyma is necessary.

The pulmonary response to acute injury whatever the cause is a progression through exudative, proliferative and fibrotic phases. In the earlier stages the appearances will be those of alveolar opacification. A variety of insults to the lung can produce an end result known as 'shock lung' or 'adult respiratory distress syndrome'. Differentiation of ARDS from pulmonary oedema or bronchopneumonia may be difficult based on radiographic appearances. There is some indication that scintigraphic assessment of pulmonary vascular permeability may assist in the diagnosis.

7 Consolidation

Consolidation, used as a radiological term, does not immediately imply infection. The term is used to describe the situation when the air within the acinus is replaced by fluid, tissue or exudate resulting in opacification of the parenchyma [39].

The plain radiographic features of consolidation are well known and described clearly in other textbooks.

Two important features are described below:

1 *Air bronchogram*. If there is consolidation without involvement of the conducting airways, the air in the bronchi will appear as a radiolucent branching pattern against the white background. This is known as an 'air bronchogram' [40].

2 *The silhouette sign* is also of interest. If the lung is opacified adjacent to a boundary, such as the diaphragm or mediastinum, the outline of the boundary will be lost. This assists in determination of the position of an opacity on the plain film.

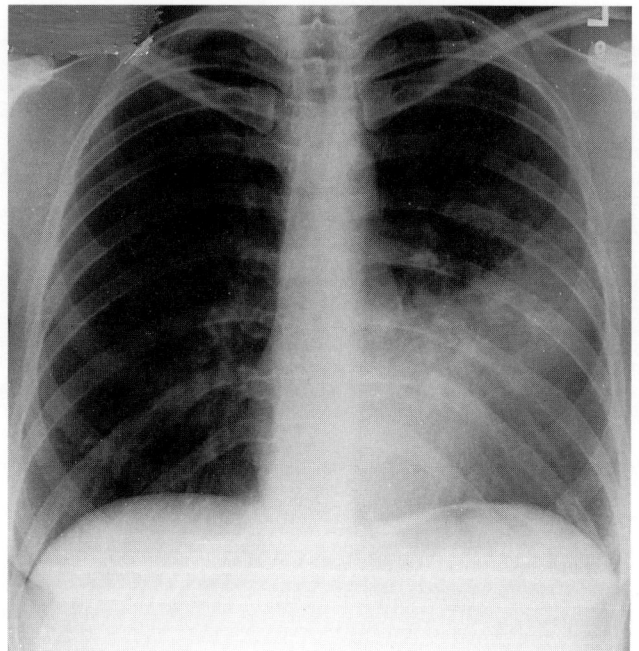

Figure 31

Case 31

Mary, aged 30, had suffered from 'flu' for the past week. She presented with a history of fever for seven days, dry cough and wheezing. Rhonchi were audible over the left side of the chest. An x-ray was performed. (See fig. 31.)

The PA chest x-ray shows opacification of the left mid and lower zone. The left heart border is obscured by the opacification and this indicates that the increased density is in lung tissue immediately adjacent to the heart.

If the opacity was not adjacent to the heart but only superimposed (for example if the opacification was posteriorly placed), the densities would be added together and the heart outline would still be visible.

The loss of a radiographic outline due to immediately adjacent opacification is known as the 'silhouette sign' since the normal silhouette is obscured.

The features in this case are due to consolidation of the lingula.

Opacification of the left lower lobe would result in loss of the outline of the left hemidiaphragm and this is particularly obvious on the PA film when the anterior basal segment is affected.

On the right side, opacification of the middle lobe will obscure the heart border, while increased density in the lower lobe will obscure the right hemidiaphragm. The site of the opacification is best revealed by a lateral chest x-ray.

The consolidation did not improve with a course of penicillin but responded to tetracycline. A radiograph two weeks later showed almost complete resolution. High antibody titres indicated that the pneumonia was due to psittacosis!

After a course of treatment, the clinical improvement often takes place before the radiological resolution. If consolidation does not, however, clear with treatment by antibiotics and physiotherapy, there may be several possible causes and they are listed in Table 9.

Table 9 Non-resolution of 'consolidation'

1 Non-sensitive organism ('wrong' antibiotic)
2 Underlying lung pathology, particularly
   (i) carcinoma obstructing a bronchus (foreign body in a child)
   (ii) bronchiectasis (and bronchopulmonary aspergillosis)
3 Repeated aspiration, e.g. oesophageal disease
4 Immunological deficiency (including acquired immune deficiency syndrome [AIDS], cytotoxic and anti-inflammatory treatment)
5 Non-infective cause of 'consolidation', e.g.:
   (i) pulmonary oedema
   (ii) pulmonary infarction
   (iii) adult respiratory distress syndrome (shock lung)
   (iv) contusion
6 Pulmonary fibrosis rather than consolidation
   (i) progressive massive fibrosis in pneumoconiosis
   (ii) post-radiotherapy pneumonitis proceeding to fibrosis
7 Opacity was *not* consolidation, e.g.:
   (i) carcinoma of the bronchus
   (ii) encysted effusion

Many of the causes of non-resolving consolidation can be distinguished by the clinical history and examination. Problems commonly exist in distinguishing between infarction and infection on plain films and in distinguishing between widespread pulmonary infection and pulmonary oedema. Luckily the clinical details allow the distinction to be made in many cases. The diagnosis of pulmonary oedema is discussed in Chapter 6 and infarction is discussed later in this chapter and also in Chapter 9.

Investigation should now be directed towards discovering the cause of non-resolution.

Sputum should be taken for microscopy, culture and sensitivity and for sputum cytology. Serum antibody titres may be requested and white cell count and in some cases white cell function studies and immunoglobulin electrophoresis can be undertaken. The diagnosis of Pneumocystis carinii pneumonia in a patient with acquired immune deficiency syndrome (AIDS) must not be forgotten. If the patient is an adult smoker, the possibility of carcinoma of the bronchus must be considered.

Bronchoscopy is then of considerable value. A carcinoma or endobronchial tumour may be directly visualized or biopsy and washings may give diagnostic

information. In children the history may suggest inhalation of a foreign body, and in such a case the foreign body may be removed bronchoscopically. Bronchoscopic samples may also reveal organisms such as Mycobacterium tuberculosis or Pneumocystis carinii. Bronchography may be performed as an adjunct to bronchoscopy or as a separate investigation.

Percutaneous needle biopsy is usually of limited value since a carcinoma would normally be proximal to the consolidation and may well be hidden within the general opacification. Needle biopsy can, however, be helpful in determining the organism causing consolidation. If the opacity is adjacent to the chest wall, mediastinum or diaphragm, *ultrasound* may assist in distinguishing between encysted pleural effusion, tumour mass and consolidation (see Case 27).

If there is a possibility of aspiration, *barium studies* may show pharyngeal or oesophageal disease and even demonstrate inhalation of barium.

Case 32

A man of 67, a heavy smoker, presented with a history of dysphagia and recurrent chest infections.

Figure 32a

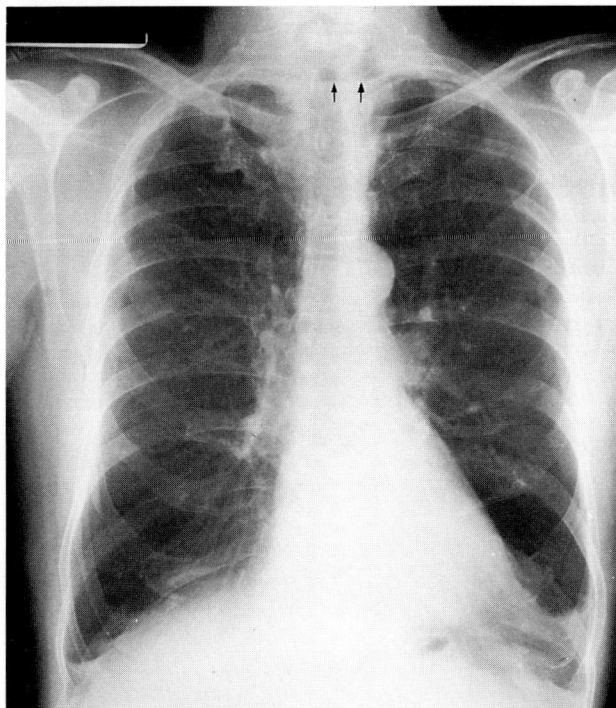

The chest x-ray shows over-expansion of the lung fields and areas of radiolucency due to pulmonary emphysema. In addition a fluid level is present in the superior mediastinum (*arrowed*). The barium swallow is shown in figure 32b.

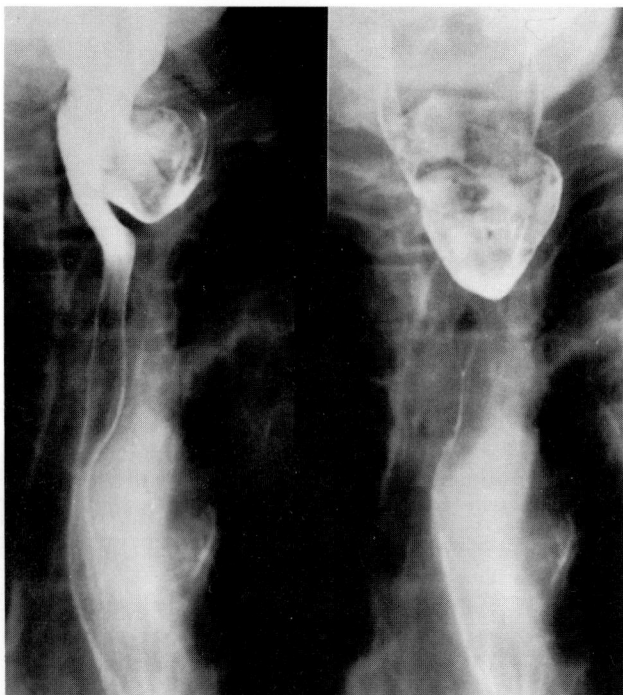

Figure 32b

There is a large pharyngeal pouch (Zenker's diverticulum). The chest infections were related both to the history of smoking and to aspiration of the contents of the pouch.

Case 33

An elderly lady had bilateral rhonchi and intermittent chest infections.

The chest x-ray showed linear opacities in both lung fields and some elevation of the left hemidiaphragm. A

Figure 33a

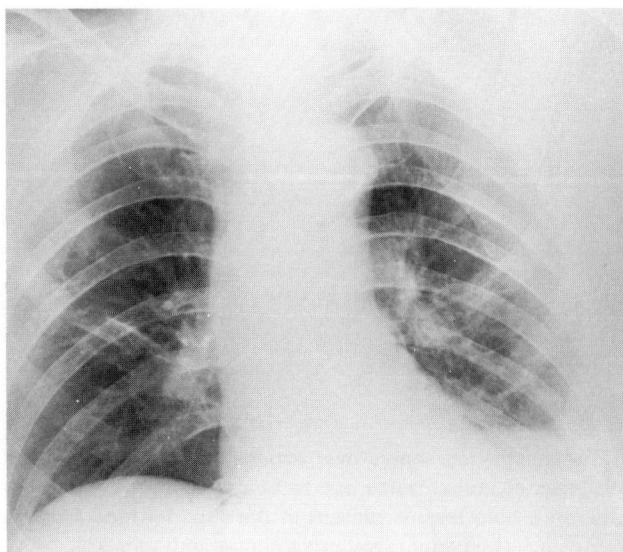

barium swallow was carried out because the patient also complained of slight dysphagia.

The barium swallow showed, on screening, that the patient had poor coordination when swallowing and there was considerable aspiration of barium. The spot film shows barium in the trachea and right bronchial tree and tertiary contractions of the oesophagus. Conclusion: recurrent aspiration pneumonia.

Figure 33b

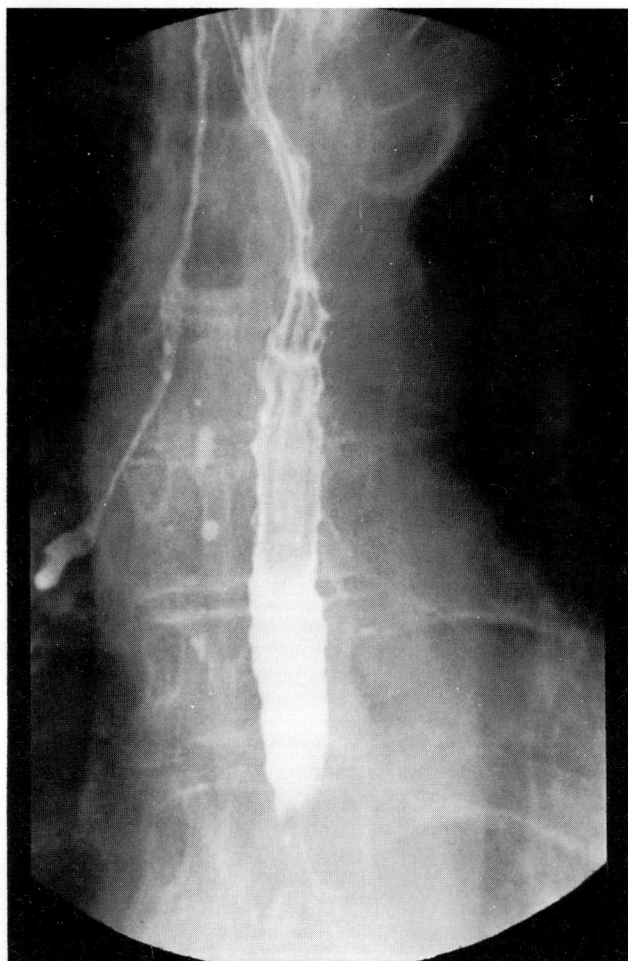

In the last two cases the diagnosis was fairly easily made by a barium swallow. The most common cause of aspiration is probably a sliding hiatus hernia. This may also be demonstrated by barium studies. Reflux and aspiration is, however, notoriously difficult to demonstrate reliably since it is an intermittent problem and may only occur when the patient is sleeping or performing a particular movement such as bending. Aspiration can cause recurrent chest infections or simulate asthma and can result in pulmonary fibrosis.

Monitoring of the oesophageal pH is now possible and can be carried out on ambulatory patients going about their normal activities. This will demonstrate whether or not there is reflux of acid stomach contents.

Various *scintigraphic* investigations can also assist in patients with non-resolving 'consolidation'.

Gallium will be taken up in any area of active inflammation but may assist by showing other sites of disease, such as the hilar nodes. It is actively taken up by lymphoma. Indium-labelled white cells act in a similar manner to gallium but are less specific than gallium in the chest.

Ventilation/perfusion studies may show mismatched defects of perfusion in the abnormality and in other areas of the lungs and thus assist in demonstrating that an area of consolidation is infarction rather than infection. The reverse is not, however, true. If there are no mismatched defects, this does not negate the possibility of infarction as a cause of an opacity. The negative result, as is often the case in radiology, is rarely of great help. Ventilation/perfusion studies matched with *computed tomography* are also useful in patients with radiation pneumonopathy (Chapter 9).

Computed tomography may be able to show whether the opacity is a solid mass or consolidated lung and can also help in showing the extent of lung and mediastinal involvement. It can demonstrate that a lesion is pleural rather than pulmonary (e.g. encysted effusion, pleural plaques). CT is replacing bronchography in the demonstration of bronchiectasis and on occasions demonstrates pulmonary consolidation that has been completely missed on the plain films.

Finally, open biopsy may be necessary in order to diagnose conditions such as Pneumocystis carinii or lymphoma.

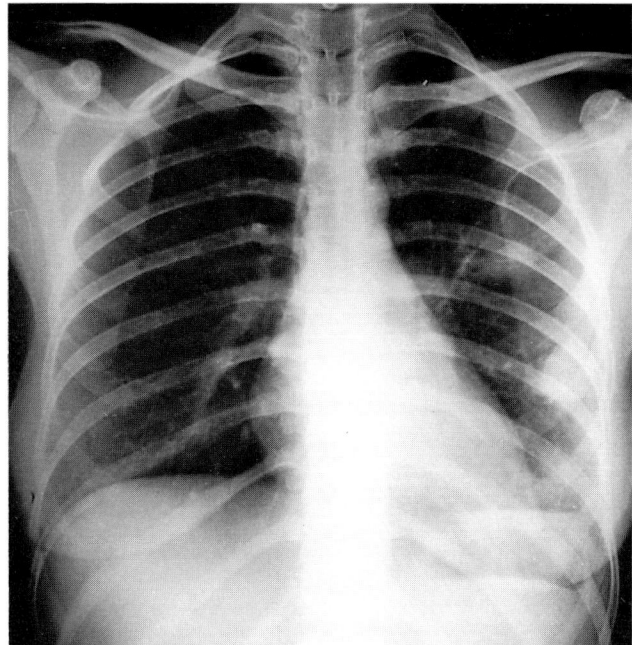

Figure 34a

Figure 34b

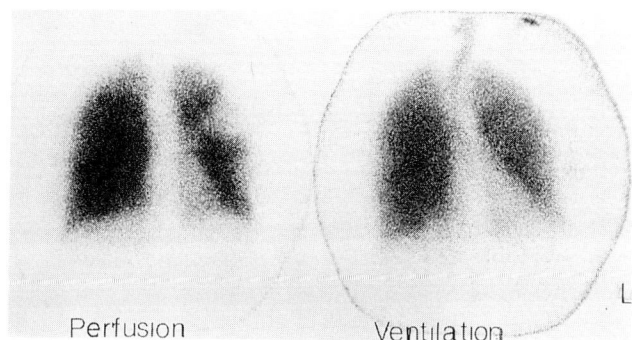

Case 34

A lady of 35 had a history of pleuritic chest pain of acute onset and deep vein thrombosis.

The chest x-ray showed two faint areas of 'consolidation' peripherally in the left lung field.

Ventilation/perfusion scanning was carried out (fig. 34b).

The ventilation/perfusion scans showed two wedge-shaped perfusion defects with very slight ventilation defect. It is always difficult to interpret ventilation/perfusion scans in the presence of chest x-ray abnormalities (see also Chapter 9, pages 91–93). In this case the mismatch of perfusion and the history were indicative of infarction rather than infection. It was concluded that the abnormalities were due to pulmonary infarction.

Case 35

A man aged 23, who had previously been treated for Hodgkin's lymphoma, presented with patchy opacification in the right lower zone on his chest radiograph.

This area of 'consolidation' persisted despite antibiotic therapy. Gallium scanning and computed tomography were done.

Gallium scanning showed marked uptake in the right lower zone. CT showed extensive dense opacification in the right lung and patchy opacification in the left lung. There were bilateral pleural effusions. Bronchoscopy and transbronchial biopsy and percutaneous needle biopsy were performed but yielded only non-specific results. Open biopsy confirmed the presence of recurrent Hodgkin's

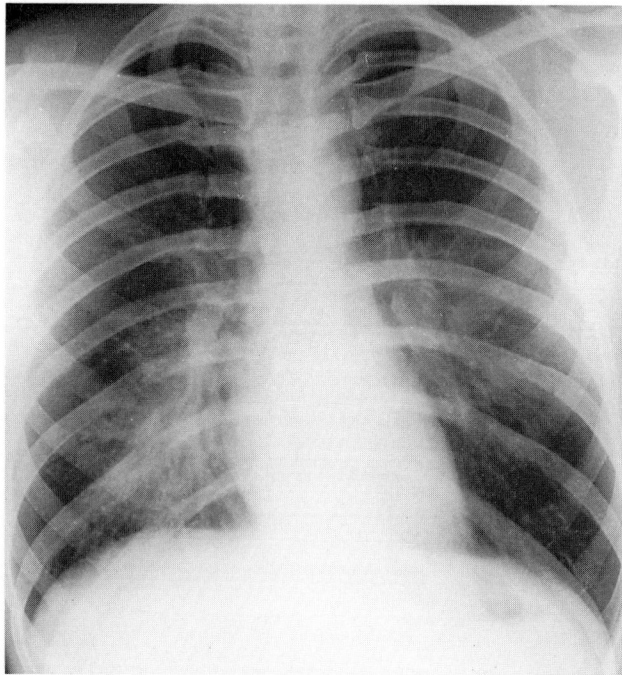

Figure 35a

Figure 35b

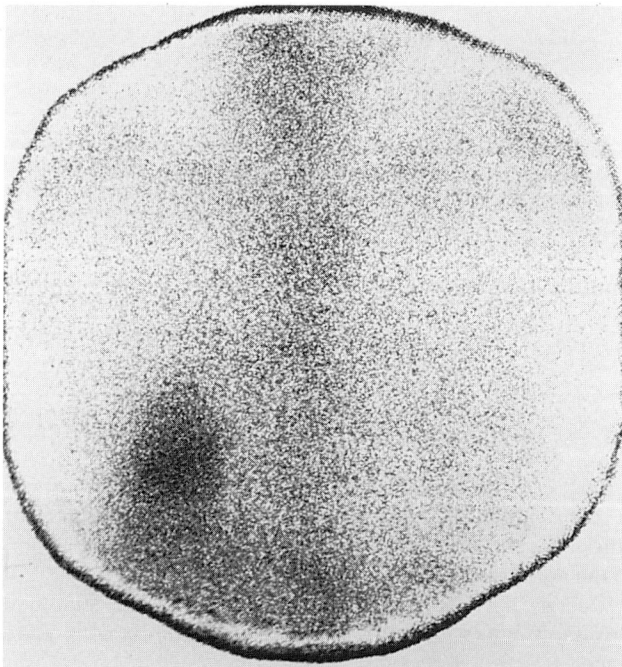

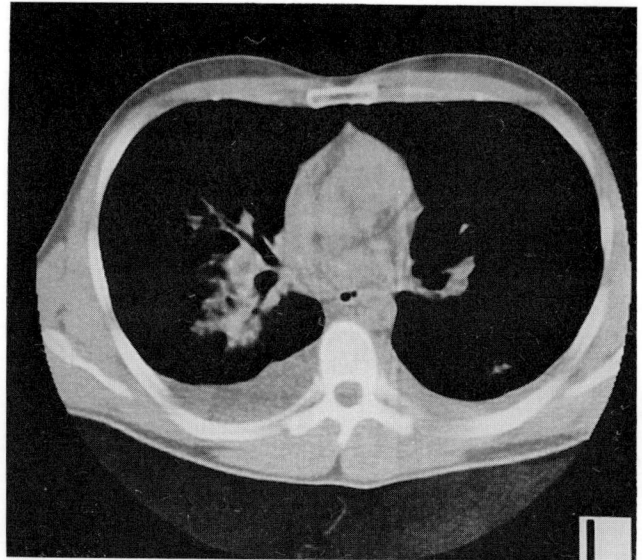

Figure 35c

Figure 35d

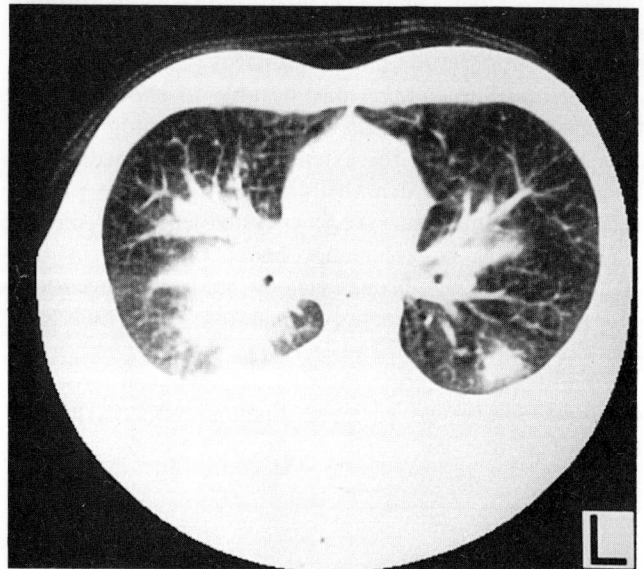

lymphoma. This case illustrates the difficulty, in cases of recurrent lymphoma, of interpretation of the cytology from needle biopsy and the value of the open biopsy. Naturally, if a more accessible lesion such as a palpable lymph node had been available, it would have been the preferable site to biopsy.

Case 36

A 33 year old lady had a history of recurrent chest infections and sinusitis.

The chest radiograph shows opacification obscuring the left heart border. The appearances are similar to those seen in Case 31 and represent consolidation in the lingula. This had been present for some months and did not clear with antibiotics. The x-ray of the sinuses shows an opaque right

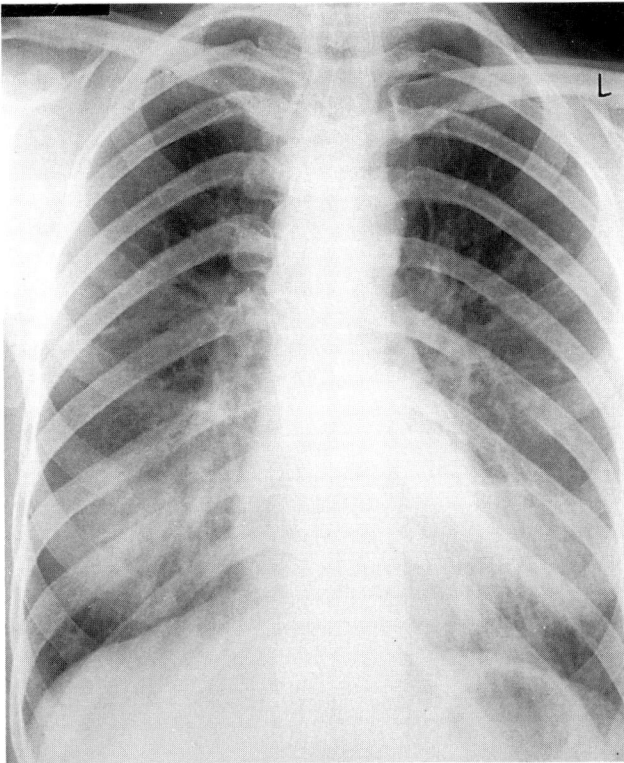

Figure 36a

Figure 36b

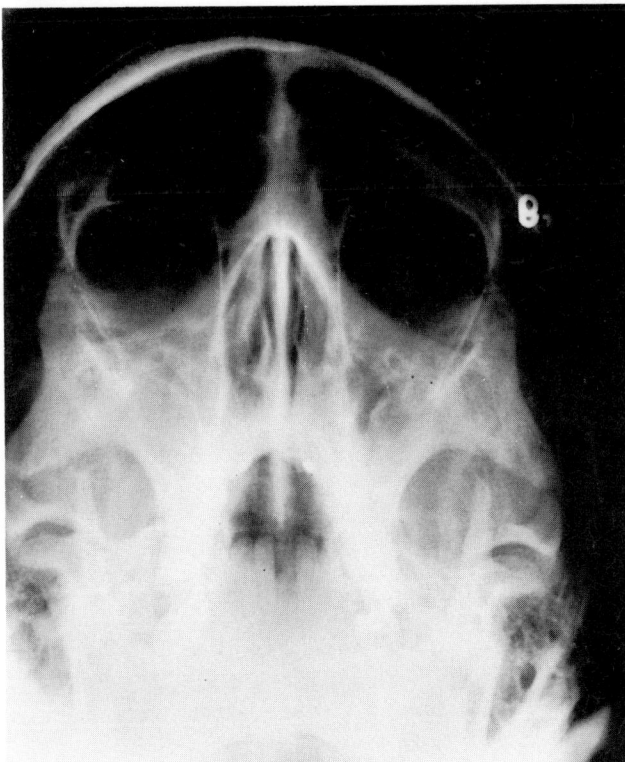

maxillary antrum and mucosal thickening of the left antrum, features that are due to chronic sinusitis.

Computed tomography of the chest was done.

Figure 36c

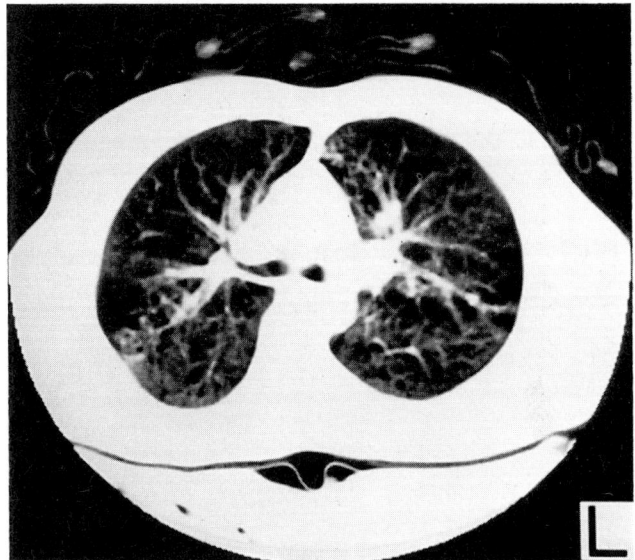

The CT scans show 'cystic' holes and dilatation of bronchi in both lung fields. On the scan shown, in the left lung the lingula is affected and on the right side there is bronchiectasis of the posterior segment of the upper lobe (the blow-up [fig. 36d] shows the changes in the right lung).

Figure 36d

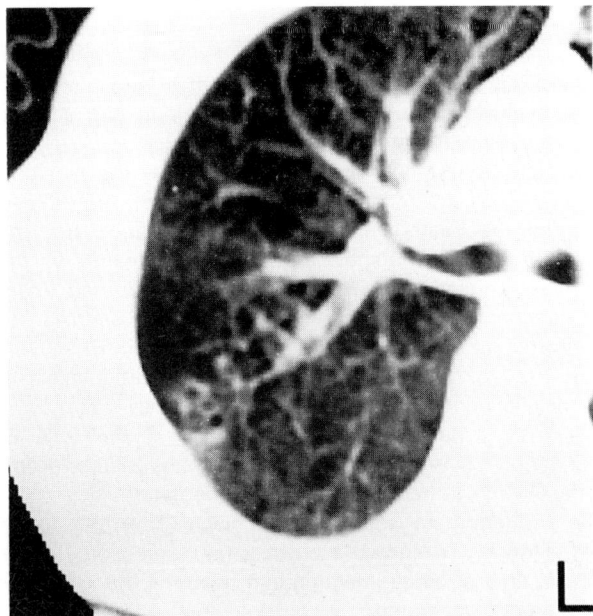

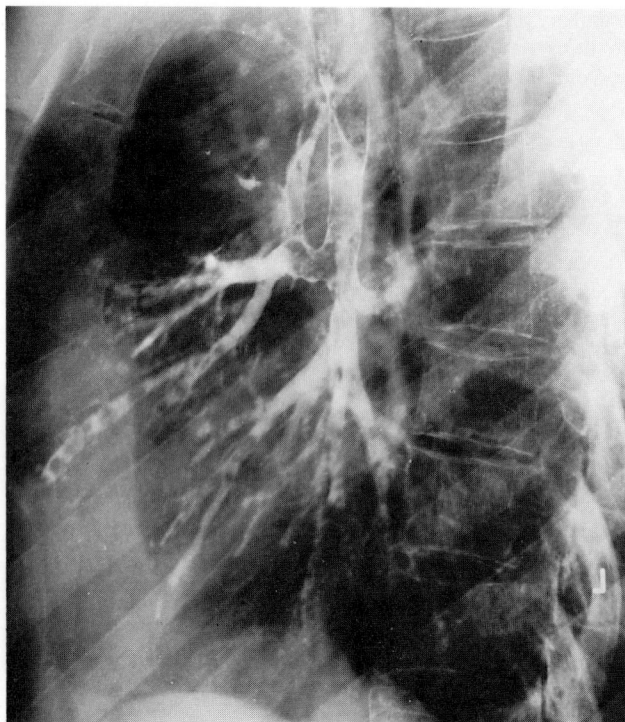

Figure 36e

A bronchoscopy was undertaken followed by a limited bronchogram to show the lingula. Bronchiectasis in the lingula was confirmed (fig. 36e).

Computed tomography is capable of showing even minor degrees of bronchiectasis. Because bronchography is an unpleasant examination, the investigation is being replaced, wherever possible, by CT or bronchoscopy.

Case 37

A young girl in her teens presented with a long history of recurrent chest infections. A chest radiograph and a sinus x-ray are shown in figures 37a and 37b.

The main abnormality on the chest x-ray is the fact that the patient has dextrocardia. The film has been reproduced such that the heart is in the normal orientation but the markers are visible and show that the heart is mainly on the right side. The other main abnormality is ill-defined linear opacification in the left mid to lower zone obscuring the heart border. In addition an endotracheal tube is in situ.

The x-ray of the patient's sinuses shows fluid levels in both maxillary antra indicative of acute sinusitis.

The patient had bronchography, since at the time of investigation CT was not available. In figures 37c, 37d and 37e the chest is turned into the normal orientation.

The bronchogram showed bronchiectasis in the lower zones. Figure 37e shows a chest x-ray taken some years later at a time of acute infection and this time the x-ray has been correctly orientated.

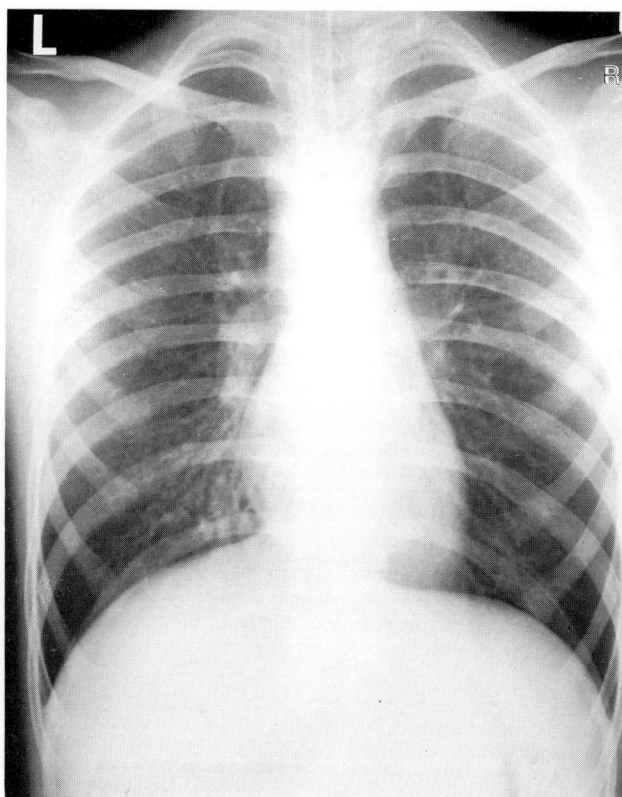

Figure 37a

Figure 37b

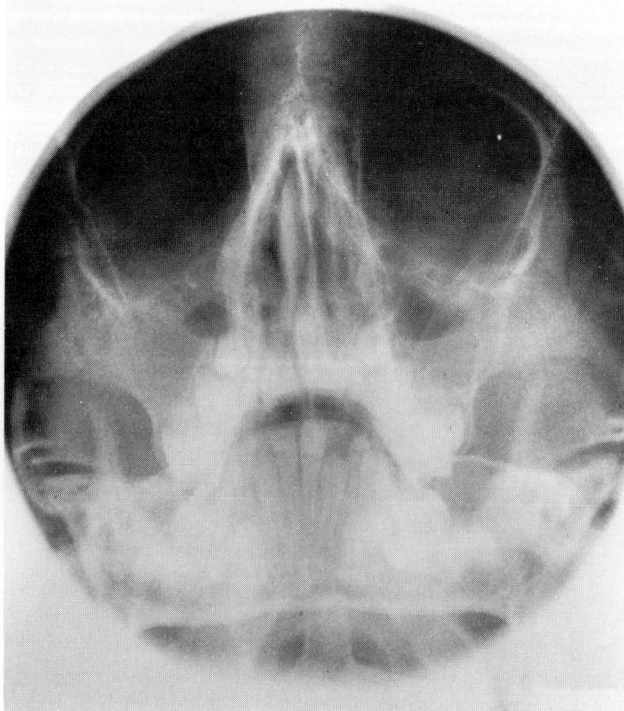

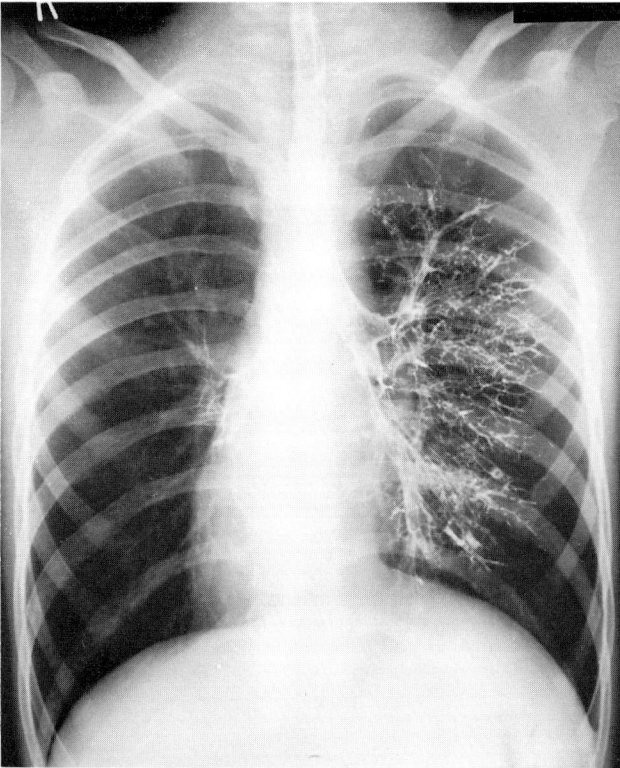

Figure 37c

Figure 37d

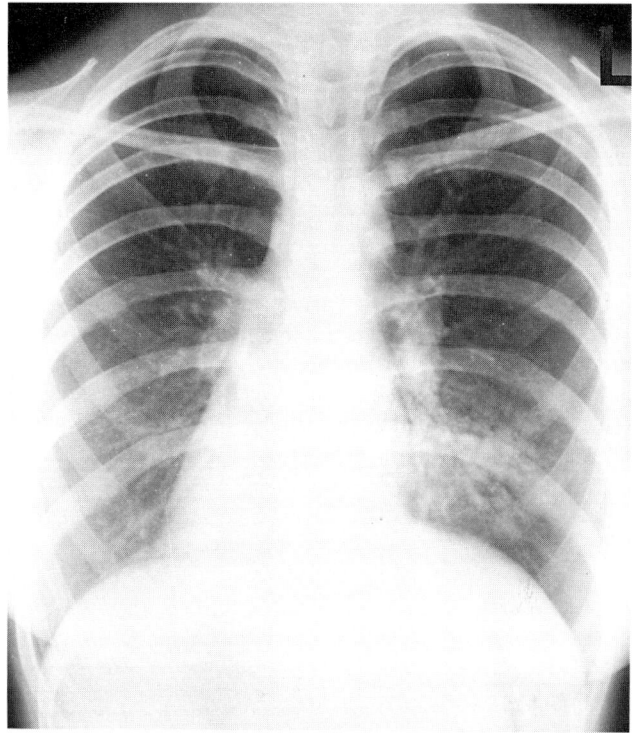

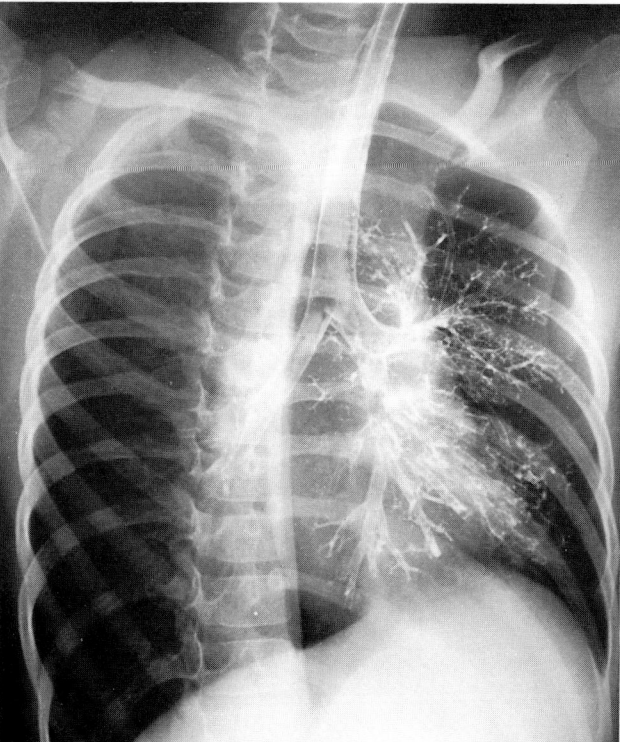

Figure 37e

The combination of dextrocardia, bronchiectasis and sinusitis make up the condition known as Kartagener's syndrome. This syndrome was first described by Kartagener in 1933 and in 1975 Afzelius, using electron microscopy, found ultrastructural defects in the cilia of patients with the condition. The main defect of the cilia is the lack of a small projection on the outer microtubules (known as a dynein arm). These abnormalities of the cilia impair mucociliary clearance leading to chronic infections, bronchiectasis and sinusitis. In men the spermatozoa also have deficient movement of their tails and it was this feature that brought attention to the ciliary abnormality in the syndrome. The discovery of the defects in ciliary structure has led to the adoption of the term 'immotile cilia syndrome' or more appropriately 'ciliary dysfunction syndrome'.

Although dextrocardia is a feature of Kartagener's syndrome, it is possible to have bronchiectasis due to abnormal ciliary movement without dextrocardia. This should be suspected in patients with chronic lung disease who have siblings with Kartagener's syndrome, or in men when the spermatozoa are living but immotile. Patients with ciliary dysfunction are uncommon, but it is possible that in the future electron microscopy of nasal biopsies will be a routine procedure for the diagnosis of ciliary dysfunction in patients with chronic sinusitis and bronchiectasis.

(This case was provided by Dr A Duncan of Bristol Children's Hospital.)

Case 38

A lady with carcinoma of the bronchus was treated with two opposing radiotherapy fields. The chest radiograph one year later is shown.

An opacity was present in the left hilar region. It was questioned whether this was recurrent carcinoma or fibrosis from radiation therapy.

CT clearly showed the 'mass' to be straight-edged in accordance with the edge of the radiation field. An 'air-bronchogram' was very clearly seen within the opacity. The lung beyond the fibrosis was reduced in lung volume and the vessels small. In retrospect these features are all visible on the plain film.

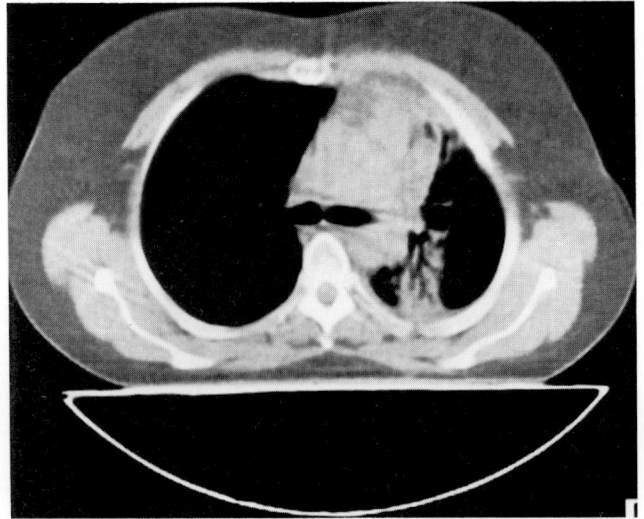

Figure 38b

Figure 38a

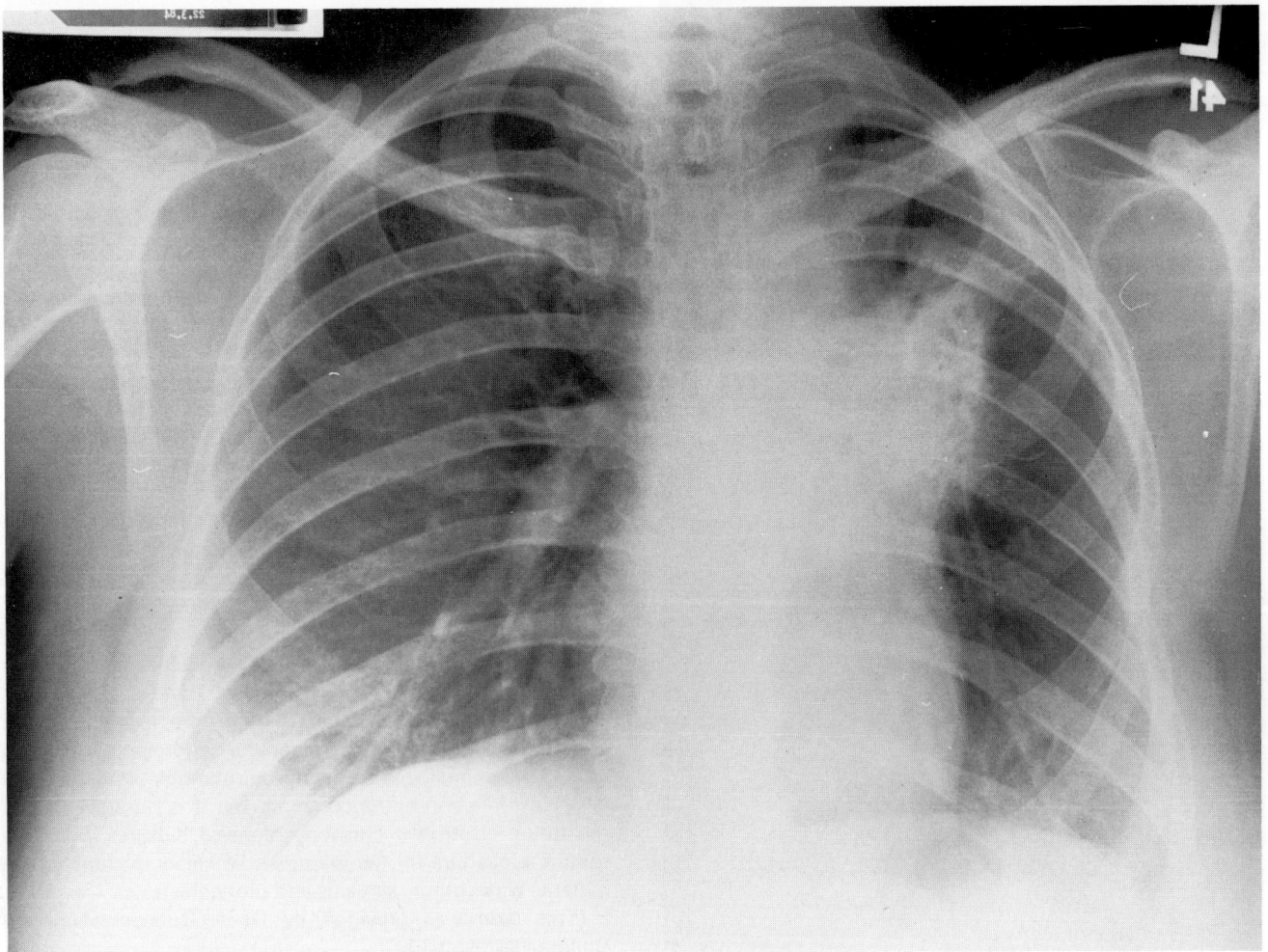

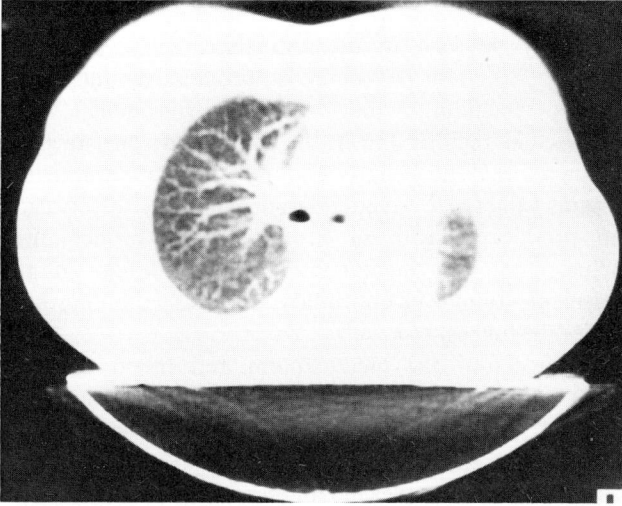

Figure 38c

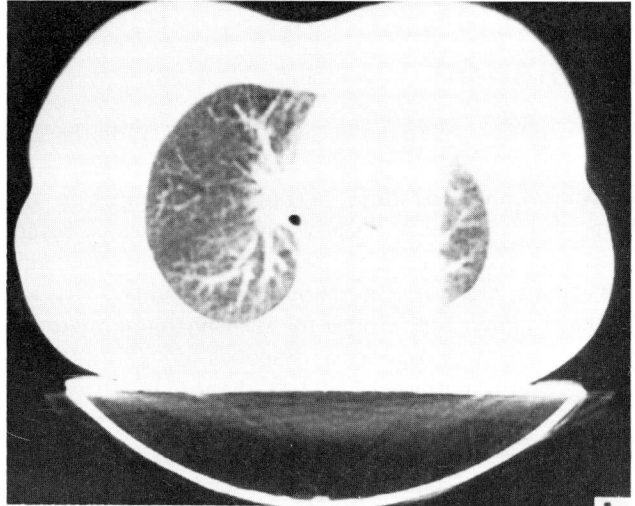

Figure 38e

Figure 38d

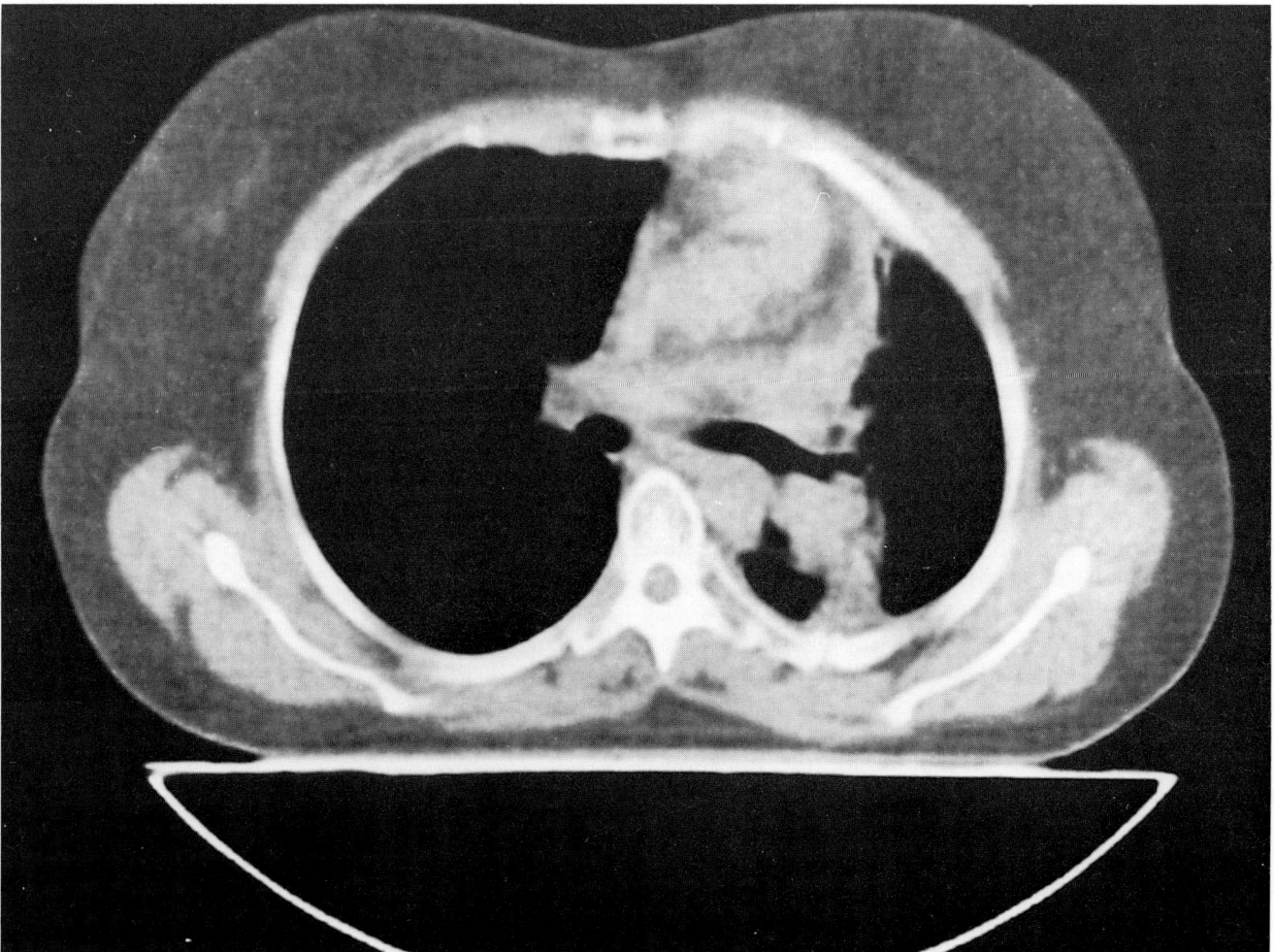

Pulmonary changes following irradiation

The majority of patients who receive radiotherapy involving the chest are effectively treated with subclinical manifestations of radiation changes in the lungs [41]. However, some patients develop severe pneumonopathy following radiation therapy and this can cause considerable morbidity and mortality.

The common time course for such pneumonopathy is for the patient to experience dyspnoea, cough and fever some two to ten weeks after radiation involving the chest. The radiograph seven to ten days later reveals the first sign of diffuse haze in the treatment zone which becomes more coalescent later and defined more precisely to the treatment portals with a straight edge. If the injury has been severe, the clinical signs may include cyanosis, orthopnoea, high fever and intractable cough. The lung changes may progress to a chronic fibrotic phase with increased pulmonary disability.

Initially the radiation changes may be misinterpreted as being due to pneumonia (particularly opportunistic infections such as *Pneumocystis carinii*), recurrent cancer, lymphangitis or metastasis. The main distinguishing features radiologically occur because the opacity is confined by the boundaries of the radiation fields. The consolidation is not confined to the normal lung architecture and thus is not segmental or lobar. The edge of the abnormal area is usually straight due to the sharp cut-off of the radiation field. Whilst this may not be apparent on the chest x-ray or lateral film it is often clearly seen by computed tomography. It follows that it is important to know the shape of the radiation fields incurred by the patient before making definitive comments on the results of the imaging investigations.

There is, however, no consistent correlation between the recognition, duration and severity of an early radiation pneumonopathy and the occurrence of late delayed pulmonary fibrosis. Moreover, progressive pulmonary fibrosis producing a scarred and retracted lung and cor pulmonale may develop seemingly with no clinical evidence of pre-existing acute radiation pneumonopathy [41].

In a few patients the exudative stage and the consolidation of fibrosis extend outside the radiation portals and this is considered likely to be due to an immune reaction. The characteristic pathology changes in the area affected directly by the radiation damage are twofold. Progressive vascular sclerosis must be considered as primarily responsible for most major lung changes, the arterioles and small arteries exhibiting the most profound changes. The changes, however, will eventually be seen in medium sized and even larger arteries. Secondarily there is progressive interstitial fibrosis including the septa, peribronchial and perivascular regions and in the subpleural zone. In most instances the bronchial and bronchiolar epithelium remains intact. However, intercurrent bacterial invasion can produce necrotizing bronchitis and bronchiolitis. Inclusion of the mediastinum or the hilum in the treatment volume in continuity with the adjoining lung carries the highest risk.

If fibrosis of the mediastinum and hilum develops following irradiation, there is often marked reduction in perfusion and ventilation of the lung beyond the confines of the radiotherapy field. This is further discussed with examples in Chapter 9, pages 87–89.

Varying opacities

In the immediately previous part of this chapter the investigation of persistent consolidation has been discussed. Many of the causes of persistent consolidation result in opacification that remains in one place with only slow change occurring from one examination to the next. Some conditions that cause recurring consolidation result in opacities that vary in position or configuration on successive chest radiographs. The common causes of this phenomenon and listed in Table 10 and a number of examples follow.

Table 10   Varying opacities

Opacification that varies in position and configuration from one chest x-ray to the next
1   Pneumonia
2   Aspiration pneumonia
3   Bronchiectasis
4   Pulmonary oedema
5   Bronchopulmonary aspergillosis
6   Eosinophilia
7   (Hyaline membrane disease – newborn)
8   Pulmonary haemorrhage

Case 39

A man aged 33 presented with a history of eczema and asthma and had the following appearances on his chest radiograph.

The chest radiograph revealed an opacity in the right

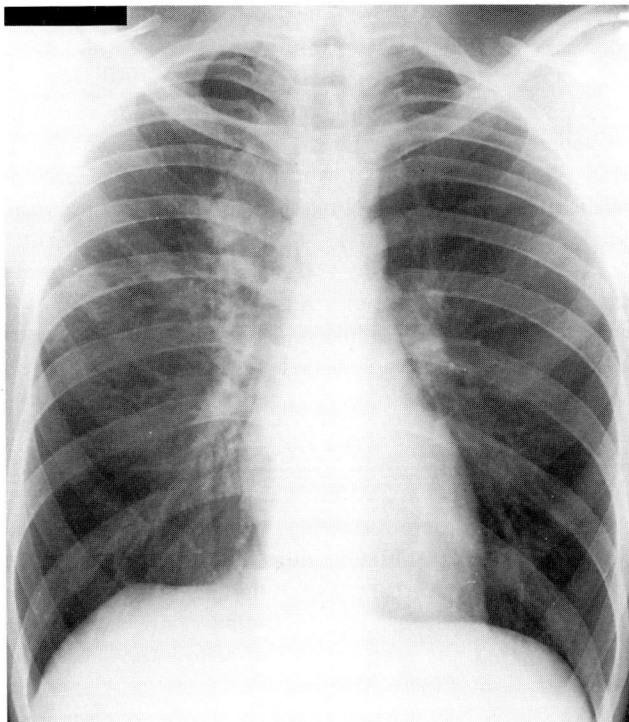

Figure 39a

Figure 39b

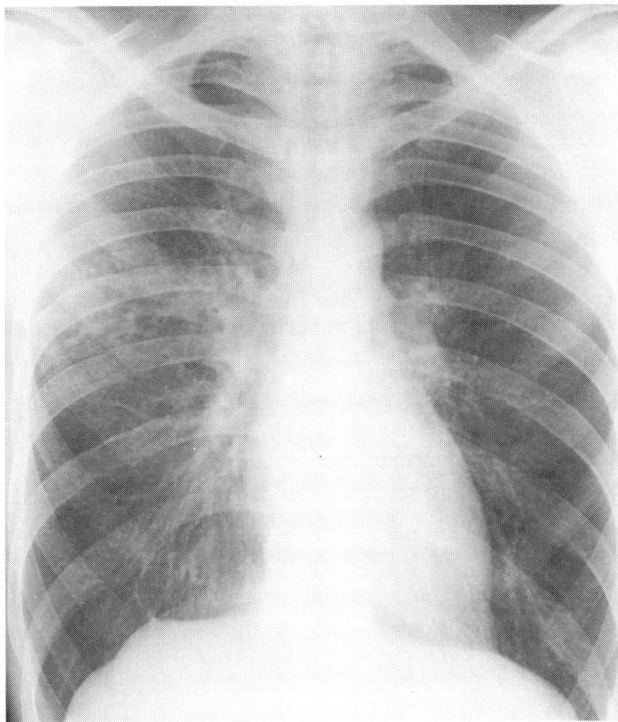

Figure 39c

Figure 39d

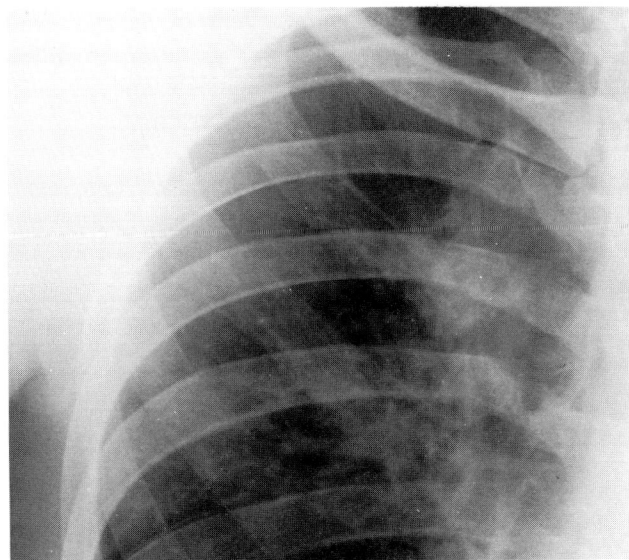

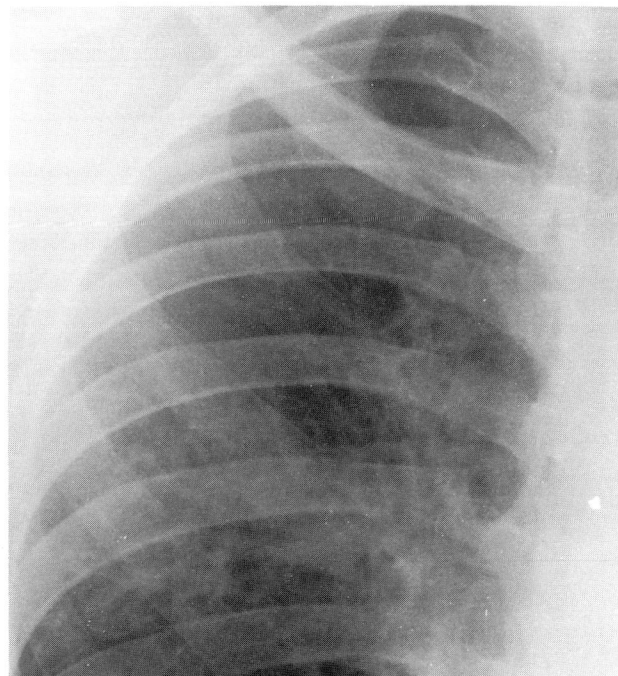

paramediastinal region. An 'air bronchogram' was visible running through the opacity indicative of consolidation. Close examination (fig. 39b) showed slight reticular shadowing above the horizontal fissure. A further radiograph was taken just two weeks later.

This showed that the paramediastinal opacity had disappeared. The changes above the horizontal fissure were more prominent. A tentative diagnosis of bronchopulmonary aspergillosis had been made on seeing the first radiograph. By the time of the second radiograph the diagnosis had been confirmed by positive precipitin tests.

Aspergillus fumigatus has now been described in this book as causing three different, but related diseases. In Case 26 there is an example of an intracavitary fungus ball or mycetoma due to *Aspergillus* growing in a pre-existing cavity. Invasive *Aspergillus* pneumonia has been discussed (Case 27). The fungus ball and the invasive pneumonia probably represent two ends of the spectrum of disease caused directly by *Aspergillus*.

The third condition, bronchopulmonary aspergillosis, has been described in the previous example and is probably the most common of the three. The condition occurs in asthmatic patients and the pulmonary changes result from hypersensitivity to *Aspergillus*. Bronchiectasis of the moderate sized bronchi is the characteristic pulmonary abnormality and there may be opacification that varies from film to film. There is usually an increase of eosinophils in the sputum and blood and positive precipitins to *Aspergillus*.

Summary: pulmonary consolidation

Consolidation is a radiological term used to describe a lung in which there is opacification of the parenchyma due to either fluid, tissue or exudate. Two of the important features on the plain chest radiograph are the air-bronchogram and the silhouette sign.

Localized areas of consolidation are usually due to infection. Further radiological investigations may be necessary if there is non-resolution of the consolidation. This may occur due to many causes but probably the most common are carcinoma obstructing the bronchus, bronchiectasis, pulmonary infarction and aspiration. Many of the causes of non-resolving consolidation can be distinguished by the clinical history and examination but, if the diagnosis is not forthcoming, further investigations should be directed towards discovering the cause. Bronchoscopy must be considered if the appearances suggest carcinoma of the bronchus. Barium studies may be of value if repeated aspiration is a possibility. Other radiological investigations that may be helpful include scanning with gallium- or indium-labelled white cells and ventilation/perfusion studies. Computed tomography may be an extremely useful investigation by demonstrating whether an opacity is a solid mass or consolidated lung, by showing whether a lesion is pleural rather than pulmonary and in some cases demonstrating a carcinoma obstructing a bronchus. CT is replacing bronchography in the demonstration of bronchiectasis.

A separate but related problem is that of recurring consolidation resulting in opacities that vary in position or configuration on successive chest radiographs. Conditions that are prone to result in such appearances include aspiration pneumonia, bronchiectasis and bronchopulmonary aspergillosis. The latter condition particularly occurs in asthmatic patients and in most cases the precipitins to *Aspergillus* are positive.

8 | The opaque hemithorax

If a hemithorax is completely opaque, the implication is that either the lung itself is completely opacified or there is opacification of the pleura. If the mediastinum is shifted towards the opaque side, there must be some loss of volume in the affected lung. In the most extreme case this may be due to agenesis (it never developed) or pneumonectomy (it's in the bucket!). In most adult patients presenting with the problem of 'opaque hemithorax' shift of the mediastinum to the affected side will imply collapse of the affected lung. This in turn is due to bronchial obstruction (see Table 13, Chapter 9) and, if the diagnosis is not forthcoming from the patient's history and simple investigations, probably the correct investigation to be performed next would be *bronchoscopy*. Many such cases are due to bronchial carcinoma.

If there is no shift of the mediastinum, the appearances may be due either to consolidation, pleural thickening (including pleural tumour) or pleural effusion. Penetrated, lateral and decubitus films may assist in differentiating between these conditions. Ultrasound is able to show pleural fluid clearly and may also demonstrate consolidation.

If the mediastinum is shifted away from the affected side, the most likely causes are either a large pleural effusion or a large tumour or, of course, a combination of the two!

Computed tomography is valuable because it will differentiate between pleural, pulmonary and chest wall lesions and measurement of the radiodensity will assist in distinguishing between different conditions.

The investigation of pleural abnormalities is discussed in greater detail in Chapter 11.

Case 40

A woman of 58 years presented with a dry cough and choking sensation. Her chest x-ray PA and lateral are shown.

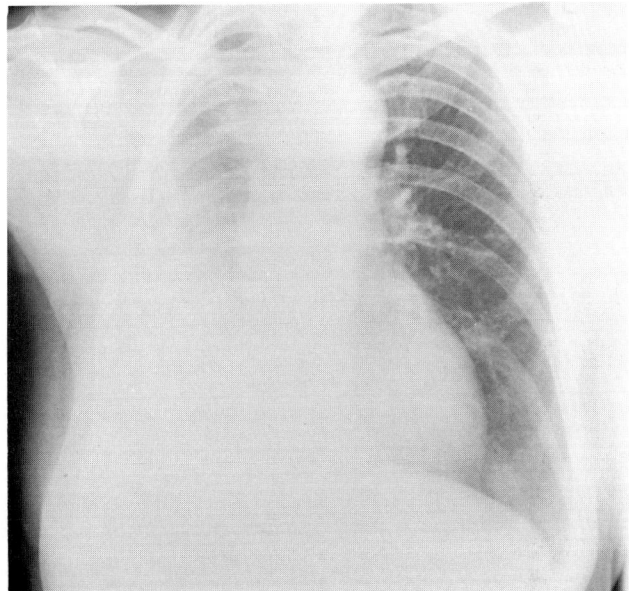

Figure 40a

Figure 40b

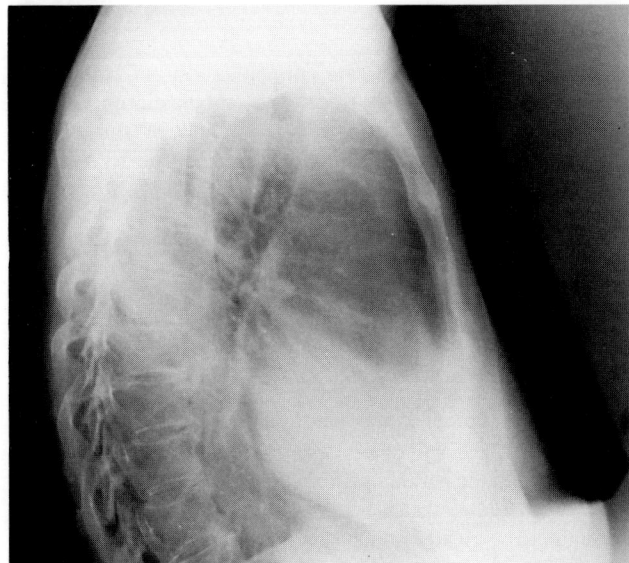

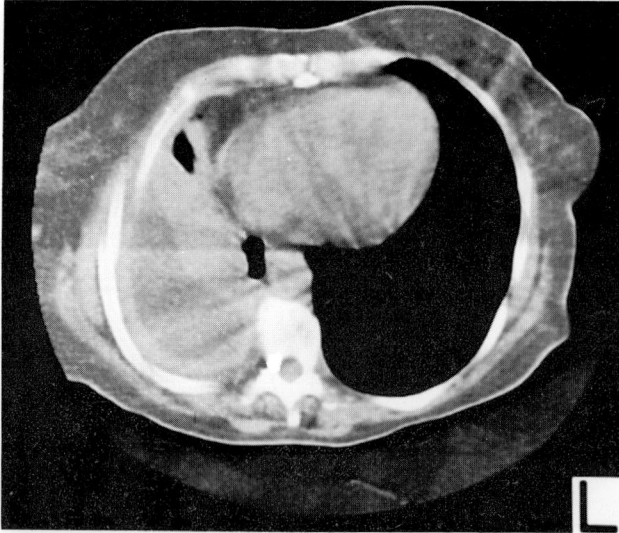

Figure 40c

Figure 40d

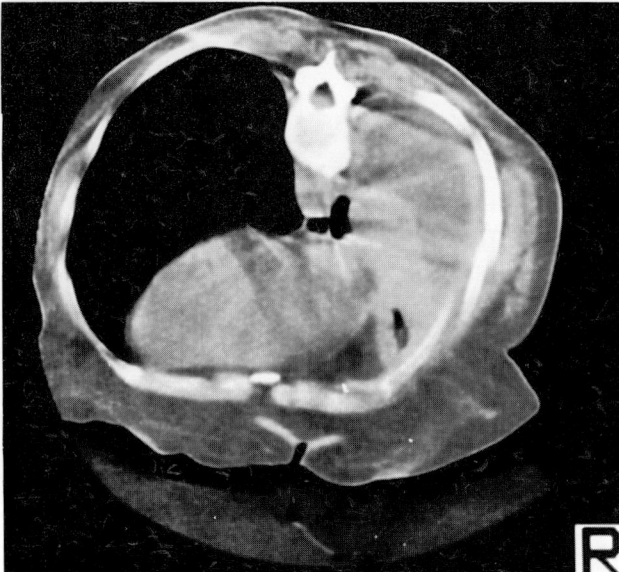

There is almost complete opacification of the right hemithorax with no shift of the mediastinum. These appearances could be due to almost any of the causes listed in Table 11 but the history was such as to exclude

Table 11 The opaque hemithorax

1 Pleural thickening
2 Pleural effusion
3 Consolidation
4 Collapse
5 Post-pneumonectomy
6 Very large tumour (pulmonary, pleural, mediastinal or chest wall)
7 Diaphragmatic hernia or traumatic rupture
8 Agenesis
9 Simulated—greater radiolucency of the opposite lung field

some of them. Thus it was known that the patient had not had a pneumonectomy and that previously she had normal pulmonary function with no evidence of agenesis or diaphragmatic hernia. There was no history of trauma.

Thus the list could be whittled down to four likely conditions: pleural thickening, pleural effusion, consolidation or collapse. If the appearances had been solely due to pleural effusion, the mediastinum would probably have been shifted away from the affected side. Conversely, if the appearances were solely due to collapse, one would expect shift of the mediastinum towards the affected side. Further investigation was necessary and the options open included ultrasound and computed tomography. CT was undertaken.

Figure 40c shows the patient in the supine position and figure 40d in the prone position. The CT revealed pleural thickening in a solid rind-like manner with a central area of fluid density. On turning the patient prone no change was observed in the solid mass or in the encysted fluid. A diagnosis of pleural malignancy with encysted effusion was made.

CT had revealed considerable detail about the opaque hemithorax. The distinction between different pleural malignancies especially mesothelioma and adenocarcinoma cannot, however, be made conclusively by CT since the appearances can be very similar [42]. This subject is further discussed in Chapter 11 under pleural and chest wall lesions.

In order to obtain a definitive diagnosis, biopsy of some form is necessary and this may either be done via a limited thoracotomy or by percutaneous pleural biopsy.

Case 41

Clive presented at birth with a respiratory distress and no air entry on the right side of his chest. After intubation a radiograph was performed (fig. 41).

The radiograph shows complete opacification of the right hemithorax. In addition the mediastinum is shifted to the right. The left hemithorax is well expanded. Bowel gas is present in the right hypochondrium and the right hemidiaphragm cannot be seen.

Complete opacification of the hemithorax can occur in the neonatal period due to collapse of the entire lung, agenesis of the lung, consolidation, pleural effusion or diaphragmatic hernia. The presence of gas in the right hypochondrium is suggestive of a diaphragmatic hernia with the liver displaced upwards into the right hemithorax. Ultrasound is a useful technique for demonstrating the diaphragm and liver in cases of opaque hemithorax and will aid differentiation between agenesis, collapse of the lung and diaphragmatic hernia.

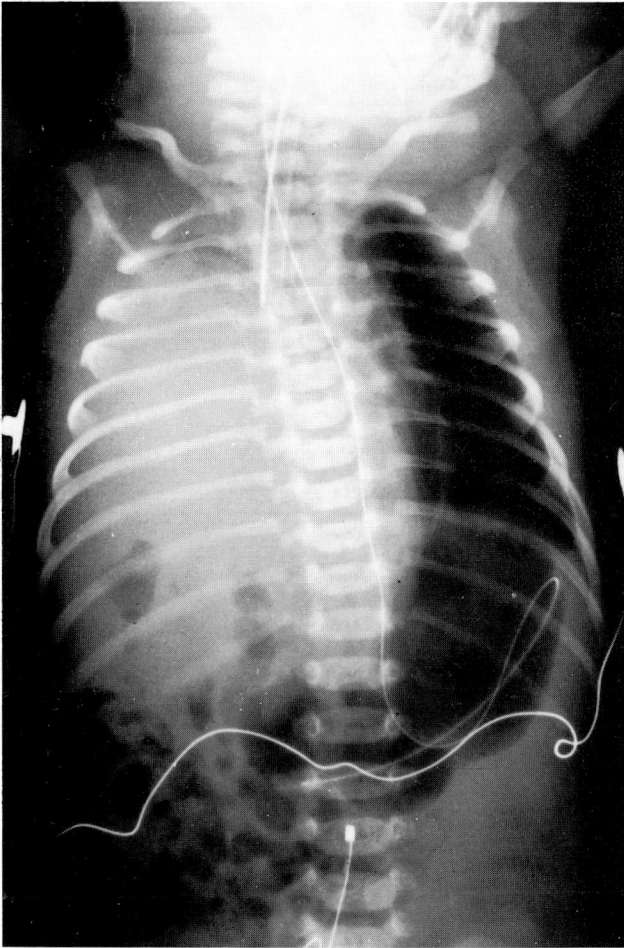

Figure 41

Figure 42a

Figure 42b

At surgery a diaphragmatic hernia of the Bochdalek type was confirmed on the right side and repaired. There was also hypoplasia of the right lung which is a common associated finding.

Right-sided diaphragmatic hernias are uncommon. Roughly 85 per cent of congenital diaphragmatic hernias occur on the left. In such cases the diagnosis is more easily made because gas-containing bowel may be present in the left hemithorax and the abdomen would be relatively devoid of gas.

Case 42

A young boy presented with a history of chest pain and cough which had followed inhalation of a peanut some months previously.

The chest PA and lateral films show almost complete opacification of the left lung field with shift of the mediastinum to the left. The appearances indicate collapse of the left lung. A bronchogram was performed.

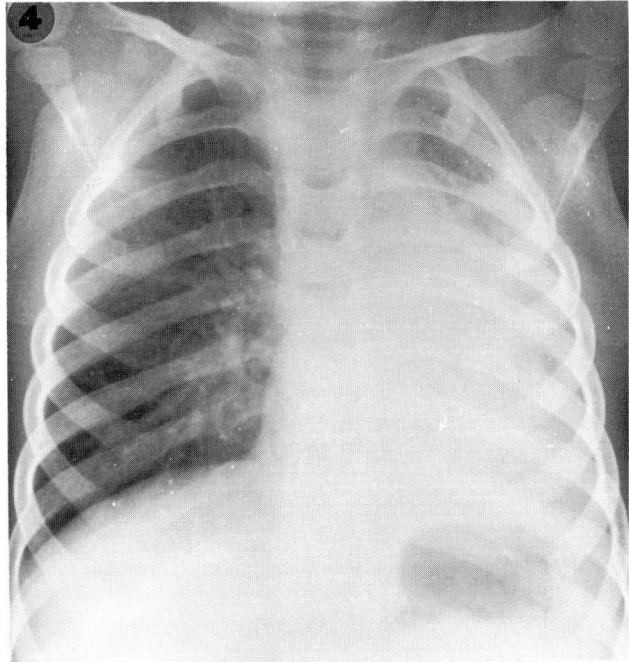

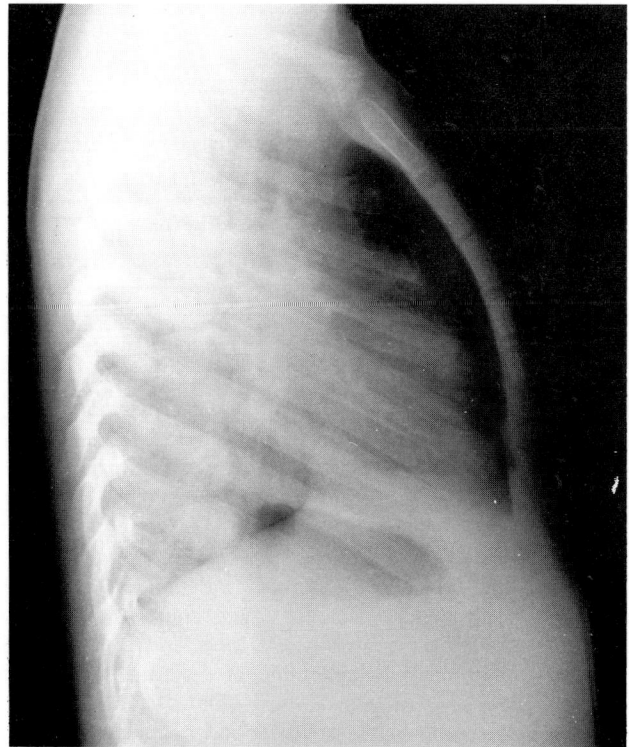

The bronchogram shows considerable resultant bronchiectasis. Initially when a foreign body is inhaled there may be obstructive over-expansion (obstructive emphysema, see Case 44). If the foreign body is not

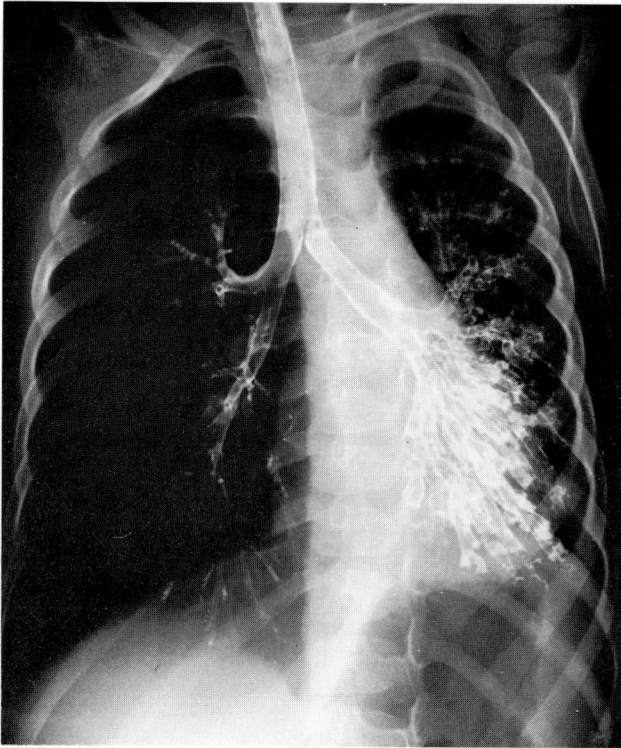

Figure 42c

removed, the air may be gradually resorbed and the lung becomes collapsed. Peanuts are particularly dangerous because they are liable to break into small pieces and, being oily and irritant, cause pneumonitis. Eventually, if untreated, bronchiectasis and chronic infection can occur, necessitating removal of the affected part of the lung.

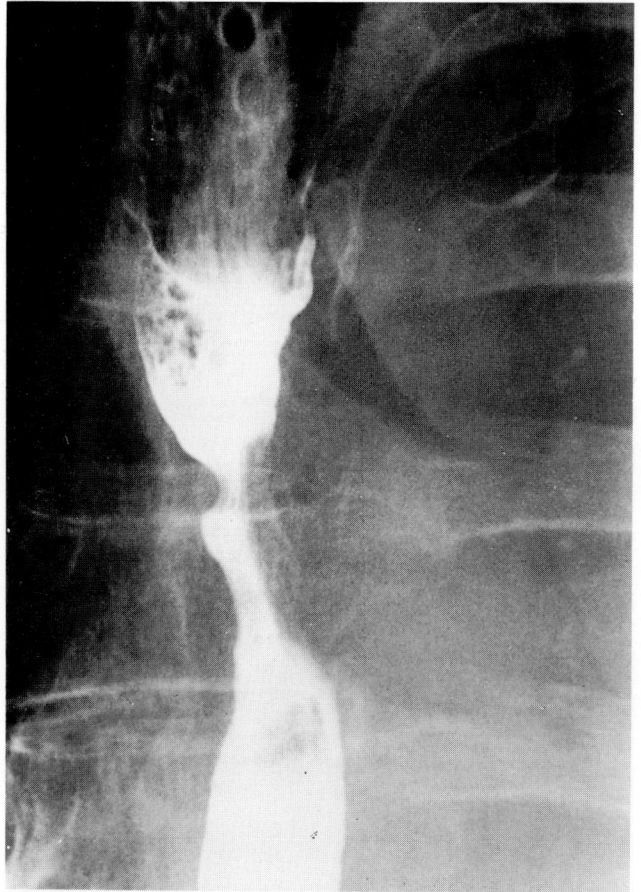

Figure 43a

Figure 43b

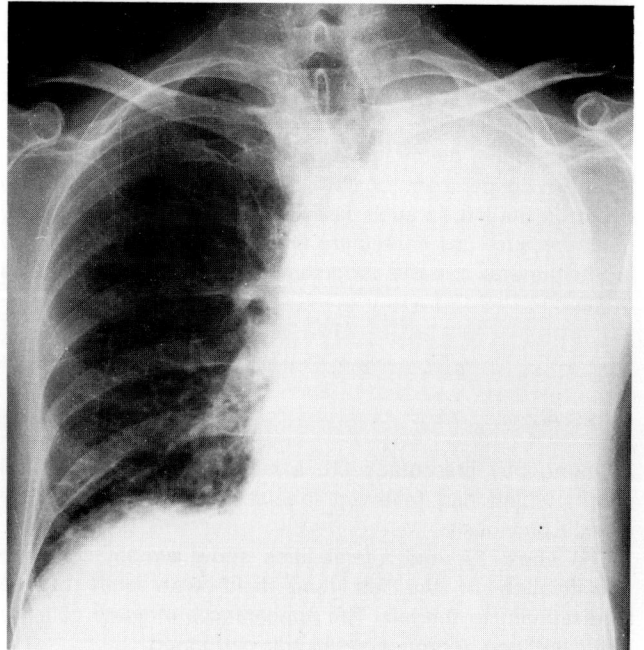

Case 43

Clive, aged 72, was referred for GP direct access radiology, with a history of dysphagia and a sensation of food sticking at the mid-oesophagus level. He also had weight loss over a period of some months and was becoming short of breath.

Barium swallow and a chest x-ray were performed.

The barium swallow shows indentation of the oesophagus by an extrinsic mass. The chest x-ray shows complete opacification of the left lung and shift of the mediastinum to the left, indicative of collapse of the left lung. On close examination of the barium swallow, the left main bronchus can be seen to taper and become occluded. The appearances are due to a large carcinoma of the bronchus obstructing the left main bronchus and spreading to mediastinal nodes. The enlarged posterior mediastinal nodes are compressing the oesophagus. Similar cases are discussed in Chapter 13.

Summary: the opaque hemithorax

Complete opacification of the hemithorax on a chest x-ray is due either to opacification of the lung itself, opacification of the pleura or a combination of the two. In many cases the diagnosis can be made at this stage. In more complicated cases investigations that are useful in distinguishing between the different causes, include ultrasound and computed tomography. If there are signs of collapse, bronchoscopy may well be indicated. In adults the most common cause would be carcinoma of the bronchus and in children inhalation of a foreign body. If a foreign body, such as a peanut, is not removed as soon as possible, there may be progression to bronchiectasis and chronic infection which can necessitate removal of the affected part of the lung.

The causes of bronchial obstruction are further discussed in Chapter 9 and pleural abnormalities are discussed in greater detail in Chapter 11.

9 Decreased density of the lung fields

Decreased density of the lung fields on chest x-ray

There are a number of causes of unequal density of one lung field compared with the other. They are listed in Table 12.

Table 12 Unilateral translucency of the chest on chest x-ray

True decrease in density
1 Emphysema
   (a) compensatory emphysema/hyperaeration
   (b) obstructive emphysema/hyperaeration
   (c) bullous emphysema
   (d) McLeod's (Swyer–James) syndrome (unilateral emphysema)
2 Pneumothorax
3 Cyst
4 Pulmonary emboli
5 Post-radiotherapy (distal to fibrosis)

Simulated *i.e. apparent decrease in density*
1 Rotation
2 Loss of soft tissue (mastectomy, Poland syndrome)
3 Denser on other side (which see—Chapter 8)

Some of the causes, including pulmonary emphysema and pulmonary emboli, can cause bilateral decreased density or patchy decreased density. Sometimes patients with conditions such as asthma, emphysema and pulmonary emboli present symptomatically but the chest x-ray is apparently normal or the findings are non-specific. The clinical presentation is very important since, unless there is a relevant history or there are relevant symptoms or signs, an area of decreased density on a chest radiograph may not warrant further investigation. Discussion is included in this section on the causes of chest pain and of breathlessness.

When presented with a chest radiograph showing greater radiolucency of one lung field compared with the other it is necessary to first determine whether the abnormality is real or apparent. The radiograph should be scrutinized to see if the patient was straight or rotated and to check for scoliosis. The breast shadows should be examined on the film for signs of a mastectomy. Moreover, it is necessary to consider whether that which is being interpreted as greater radiolucency of one lung field (or part of the lung field) may in fact be due to the relative increase in density of the rest of the chest, or, in other words, which is the abnormal area? Is the area of decreased density abnormal or the area of increased density?

The pulmonary vessels are a helpful pointer to abnormalities causing a true decrease in density. They may be splayed apart and displaced in position in compensatory 'emphysema' (expansion) and considerably diminished or truncated in bullous emphysema, pulmonary embolism, obstructive over-expansion and Macleod's syndrome.

Clinical examination may suggest the cause of the decreased density. Loss of soft tisue is apparent on examination. Reduction in volume of a hemithorax, as for example in Macleod's syndrome, can also be detected clinically. Breath sounds may be decreased on one side compared with the other, suggestive of decreased air entry. There may be a history of choking whilst eating food, resulting in inhalation of a foreign body. The patient may have a long history of heavy smoking and chronic obstructive airways disease indicating that emphysema is a likely problem, or may have recent onset of severe chest pain suggestive, perhaps, of pulmonary embolism or pneumothorax.

Further radiological examination should start with the simpler investigations such as inspiration and expiration films to show air trapping, or decubitus films to the same end. They may also assist in showing a small pneumothorax. These investigations may demonstrate whether or not the abnormality is due to obstruction.

High KVp chest films should adequately demonstrate areas of collapse, but it is necessary to be aware of the patterns of lobar collapse and the pitfalls, such as the collapsed left lower lobe hidden behind the heart.

Ventilation/perfusion scans are helpful if pulmonary embolism is suspected as a cause of the radiolucency and will also be abnormal in a variety of other conditions, including emphysema and asthma, in which the chest x-ray may be normal or near normal.

Computed tomography is able to show many of the causes of radiolucency. The lung fields can be seen on CT without the problem of overlying tissues and it is therefore possible to tell whether or not the lungs are truly reduced in density. With compensatory expansion the area of collapse can be clearly seen and the remaining lung will be of decreased density and the vessels splayed. Specific features are also seen in pulmonary emphysema and in Macleod's syndrome and a small pneumothorax can be clearly demonstrated by CT.

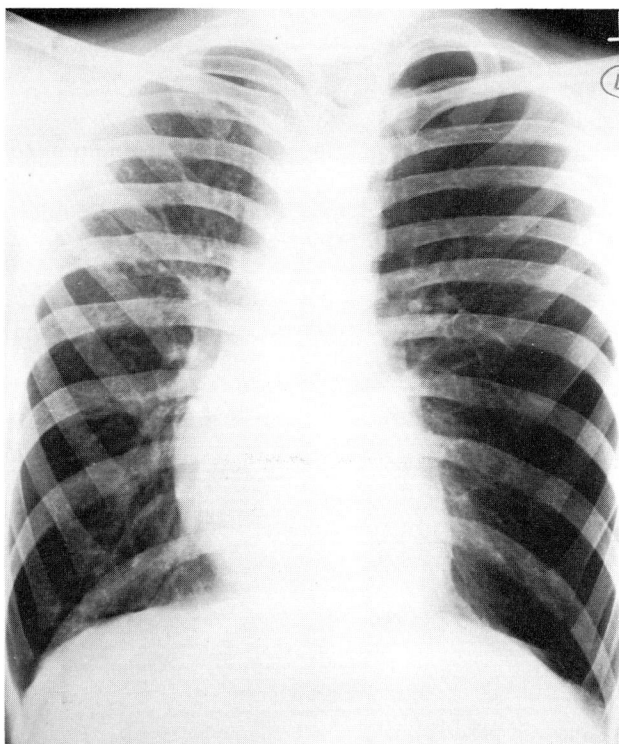

Figure 44a

Figure 44b

Case 44

The patient presented with a history of choking whilst at a party. The PA (inspiration) chest film on admission is shown.

The left lung is more radiolucent than the right and the mediastinum is slightly shifted to the right. It is not, however, possible on the one film to tell whether this is due to greater density on the right (due perhaps to collapse) or to decreased density on the left (due to obstructive emphysema). The PA film taken on expiration is shown in figure 44b.

On expiration the mediastinum has swung to the right and the left lung looks relatively more radiolucent. This is due to air-trapping in the left lung. The mediastinum always moves away from the abnormal side on expiration whether the abnormality is due to collapse, obstructive emphysema or whatever. Thus it is easy by paired films or by fluoroscopy to determine which side is abnormal. Note also that there is considerable decrease in vascularity in the left lung. This is mainly due to reflex shut-down of pulmonary vessels as the result of anoxia.

The diagnosis was made of obstructive emphysema due to inhalation of a foreign body. A peanut was removed successfully at bronchoscopy.

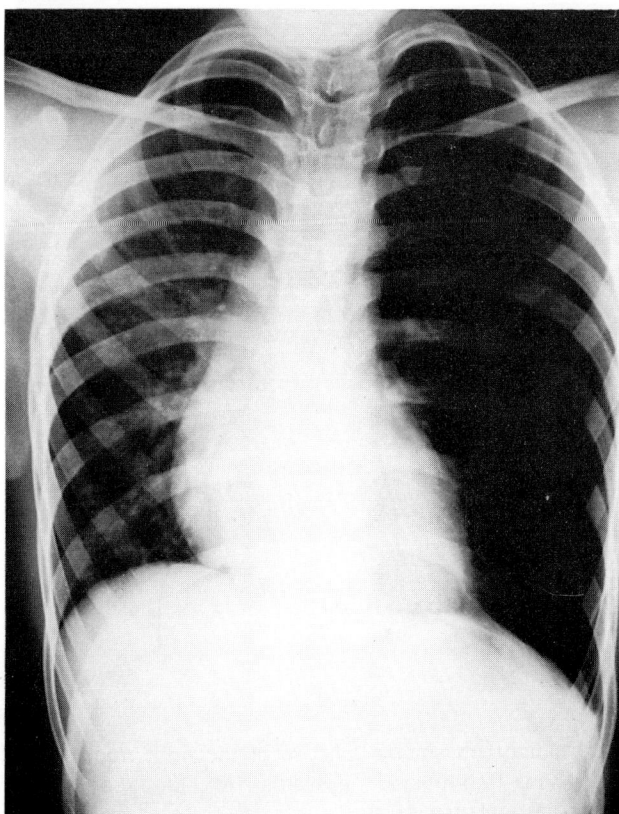

Case 45

Maria, aged five, complained of a cough and wheezing. Examination revealed bronchial breathing in the right upper zone.

She was apyrexial and gave a strongly positive Heaf test. Her father was found to have pulmonary tuberculosis.

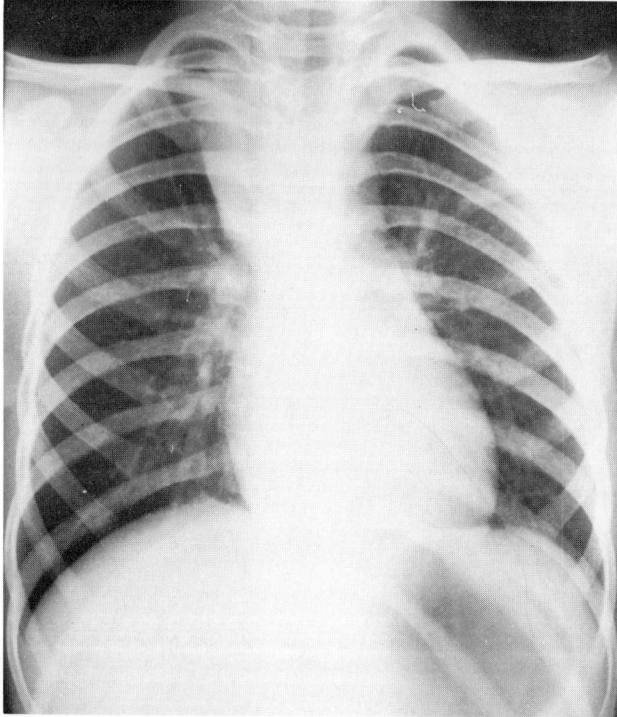

Figure 45a

Figure 45b

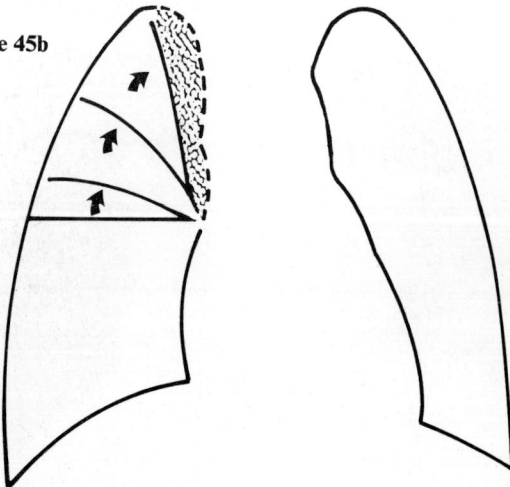

The radiograph shows collapse of the right upper lobe, which has contracted upwards to form a dense paramediastinal opacity.

Compensatory emphysema of the right, middle and lower lobes is shown by splaying of the pulmonary vessels, translucency of the right lung field, and elevation of the right hilum.

To diagnose collapse there must be evidence of loss of volume and the best guide to the volume of the right upper lobe is the position of the lesser (horizontal) fissure.

Bronchial obstruction is usually the cause of lobar collapse. This can be due to foreign bodies or mucus, lesions in the wall, such as carcinoma of the bronchus or fibrosis due to tuberculosis, or lesions outside the bronchus, such as carcinoma, tuberculosis, or aortic aneurysm.

The radiograph also shows the trachea to be shifted to the left. This was due to enlarged lymph nodes.

Tubercle bacilli were isolated from Maria's sputum. She was treated with rifampicin, isoniazid and ethambutol, resulting in a good recovery.

Collapse of the lobe or whole lung can normally be diagnosed from plain chest x-rays. Shift of structures, such as fissures and hilum, and opacification of the affected lobe are the main signs. These features are described well in standard books on chest radiology.

Table 13 Causes of collapse of a lobe or whole lung

1 Bronchial obstruction
   (i) lesion in the lumen
      foreign body, endobronchial adenoma
  (ii) lesion in the wall
      fibrosis due to TB
      carcinoma of the bronchus
 (iii) lesions outside but compressing the bronchus
      carcinoma of the bronchus
      enlarged left atrium

2 'Relaxation' collapse
   (i) pleural effusion
  (ii) pneumothorax

The most commonly missed lobar collapse is that of the left lower lobe because the main signs (increased opacity and shifted oblique fissure) are superimposed on the heart shadow on the PA film. Secondary signs such as depression of the left hilum and splaying of pulmonary vessels in the left mid and upper zones (compensatory 'emphysema' or expansion) are usually noticed first. Right upper lobe collapse is sometimes misdiagnosed as mediastinal widening. Tomography (linear and computed) can be used to demonstrate the collapsed lobe and may show the cause such as narrowing of the bronchus due to carcinoma or an inhaled foreign body. (See also increased density and decreased density of whole lung (Chapters 8 and 9).

Bronchoscopy and occasionally bronchography may be required to obtain the diagnosis of the cause of collapse. If a foreign body is demonstrated, this can often be removed bronchoscopically.

Case 46

The plain chest film of a woman aged 55 is shown in figure 46a. A close-up of the left lower zone is shown in figure 46b.

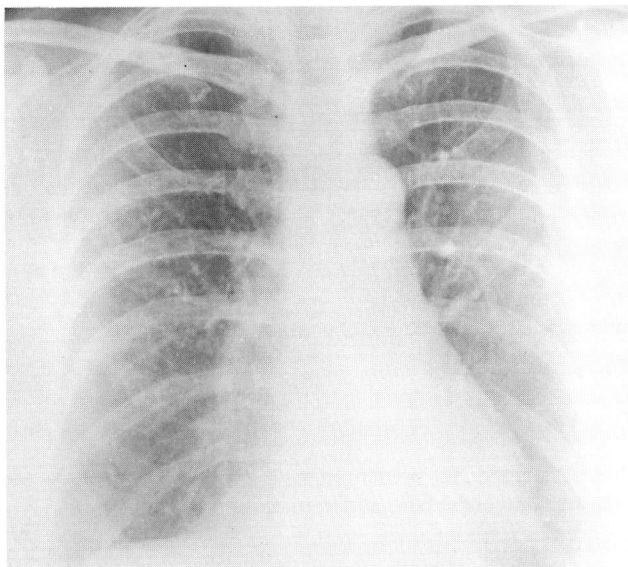

Figure 46a

Figure 46b

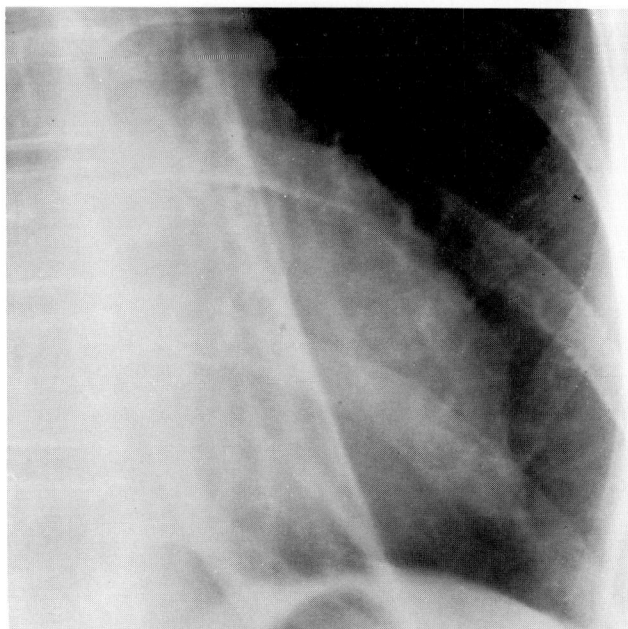

There is depression of the left hilum and splaying of the pulmonary vessels in the left mid and upper zones (compensatory expansion). On the close-up of the high KV film (fig. 46b) it can be seen that there is an opacity behind the heart which represents a collapsed left lower lobe.

Case 47

CT was performed in a patient with a known carcinoma of the bronchus. Scans of the lower part of the thorax are shown in figures 47a and 47b.

There is a lenticular shaped opacity posteriorly in the right lung field. This represents a collapsed right lower lobe. There is splaying of vessels in the rest of the right lung due to compensatory expansion.

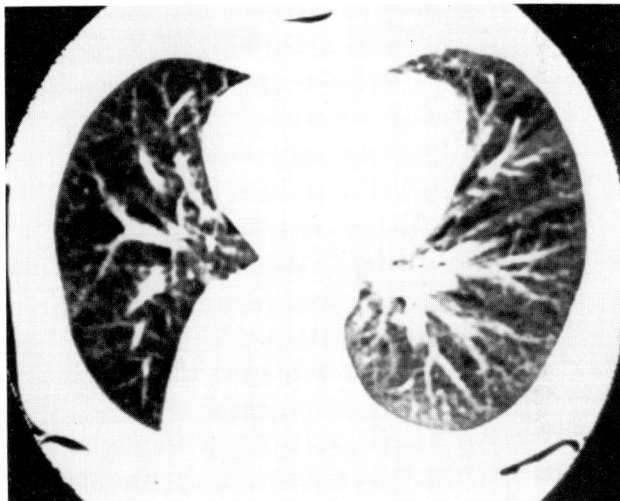

Figure 47a

Figure 47b

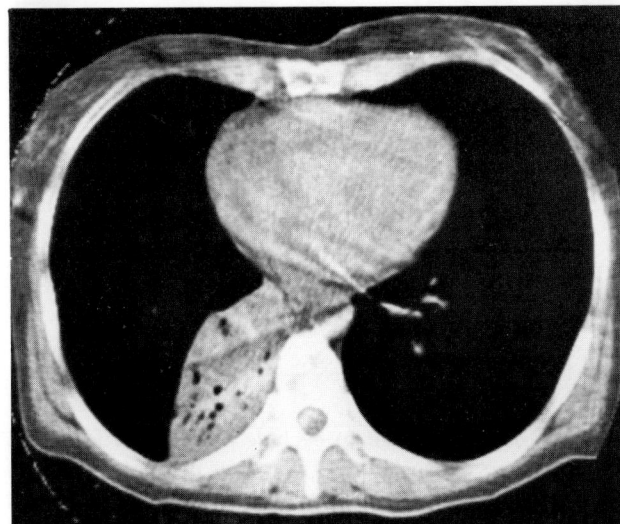

Case 48

A young boy presented with a history of previous chest infections and radiolucency of the left lung field.

The chest x-ray is shown in figure 48a and CT in figures 48b and 48c.

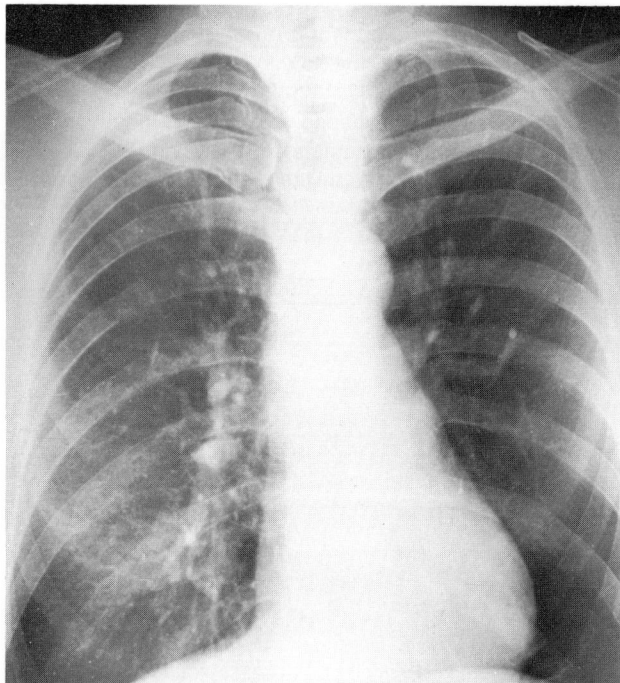

Figure 48c

is decrease in density of the left lung field. All major branches of the pulmonary arteries and veins are present on the left side but they are reduced in size and there is peripheral pruning of vessels. These are all features of Macleod's (Swyer-James) syndrome. The aetiology of this condition is not known but childhood infection is probably implicated. Pathologically there is usually emphysema and obliterative bronchiolitis in the affected lung.

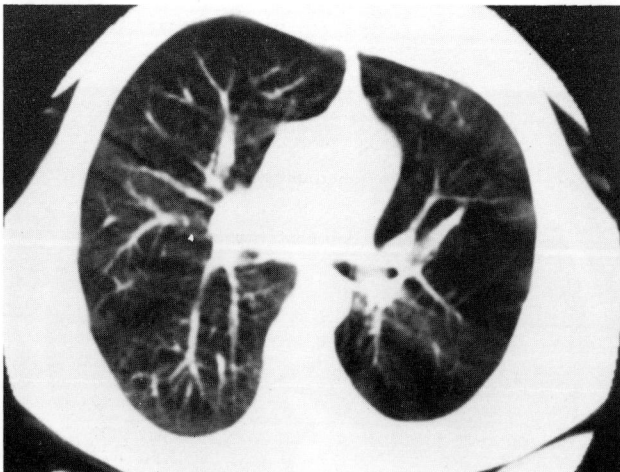

Figure 48a

Figure 48b

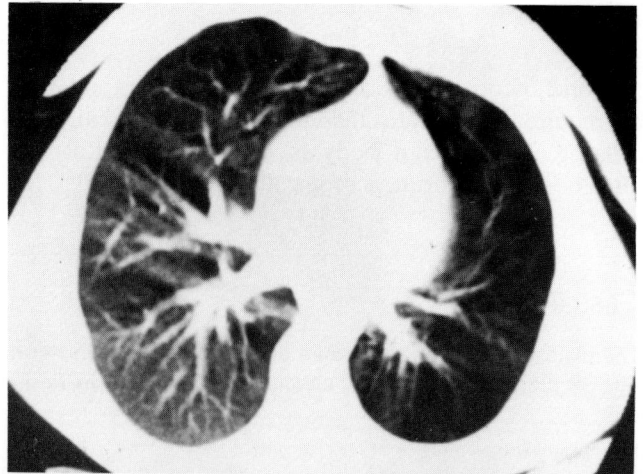

The CT was performed to exclude a collapsed lobe and compensatory expansion as a cause of the decreased density. No area of collapse was seen but the left hemithorax is considerably smaller than the right and there

Case 49

Peter W., aged 34, presented with a history of rapid onset of right sided chest pain and breathlessness.

There is radiolucency of the right hemithorax and no blood vessels beyond a centrally placed opacity. The appearances are those of a large right-sided pneumothorax.

Figure 49

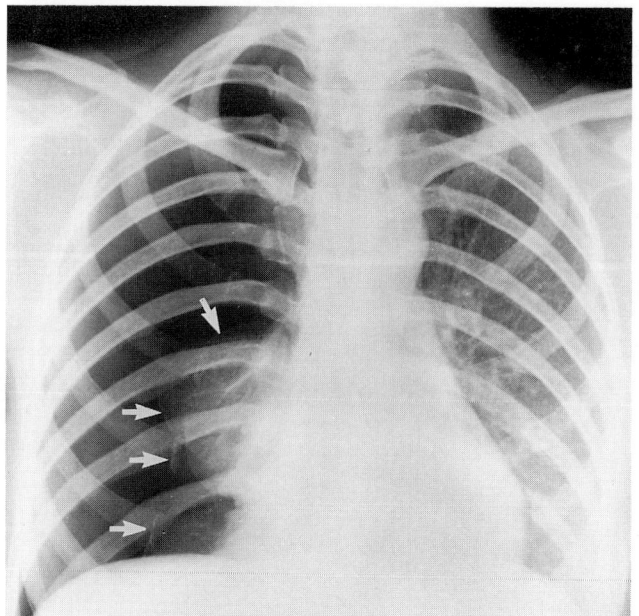

In Case 49 the diagnosis is obvious on the PA *inspiratory film*. In some cases the pneumothorax is small and if the condition is suspected it is useful to perform an *expiratory* PA film in addition to the inspiratory film. The expiratory film is able to show a small pneumothorax to greater advantage than an inspiratory film since the air in the pleura will be less compressed by the lung.

Another view that can be used is the *lateral decubitus* film.

A film is taken with the patient lying on his side, and the x-ray beam horizontal. It is of considerable value in children where obtaining an expiratory film may be difficult. It is also used to show pleural fluid.

The *lateral* film can also be useful and may, for example, assist in showing an anteriorly placed pneumothorax. Interpretation may be difficult because of the vessels on the other side being superimposed on the pneumothorax.

In rare cases computed tomography may be used to show a pneumothorax.

Case 50

CT showing collapse of the left lung and air in the pleural cavity. A small effusion is seen in the scan of the lower part of the chest.

Figure 50a

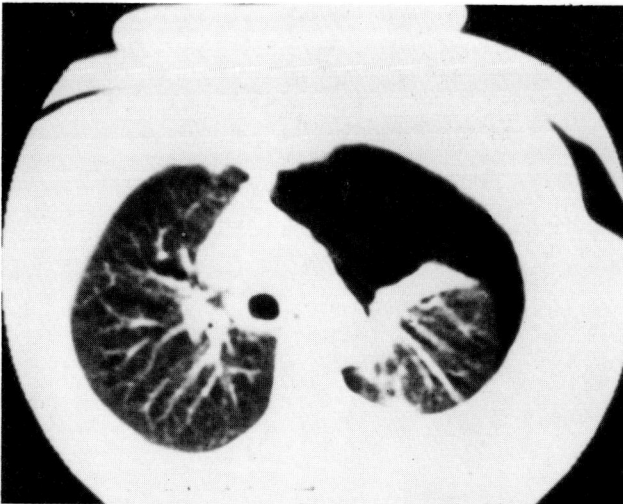

Figure 50b

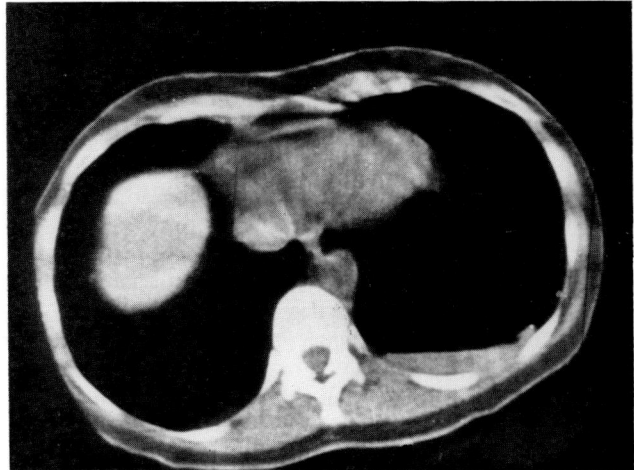

Spontaneous pneumothorax, as in Case 49, may occur in any age group, but most commonly in young male patients who apparently have normal lungs. It is likely that in these patients small pleural blebs or defects rupture and allow air to escape from the lungs. Spontaneous pneumothorax also occurs as a complication of chronic bronchitis and emphysema, pulmonary fibrosing conditions and any cause of pulmonary cavitation, including tuberculosis. Spontaneous pneumothorax is a complication of respiratory distress syndrome in premature infants and may be a serious complicating factor in acute asthma.

Tension pneumothorax is a term describing the situation where the pneumothorax develops positive pressure. This is assumed to be due to a flap valve mechanism formed by overlapping pleura allowing entry of air but not exit.

In most cases of tension pneumothorax the mediastinum is shifted away from the pneumothorax due to the pressure. Tension pneumothorax may be present, however, even if the mediastinum is not shifted and the whole pleural space not involved since the pleura and mediastinum may be tethered by adhesions. Moreover, there may be shift of the mediastinum, especially on expiration films, even when tension is not present. The importance of diagnosing a tension pneumothorax is that it causes mediastinal vessel compression, reducing return to the heart and hence causing circulatory collapse, and also causes respiratory embarrassment. The diagnosis is made on clinical grounds in association with the x-ray findings and the condition requires immediate emergency treatment by introduction of a wide bore needle or intravenous cannula into the pneumothorax.

Case 51

Figures 51a and 51b show the chest radiograph and a penetrated film centred on the diaphragm of a patient following a road traffic accident.

There is radiolucency of the right side of the chest compared with the left and the penetrated film at the level of the diaphragm shows a fluid level which is arrowed. A decubitus film was performed (fig. 51c) and showed shift of the fluid and air in the right hemithorax.

The conclusion was made that the patient had a haemopneumothorax. The possibility of a ruptured hemidiaphragm was considered but there was no further evidence to suggest this.

Figure 51a

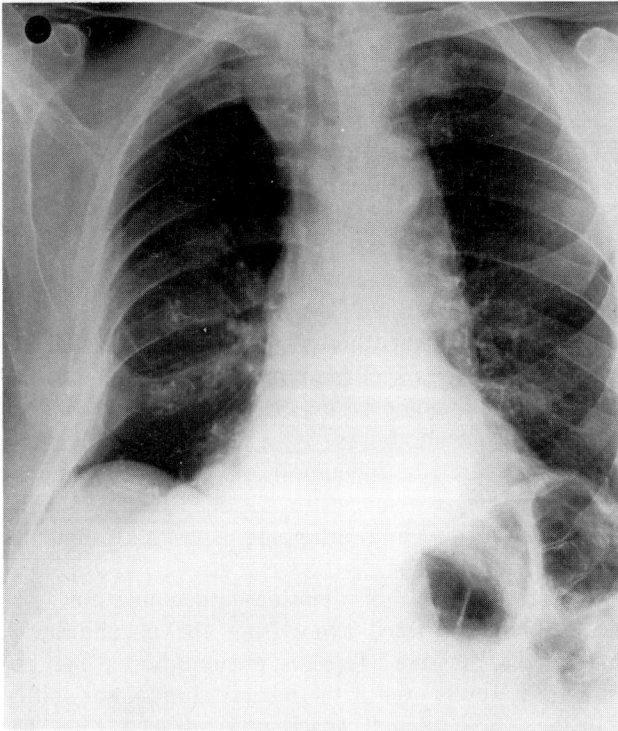

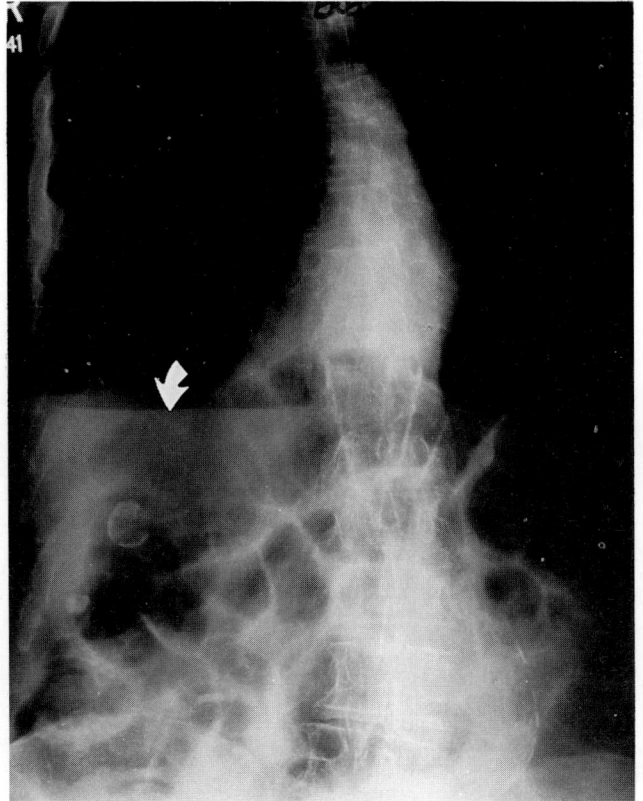

Figure 51b

Figure 51c   Lateral decubitis film

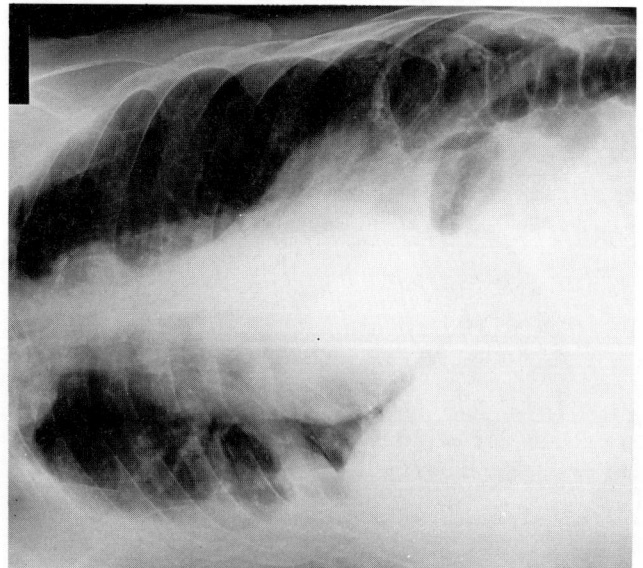

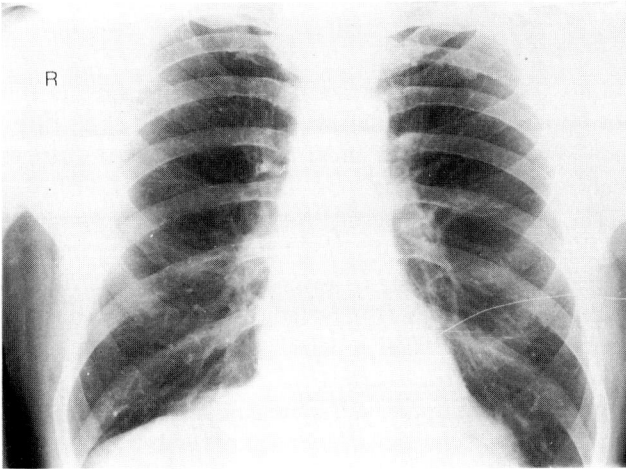

Figure 52a

Case 52

A man of 65 years of age had been a smoker for many years. He presented with a history of breathlessness.

The chest x-ray shows over-expansion but little else.

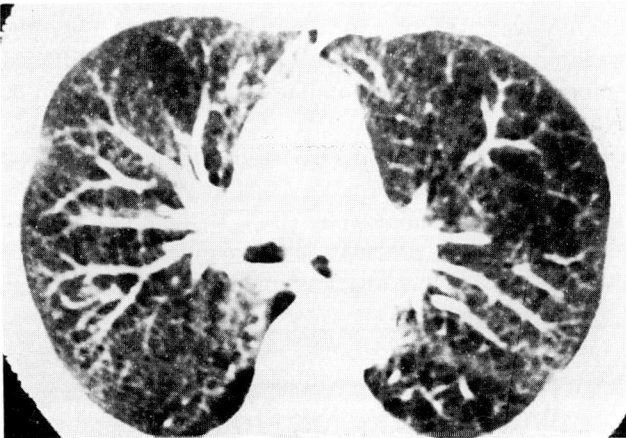

Figure 52b

Figure 52c

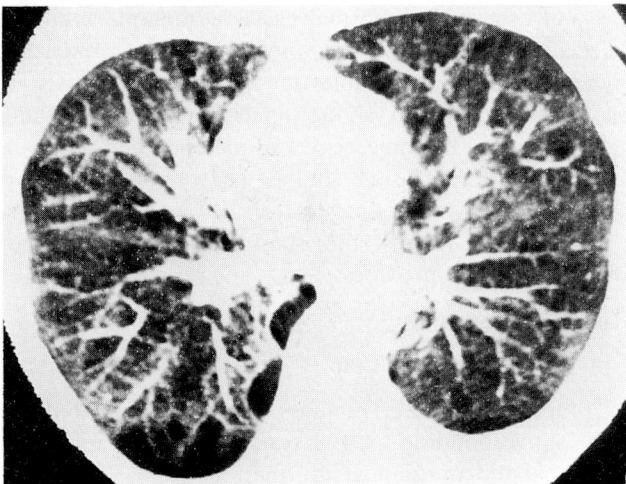

CT shows peripheral bullous emphysema and patchy vascularity throughout both lungs due to pulmonary emphysema.

Another example of emphysema is shown in Case 53.

Case 53

There are areas of low attenuation (radiodensity) situated around the periphery of the lung fields. This is the pattern of peripheral emphysema and is described further below.

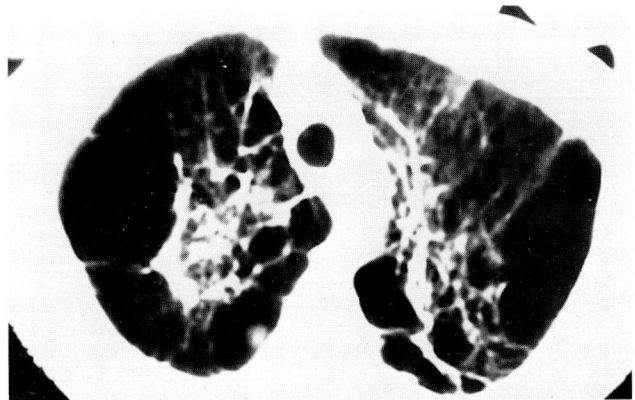

Figure 53a

Figure 53b

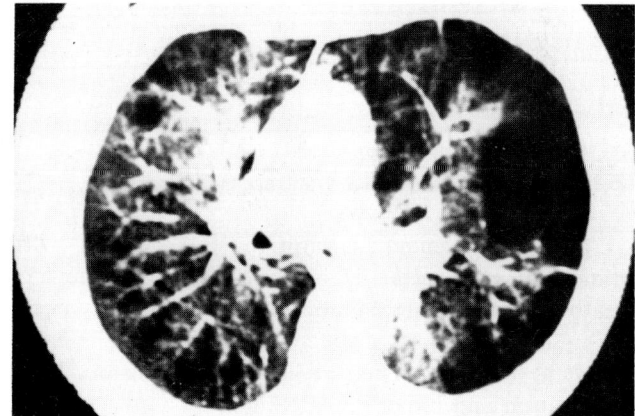

Pulmonary emphysema

(Note: CT numbers in figures H, I and J are given in EMI units. Multiply by 2 to give Hounsfield units.)

The chest radiographs of patients with gross pulmonary emphysema are often abnormal (figs. G and H). In patients with a lesser degree of disease the radiographs may be normal or equivocal.

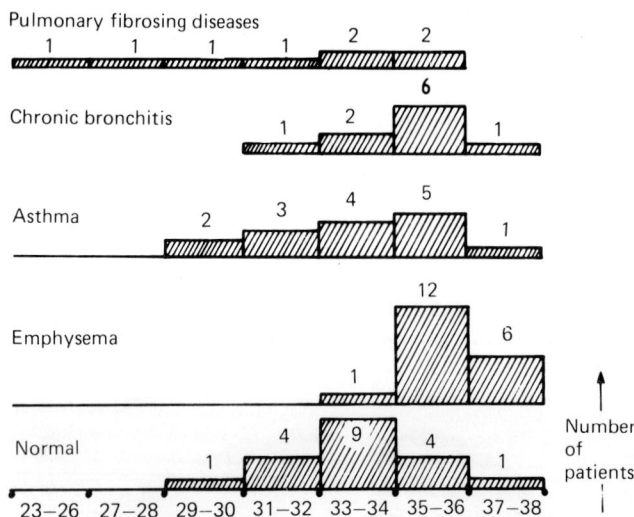

Figure G Height of diaphragm on arrested inspiration compared with clinical diagnosis

Figure H Chest radiograph compared with computed tomography

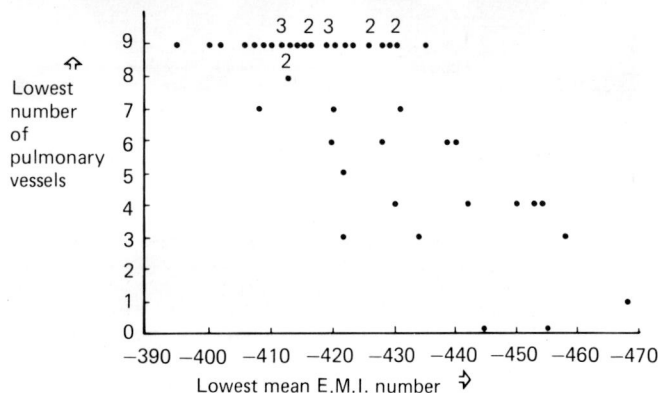

The most common symptom in patients with pulmonary emphysema is breathlessness. Shortness of breath is, however, a common symptom that may occur due to a large variety of different conditions. The cause is often rapidly discerned from the history and examination and initial investigations such as a chest x-ray and ECG. The common causes are either cardiac or pulmonary. Many of the different cardiac conditions, ranging from myocardial infarction to congenital heart disease can result in breathlessness. Detailed discussion about cardiac disease is outside the scope of this book. It is, however, usually possible to distinguish cardiac causes of dyspnoea from pulmonary by the presence of other clinical pointers and the results of the chest x-ray and ECG. Real-time ultrasound of the heart is also useful as a non-invasive technique for demonstrating cardiac disorders.

In a few cases the cause of the breathlessness is still not apparent after these investigations. The chest x-ray may appear normal or there may be equivocal changes such as minimal fibrosis.

The next line of investigation may include respiratory function studies and/or blood gases. These may indicate a treatable cause, such as reversible airways obstruction (asthma). The findings may indicate a defect mainly of perfusion or a restrictive defect, or of course, they may be normal.

If the condition is still undiagnosed after all these tests but the symptoms are genuine and troublesome, ventilation/perfusion studies and/or CT should be considered as the next line of investigation.

If the chest x-ray appears normal, if would seem advisable to proceed to ventilation/perfusion scans. These may show definite segmental defects of perfusion without a matched ventilatory defect, thus making pulmonary embolism diagnosable as the cause of breathlessness. This is further discussed on pages 91-94. If, however, there are matched defects or the appearances are equivocal, emission computed tomography with corresponding transmission CT can be helpful.

If there are equivocal chest x-ray findings, the best radiological investigation to assist in interpretation is again computed tomography (CT). If there is a fibrotic lung condition present, abnormalities should be discernible by CT. Causes of pulmonary fibrosis were discussed in Chapter 4.

Ventilation/perfusion studies

Ventilation/perfusion studies show matched defects in emphysema with great sensitivity. But the specificity is low and even with a normal chest radiograph, matched defects occur in emphysema, asthma, radiation pneumonopathy, early infection and bronchiectasis. If the chest radiograph shows opacification of the lung field, there will be some degree of matched deficiency on the ventilation/perfusion studies whatever the cause of the opacity.

Emission CT of the perfusion study is an investigation that provides:

1 increased sensitivity,

2 greater spatial resolution.

Comparison of ECT images in the transaxial plane with corresponding CT scans provides increased functional and anatomical information.

CT in pulmonary emphysema

The CT signs of emphysema [10] include:

1 Alteration in the configuration of the pulmonary vasculature shown by:

(a) pruning of small branches resulting in a simplified vascular tree with fewer orders of branching,

(b) distortion of blood vessels around areas of low attenuation value,

(c) enlargement of the main pulmonary arteries.

2 Areas of low attenuation value in the lung fields detected visually as ill-defined or well-defined regions of low density considered to represent emphysematous bullae.

The changes listed above may be present in two patterns. Firstly, a 'central pattern' in which the intermediate pulmonary vessels are deficient and the more peripheral lung well supplied with vasculature. Secondly, a 'peripheral pattern' with areas of altered vascularity or low attenuation affecting the edge of the lung. The two patterns are also seen together.

3 Overall measurable lowered radiodensity of the lungs and shift of the 'mode' towards the density of air (fig. I).

4 Loss of the normal gravitational pooling effect that causes increased radiodensity in the dependent part of the lungs (fig. J).

(Note: CT numbers in figures H, I and J are given in EMI units. Multiply by 2 to give Hounsfield units.)

Many of these changes are more noticeable if scans are performed in different phases of respiration and in both supine and prone positions.

Figure I Lowest mean lung attenuation on arrested inspiration compared with clinical diagnosis

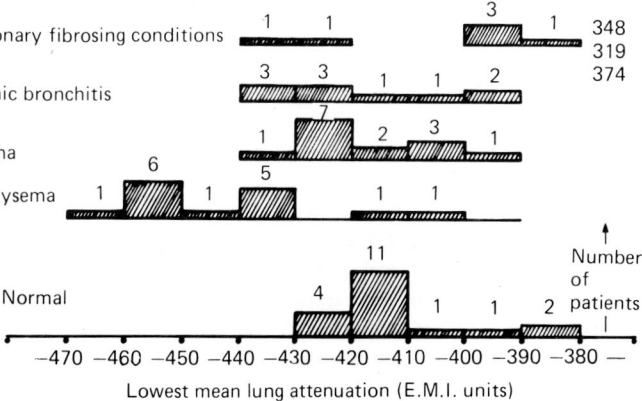

Figure J Lowest density gradient from anterior to posterior in the lung fields compared with clinical diagnosis

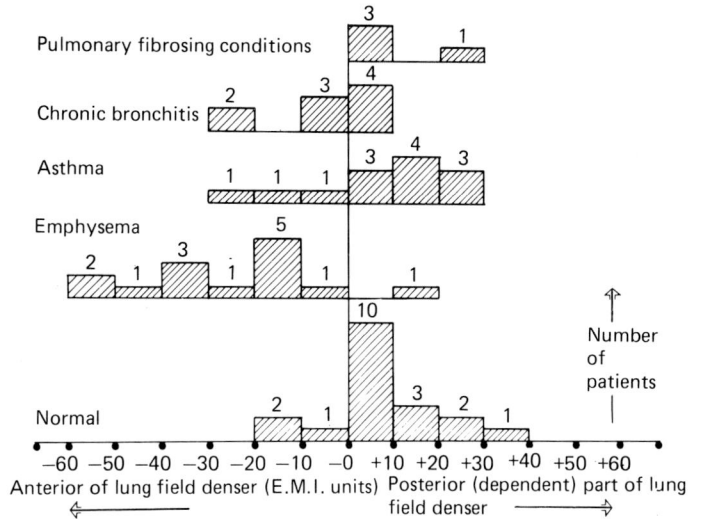

CT can be used to diagnose emphysema at an earlier stage than is possible by chest radiography and the findings correlate with respiratory function studies and pathology.

When a large bulla is causing compression of lung, surgery may be one of the therapeutic options considered. CT can be of great help in presurgical assessment since the bulla in question will be displayed in precise anatomical detail. Even more important the CT will demonstrate whether or not the remaining lung is normal. If both lungs are shown to be grossly abnormal and the bulla in question is only one of many, surgery is contraindicated. If, on the contrary, the bulla is shown to be a solitary abnormality, the results of removal may be very beneficial. Difficulty still arises in assessing the intermediate cases.

Case 54

A man, aged 57, had been a life-long smoker and consequently had severe chronic obstructive airways disease. Chest radiographs showed decreased vascularity and decreased density in the upper and mid zones bilaterally. The ventilation/perfusion study is shown below.

Figure 54a

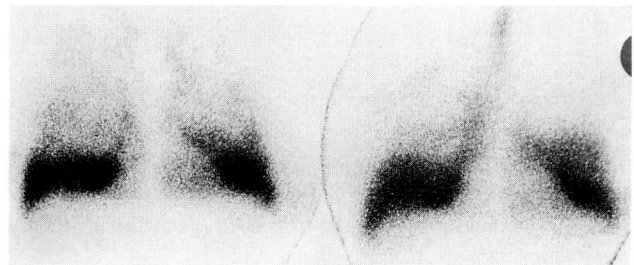

There are bilateral mid and upper zone matched defects of ventilation and perfusion. The lower zones appear normal.

Figure 54b Transmission CT

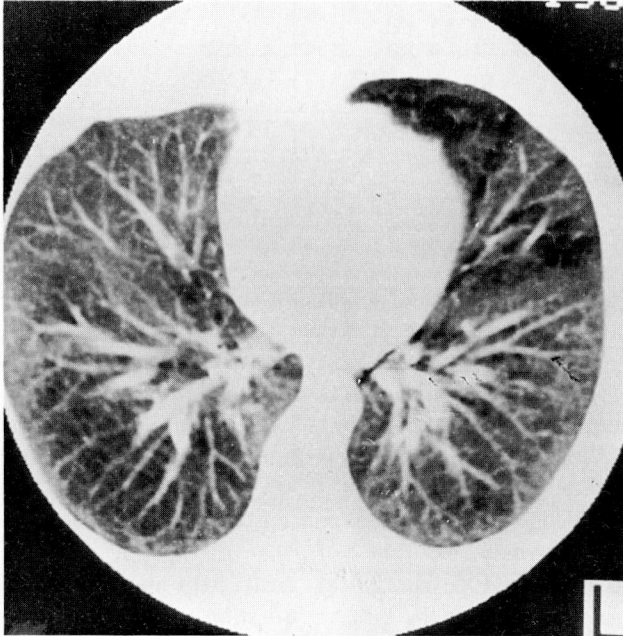

Emission CT of the perfusion study was undertaken to assist in analysis of the lower zones. Comparison was made with transmission computed tomography (CT).

Figure 54c Emission CT

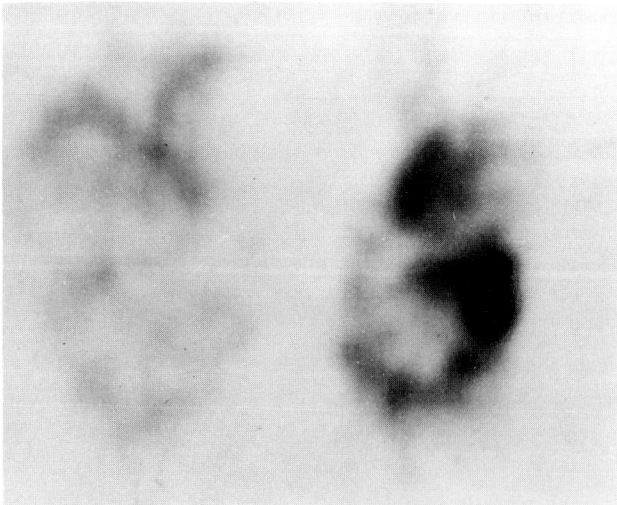

The transmission CT scan shows a central pattern of pulmonary emphysema as described earlier. There is a lack of side branches in the middle of the lung but the periphery is well supplied.

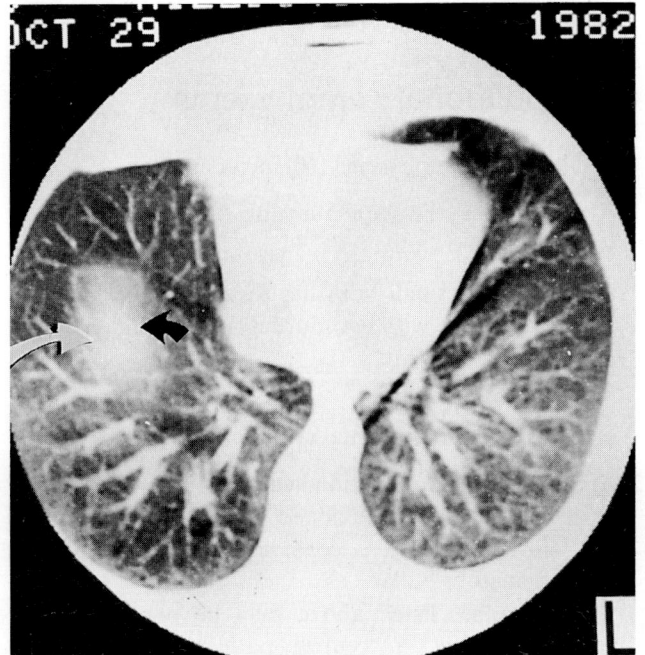

Figure 54d Transmission CT

The perfusion emission CT shows a rim of perfused lung and central lack of perfusion correlating perfectly with the transmission CT. (*The arrows indicate the top of the right hemidiaphragm*).

Figure 54e Emission CT

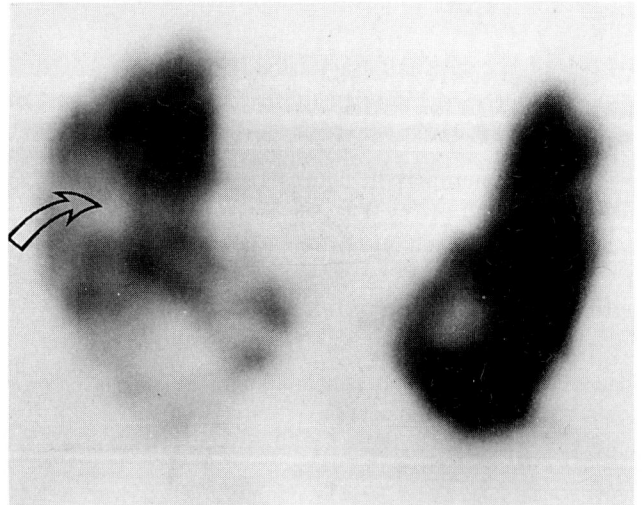

Case 55

A further example of pulmonary emphysema shown on CT scanning and emission CT of perfusion.

The areas of low attenuation and paucity of blood vessels are seen to correlate with defects in perfusion. Note also there are two pleural plaques in the left hemithorax. This patient had documented exposure to asbestos and was a smoker.

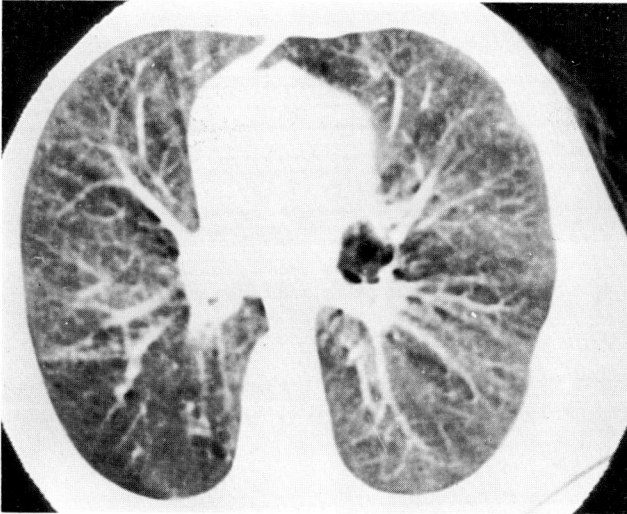

Figure 55a

Figure 55b

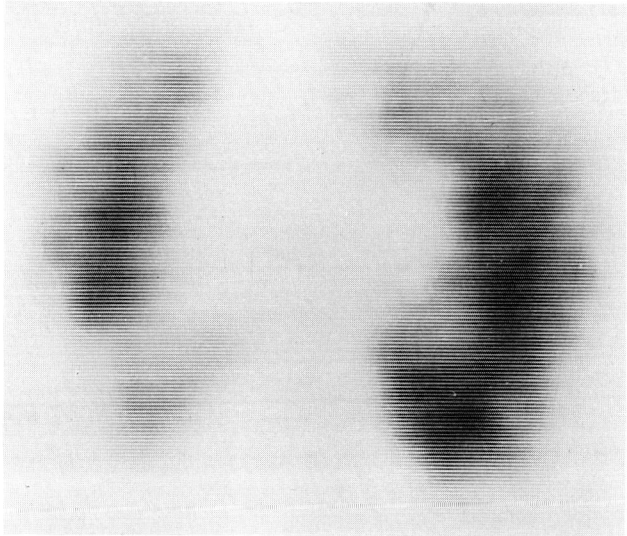

Case 56

The CT scans of a patient with emphysema are shown. There is no shift of the opacification on turning the patient prone and no gravity pooling because the vascular bed has been destroyed.

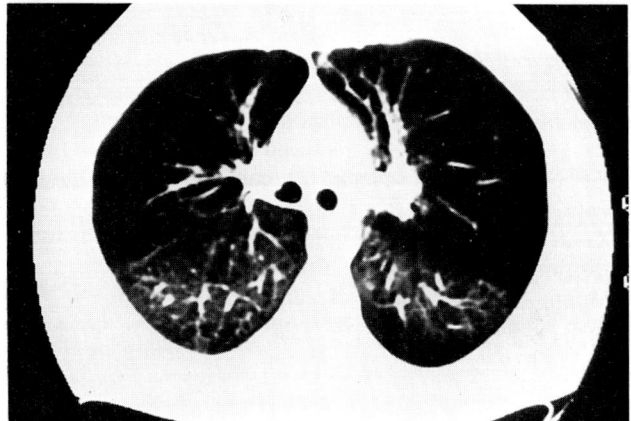

Figure 56a

Figure 56b

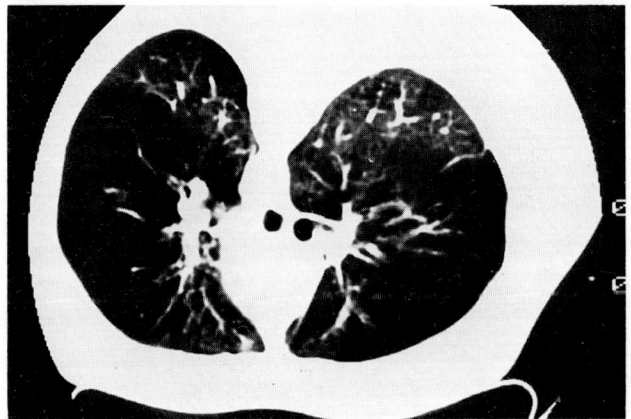

Figure 56c

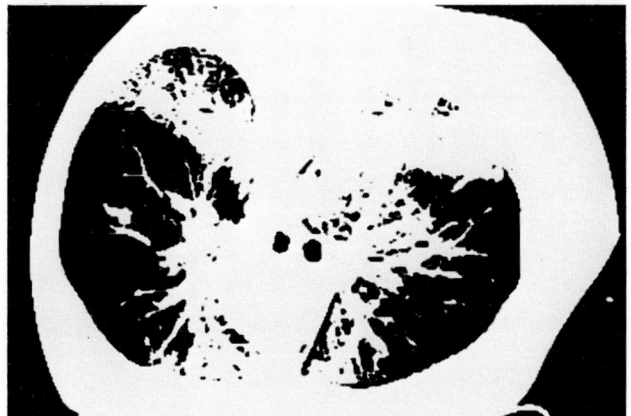

Emission CT is even more sensitive than transmission CT for showing functional disturbances in the pulmonary vasculature but the scans are hard to interpret anatomically and defects are non-specific. Comparison with transmission CT provides the combination of good functional information with fine anatomical detail. If the scans are viewed on the same console it is possible to overlay the functional information on the anatomical display thus facilitating interpretation.

The lack of pulmonary vasculature that results from emphysema also causes a lack of 'gravity pooling' in dependent regions on the CT scan. Thus the normal gradient may be absent (fig. J). When the patient is turned from supine to prone there is normally a shift of fluid resulting in vascular pooling in the dependent part.

Correlation of CT findings with pathology is important. One method is to take the lungs at post-mortem and inflate them with formalin vapour. The inflated lungs may then be scanned, sliced, x-rayed and finally mounted as Gough sections [43].

Case 57

Correlation of CT with pathology slices.

CT scan of previously removed emphysematous lungs, inflation fixed before scanning. A carcinoma is also present (*arrow*).

X-ray of separated 13-mm axial slice of lung tissue corresponding to that seen in figure 57a.

Mounted thin section of lungs taken from the slice shown in figures 57a and 57b.

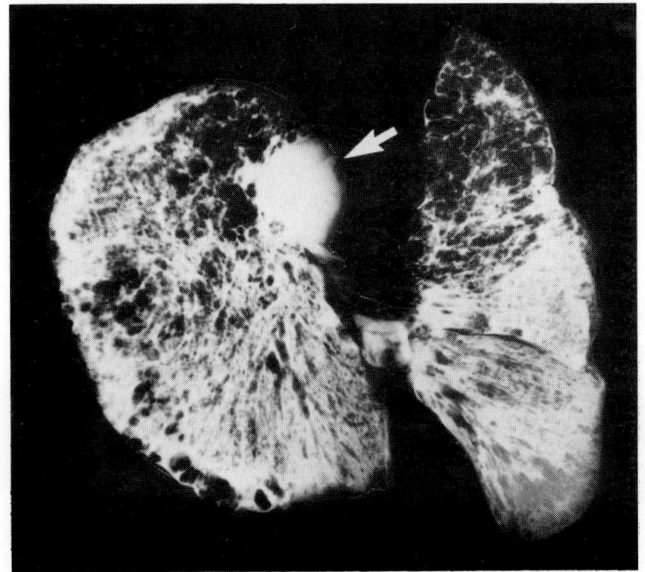

Figure 57b

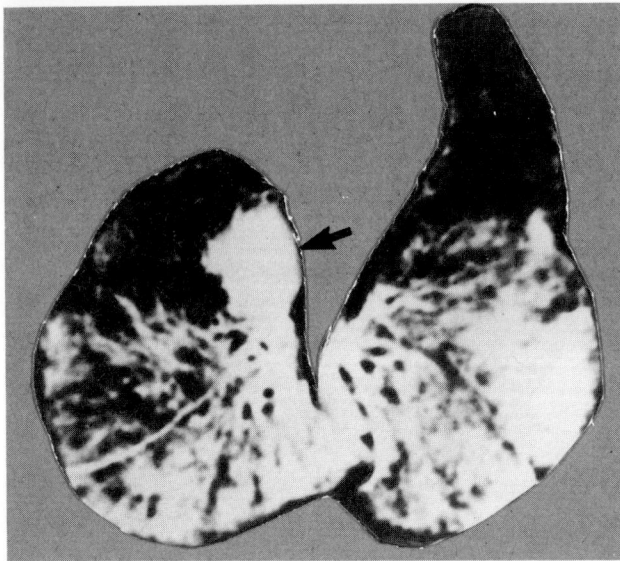

Figure 57a

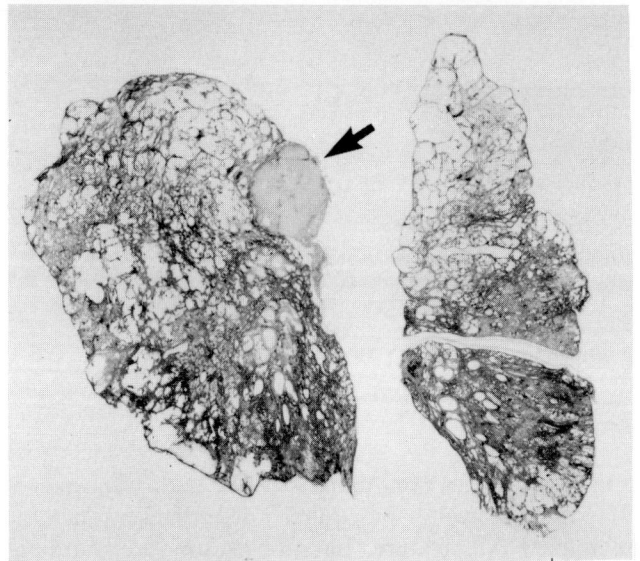

Figure 57c

Case 58

A man aged 59 had a curious history of ten years previously syphoning petrol from a lawn mower. Unfortunately for the clandestine syphoner, the owner of the lawn mower had 'spiked' the petrol with formaldehyde. The inhalation of petrol and formaldehyde fumes caused a severe chemical pneumonitis. The acute episode had resolved over a period of some months but considerable dyspnoea had persisted. On evaluation ten years after the initial problem, he had a one second forced expired volume (FEV1) of 1.0 litre (36% pn) and vital capacity (VC) of 1.3 litres (35% pn).

A chest radiograph was performed.

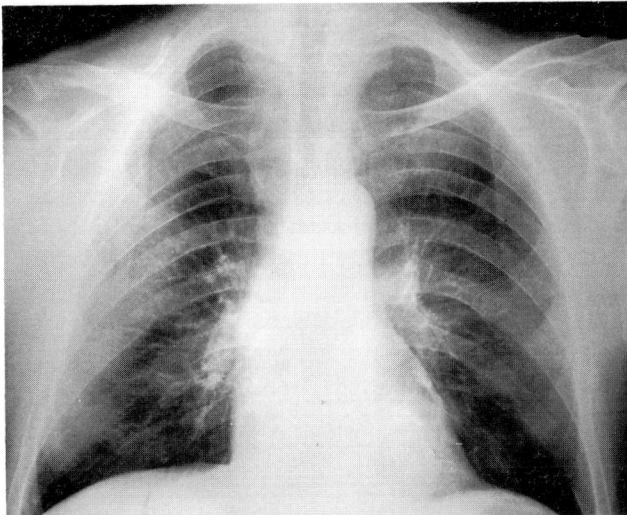

Figure 58a

Figure 58b

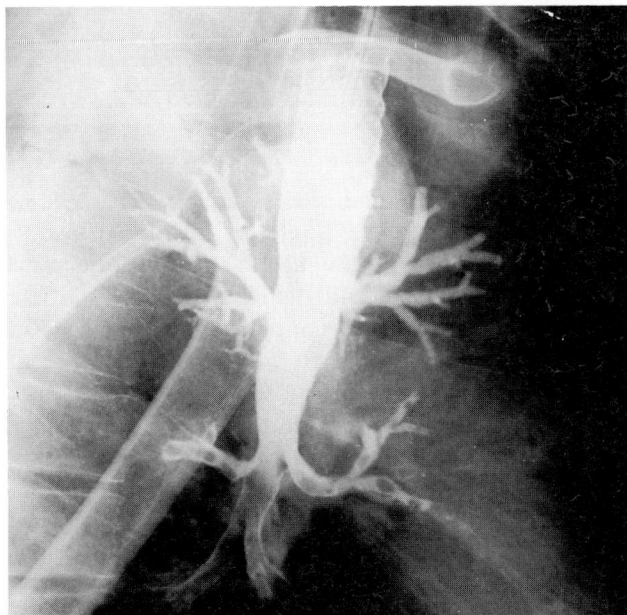

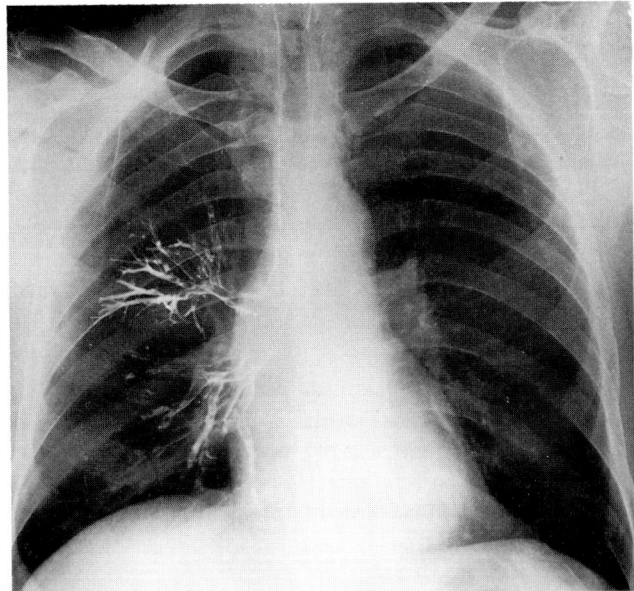

Figure 58c

The chest x-ray shows diminished pulmonary vasculature.

The main feature on the bronchogram is that there is cut-off of many of the subsegmental bronchi. The ends of the terminated bronchi are squared. These features are typical of obliterative bronchiolitis.

CT shows normal main pulmonary arteries but confirms the chest x-ray appearances of small peripheral vessels. The overall mean lung density was in the normal range (−820 HU) in contradistinction to most cases of emphysema.

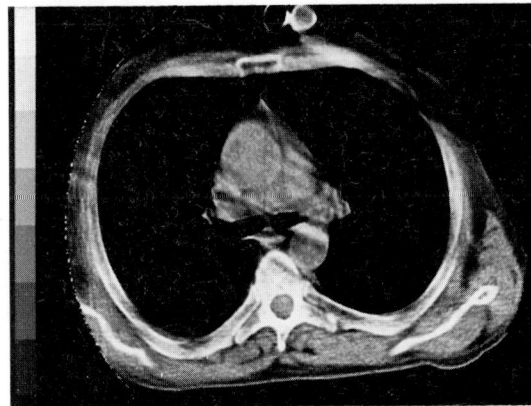

Figure 58d

Figure 58e

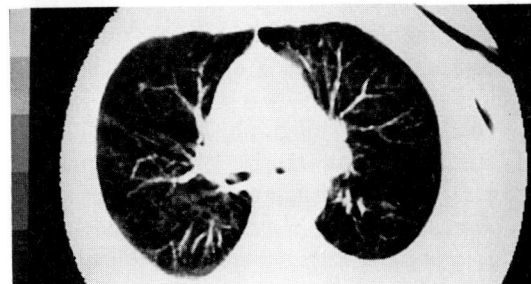

Obliterative bronchiolitis

Obliterative bronchiolitis is a rare condition that has previously been described almost solely at pathology [44]. The main feature is simply, as described in the name, obliteration of the smaller airways. It is an extreme form of chronic severe bronchiolitis. It is rare and has mainly been reported occurring as the result of inhalation of poisonous gases (war or industrial) such as oxides of nitrogen or chlorine. The obliterative bronchiolitis is the end-result of the ensuing chemical pneumonitis. A few cases have been reported in association with severe infections, including whooping cough, and with inhalatibn of foreign bodies. It is also one of the pathological features of Swyer-James or Macleod's syndrome [45].

The condition has been recently described as occurring spontaneously with no known cause. The cryptogenic form of the condition occurs mainly in female patients in association with rheumatoid arthritis [46]. With the use of bronchography the condition has been diagnosed during life but the investigation is associated with considerable morbidity, particularly in the patients with rheumatoid arthritis.

Respiratory function studies yield certain characteristic results in obliterative bronchiolitis. There is usually airflow obstruction which is irreversible with bronchodilators and corticosteroids. The transfer coefficient, KCO, is normal or high as opposed to emphysema in which it is low. These findings are not specific but should alert one to the possibility of the diagnosis of obliterative bronchiolitis.

The symptoms in the acute stages, if due to inhalation of toxic gases, include cough, chest pain, dyspnoea and haemoptysis. Because the condition has usually been described after death it has gained a reputation as a fatal disease. However, minor or patchy changes could occur with little symptomatology and this may well be the case in a condition such as Macleod's syndrome. In the early stages the appearances on the radiographs may be those of alveolar pulmonary oedema particularly with a degree of nodularity. The heart would not usually be enlarged nor the upper zone veins distended enabling the distinction from heart failure to be made. Later there is diffuse hyperinflation or appearances similar to Macleod's. On careful examination of the chest radiograph, if the condition is widespread, the diminution in size of the pulmonary vessels can be seen, although there is preservation of all the major branches. There may also be generalized increase in radiolucency. These changes are more easily seen by computed tomography. Bronchography will show the obliteration of the bronchi with startling detail but as stated above is associated with a level of morbidity that may not be acceptable.

Chest pain

In patients over ten years of age chest pain is almost as frequent as abdominal pain and backache and is a more common presenting symptom in general practice than headache [47]. Many of the patients are worried that they may be suffering from cardiac disease but in General Practice the vast majority are due to musculoskeletal causes—in particular rib or intercostal muscular injury resulting from coughing. The hospital doctor sees a selected group of patients referred either because of difficulty in diagnosis, or because special tests or hospital treatment are necessary.

The most probable cause of chest pain can be ascertained with some accuracy from the exact history of the type of pain and an electrocardiogram.

The causes of chest pain presenting to a general practitioner in one survey [47] were:

Musculoskeletal and neurological (particularly chest wall)	44.4%
Cardiac (particularly ischaemic heart disease)	19.3%
Alimentary tract pain (mainly oesophageal)	17.6%
Respiratory tract (including infection, infarction and pneumothorax)	13.4%
Neurosis	5.3%

The type of pain and the severity will determine whether or not the patient is referred for further investigation. Clinical history is the most essential feature in the diagnosis of chest pain and the electrocardiograph is a major factor in the diagnosis of patients with cardiac-like pain (i.e. pain on exertion etc). The high incidence of oesophageal pain was a finding that had not previously been reported and is of great importance in view of the considerable similarity between cardiac and oesophageal pain. Barium swallow and meal may well be tests to consider early in the investigation of chest pain following ECG and chest radiograph. The most common positive findings are hiatus hernia, gastro-oesophageal reflux and oesophagitis.

Severe chest pain and breathlessness

Patients who present with very severe chest pain and shortness of breath represent a separate subgroup of the patients discussed above. The major differential is between cardiac and respiratory disease with the latter including pulmonary embolism/infarction and pneumonia.

Table 14 Some causes of severe chest pain, and breathlessness

Condition	Diagnostic investigations
Pulmonary embolism/ infarction	Chest x-ray, ventilation/ perfusion scan (ECG, enzymes)
Myocardial infarction	Chest x-ray, ECG, enzymes
Pulmonary infection	Chest x-ray, WBC, sputum (viral etc antibodies)
Dissecting aneurysm	Chest x-ray, aortography
Pneumothorax	Chest x-ray

Case 59

Arnold, aged 60, had a history of obesity and chronic bronchitis. Seven days after a herniorrhaphy he complained of right-sided chest pain. He also had a cough productive of yellow/green sputum flecked with blood. A chest x-ray showed old inflammatory changes at the left base which were unchanged compared with the preoperative film. Ventilation/perfusion scans were performed.

Figure 59

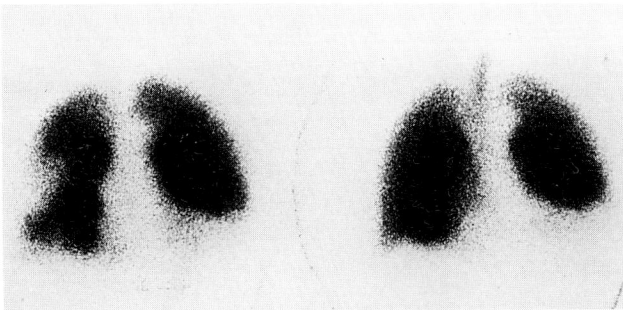

The ventilation/perfusion scans show a matched defect at the left base which is due to the chronic inflammatory changes and a mismatched defect of perfusion in the right mid zone which is a result of pulmonary embolus.

The investigation of suspected pulmonary embolism and infarction

Pulmonary emboli most commonly arise from thrombi in leg veins. Patients at most risk of developing pulmonary emboli are therefore those in whom leg vein thrombosis is likely to occur. The group includes patients following surgery, during pregnancy, patients on prolonged bed rest and in association with severe heart failure.

If death is not immediate from severe pulmonary embolism, the resulting symptoms include acute shortness of breath with a sensation of tightness across the chest or severe retrosternal pain. The patient may be agitated, breathless and cyanosed. The list of possible causes of these particular signs and symptoms includes pulmonary embolism, myocardial infarction, pulmonary infection, dissecting aneurysm and pneumothorax.

The diagnosis of pulmonary embolism and infarction may be made by assessment of clinical signs and symptoms and by radiological tests. The latter usually include a chest radiograph and some form of radionuclide ventilation/perfusion scan. Some centres also use pulmonary angiography to confirm the diagnosis. The radiological studies will be further discussed later in this chapter.

Other investigations of value include ECG and laboratory tests. In pulmonary embolism the ECG is often normal but may reveal evidence of right axis deviation or right ventricular strain. A pattern similar to a posterior myocardial infarction may occur, although a significant O wave in lead 11 occurs only rarely in pulmonary embolism.

The most useful differentiating feature between myocardial infarction and pulmonary embolism is that the ECG changes in the latter are only transient (perhaps lasting only for a few hours) whilst in myocardial infarction they may persist for several weeks.

The diagnosis of pulmonary embolism can be supported by laboratory investigations. There may be a raised ESR and plasma viscosity, neutrophilia and increased serum lactase dehydrogenase activity. There is moderately slow rise in plasma fibrinogen but serum creatine phosphokinase activity is not increased which is in direct contrast with myocardial infarction [48].

Radiological investigation

Chest x-ray

Patients with severe chest pain require a chest radiograph at some stage. Important differential diagnoses may be revealed or virtually excluded by the chest x-ray. Thus the chest radiograph may reveal a widened mediastinum due to dissecting aneurysm or peripherally placed radiolucency due to a pneumothorax. The chest x-ray is only rarely of value in acute myocardial infarction but later may show changes due to left-sided heart failure or even a left ventricular aneurysm.

In the absence of infarction, the chest x-ray of a patient with pulmonary embolism may show no abnormality whatsoever. In some cases there is 'cut-off' of pulmonary vessels and increased radiolucency in the affected area. In a few cases cardiomegaly and dilatation of the main pulmonary artery may be seen.

With infarction there may be a small area of linear opacification or a peripheral opacity. The latter is often described as wedge-shaped or triangular but in reality is usually rather rounded with the wider 'base' laterally, or the opacity is linear. Multiple small infarcts can present as peripherally placed rounded opacities (see Case 13).

The difficulty in the radiological diagnosis of infarction lies in distinguishing between infarction and infection, since both can cause the linear, subsegmental collapse and opacification. The other signs of a small pleural effusion and a raised hemidiaphragm can also occur in both conditions.

Case 60

A man of 42 years of age presented with pleuritic chest pain. There was reduced air entry at the right base and he was hypoxic (PO$_2$ 77). His chest x-ray is shown.

Figure 60a

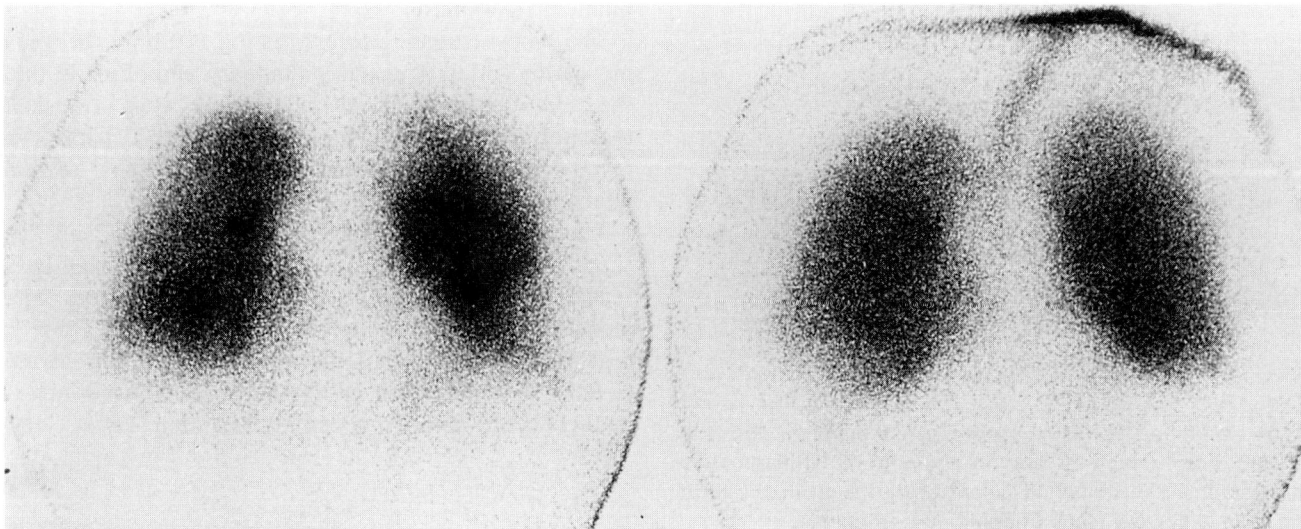

The chest radiograph shows linear opacification in both lower zones with the right base being more affected than the left. Ventilation/perfusion scanning was performed.

There is a matched defect at the right base. There are in addition in both lungs several mismatched defects of perfusion compared with ventilation.

On the strength of this evidence the diagnosis of multiple pulmonary emboli was made.

Figure 60b

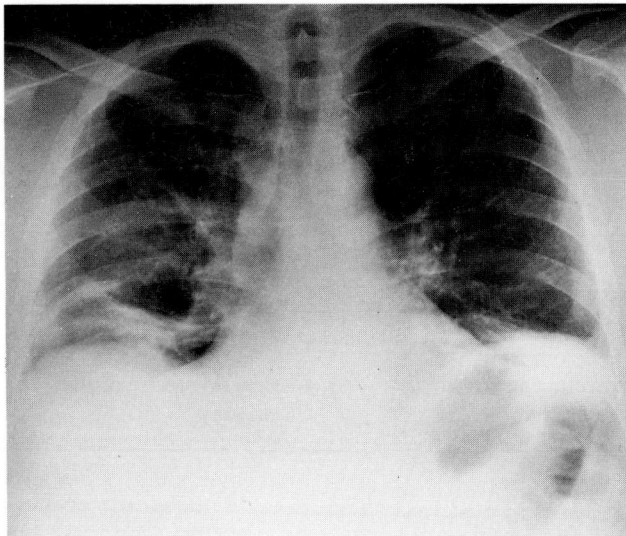

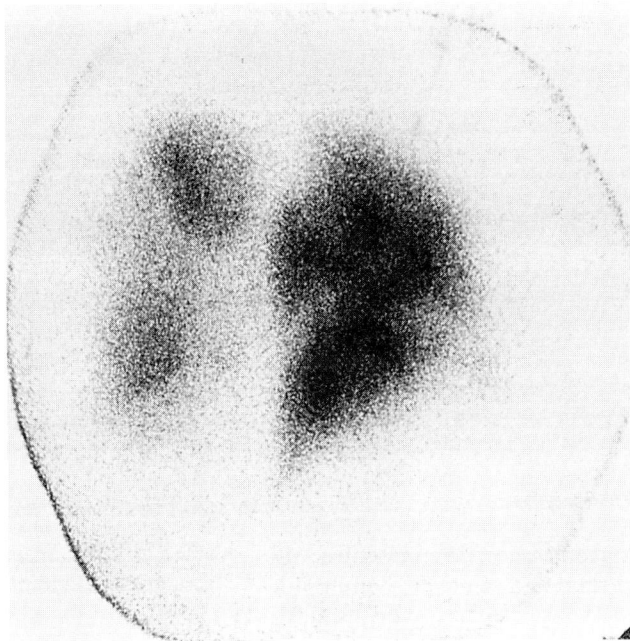

Figure 60c Oblique (perfusion)

In the presence of an opacity on the chest x-ray the matched defect could have been due to almost any cause but particularly infarction or infection. If the mismatched defects of perfusion had not been present, the presumed diagnosis of infarction would therefore have been neither supported nor refuted by the ventilation/perfusion scanning. If there is an abnormality on the chest x-ray, the findings on ventilation/perfusion scanning are much harder to interpret. Thus it is the normal areas on the chest x-ray which are often able to provide the most information on ventilation/perfusion scanning.

Figure 60d Oblique (ventilation)

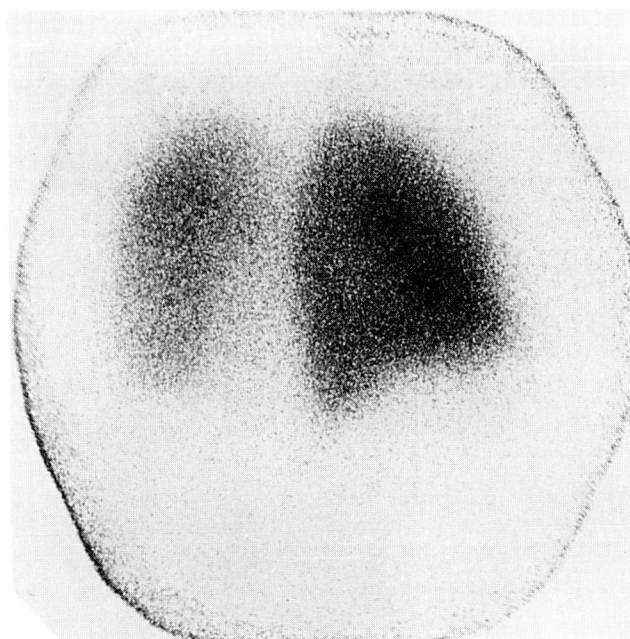

Ventilation/perfusion scanning

Because of its safety and accuracy, ventilation/perfusion (VQ) scintigraphy is the primary method of evaluating patients with suspected pulmonary embolism [49].

Perfusion scanning alone is sensitive but lacks specificity. It is best, therefore, to perform ventilation scans in addition to the perfusion scan. A chest x-ray at the time, or at least within 24 hours of the study, must also be regarded as part of the investigation.

In Bristol, macroaggregates of albumin labelled with technetium-99m are injected intravenously for the perfusion studies. The radiopharmaceutical is injected whilst the patient is lying supine and breathing deeply, but the imaging is undertaken with the patient upright since this provides better visualization of the bases. Krypton-81m gas is used in Bristol for ventilation studies, although in other centres xenon is commonly used. The use of a technetium labelled DTPA aerosol is gaining acceptance in centres that do not have access to krypton.

In pulmonary embolism, the characteristic scintigraphic appearance is a segmental perfusion defect in a normally ventilated lung that is apparently normal on chest x-ray. This is known as a mismatched defect of perfusion. Defects in the perfusion scan that are precisely matched by ventilation defects almost never represent pulmonary emboli if the chest radiograph is normal but can represent infarction if there is opacification on the chest x-ray.

Absolute specificity is rarely possible and the interpretation of ventilation/perfusion studies for pulmonary emboli is best approached by assigning a probability to the correct diagnosis. The probability of pulmonary emboli is high if there are perfusion abnormalities of at least two full lung segments with no corresponding ventilation abnormalities or disease on chest films, whereas the probability is low if there are fewer than two subsegmental perfusion defects in lung zones with normal ventilation and a normal radiograph. A subsegmental defect is a perfusion defect in the distribution of a lung segment that has a smaller volume than a full segment and is clearly segmental in shape. On at least one view of the perfusion scan the defect should extend to the periphery if it is a pulmonary embolus. This can be shown particularly well by single photon emission computed tomography (SPECT) [50]. Non-segmental defects that are small, rounded and do not reach the periphery of the lungs cannot be diagnosed with any degree of certainty as being pulmonary emboli even if there is no matched ventilation defect. This is because in patients with emphysema the defects are not always associated with air-trapping on ventilation study. The fact that a defect does not reach the periphery is therefore a good discriminating feature. (See also Pulmonary emphysema, page 77.)

Causes of mismatched defects other than pulmonary embolus

Although mismatching of the perfusion scan with the ventilation scan has classically been associated with pulmonary embolism since ventilation/perfusion scanning started, there are several other causes of mismatched defects.

When talking about mismatched defects it is of course important to qualify whether the defect is of perfusion or of ventilation. A number of inflammatory conditions including pneumonia may cause mismatched defects of ventilation with a relatively increased perfusion. This physiologically results in shunting and is a cause of cyanosis in patients with pneumonia.

Mismatched defects of perfusion are very uncommon in pneumonia but can occur in acute on chronic bronchitis, as stated above in patients with emphysema (although on careful inspection the defects often do not reach the periphery), in patients with primary bronchogenic carcinoma, pulmonary vascular anomalies, pulmonary artery sarcoma and tumour embolism from distant site [51, 52]. Mismatched defects of perfusion are also seen in mediastinitis due to histoplasmosis [53] and due to radiotherapy. In fibrosing alveolitis and probably in other fibrosing lung conditions it is possible to have mismatches in both directions—there can be mismatch of perfusion or mismatch of ventilation both occurring in the same patient. The distinction from pulmonary emboli can be made from the fact that the plain film is usually considerably abnormal but it does mean that detection of pulmonary emboli by ventilation/perfusion scanning in patients with fibrosing lung conditions is of limited value unless a very large mismatched perfusion defect is discovered that was not previously present. In the case of histoplasmosis, Park et al [53] suggest that gallium-67 scanning may occasionally be of use in distinguishing between pulmonary embolism and the fibrosing condition.

In patients with pulmonary infarction there is again a relative mismatch with decreased perfusion compared with the ventilation. Thus, although ventilation is slightly decreased, the corresponding defect of perfusion is usually profound. Some of these principles are discussed in the preceding and following cases.

Case 61

A middle-aged lady presented with a history of acute onset of shortness of breath and chest pain. The chest radiograph was considered to be normal.

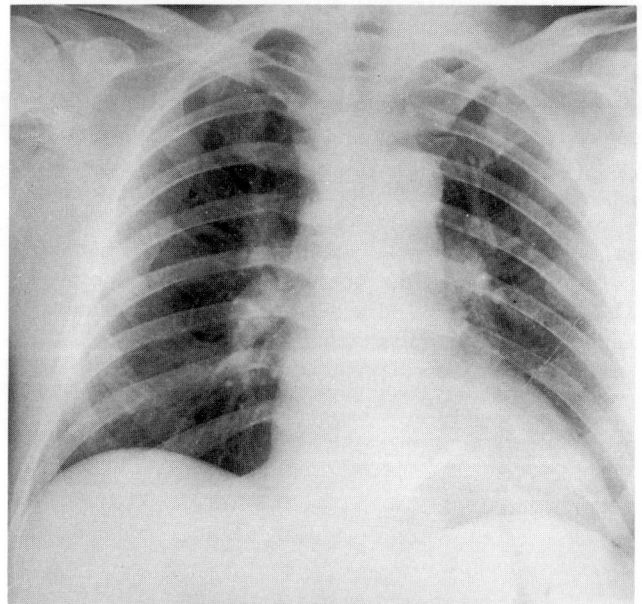

Figure 61a

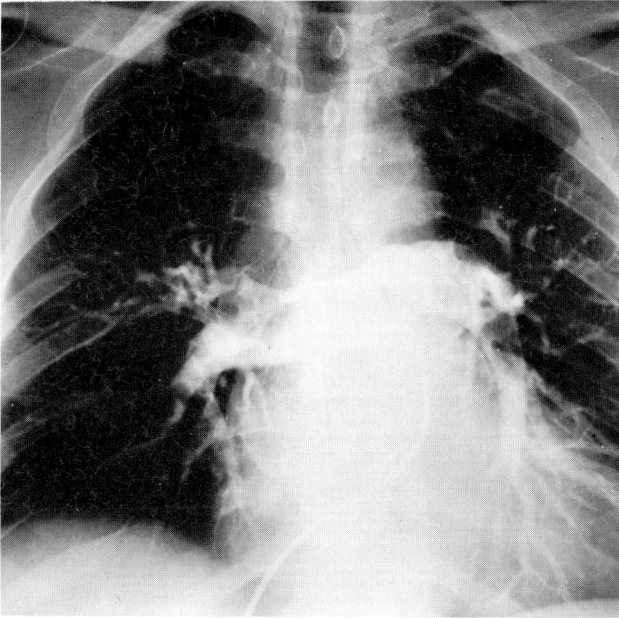

Figure 61b

Pulmonary angiography revealed multiple intraluminal filling defects due to pulmonary emboli.

Pulmonary angiography in the diagnosis of pulmonary embolism

Pulmonary angiography is possibly the most accurate method for the diagnosis of pulmonary embolism. Many centres would advocate the use of angiography for patients in whom the ventilation/perfusion scans are indeterminate. In such cases the perfusion scan can be used as a form of 'road map' and the areas of abnormal perfusion would be the areas to be studied by angiography. In other centres it is felt that, if the lesions are so small as to be indeterminate or equivocal, it is unlikely that the patients will need treatment with anticoagulation and therefore angiography would not usually be recommended. If further investigation is required, one could perhaps perform computed tomography and emission computed tomography rather than pulmonary angiography. If, however, there is a question of surgical intervention to remove the thrombus, then angiography is essential.

Detection of venous thrombi and pulmonary emboli with 111 indium-labelled platelets

Indium-labelled platelets injected intravenously may be incorporated into thrombi and emboli. Several reports have indicated that imaging remains productive with thrombi aged in vivo for ten hours if heparin is not given. This raises the possibility that pulmonary emboli could be detected if scanning is performed quickly enough and before anticoagulation therapy has been started. Reports show that the method is successful in dogs but in human beings, because most of them have already been put on heparin therapy, the detection of pulmonary emboli has been disappointing. Much work needs to be done before the sensitivity and specificity of this test in human beings can be assessed.

Magnetic resonance imaging

Magnetic resonance has been used experimentally to show emboli in the pulmonary arteries of dogs [54] and in one patient [55].

Pulmonary scintigraphy in fibrosing mediastinitis due to histoplasmosis

Histoplasmosis can result in fibrosing mediastinitis. This in turn can give rise to entrapment of pulmonary vessels and large perfusion defects with normal ventilation. These will therefore mimic ventilation/perfusion scan mismatch of pulmonary emboli. The mediastinal fibrosis can even be severe enough to lead to superior vena cava obstruction with minimal findings on the chest radiograph. In these cases, if there is a suggestion of histoplasmosis, gallium-67 scanning can be quite helpful and show intense uptake in the areas affected by the histoplasmosis [53].

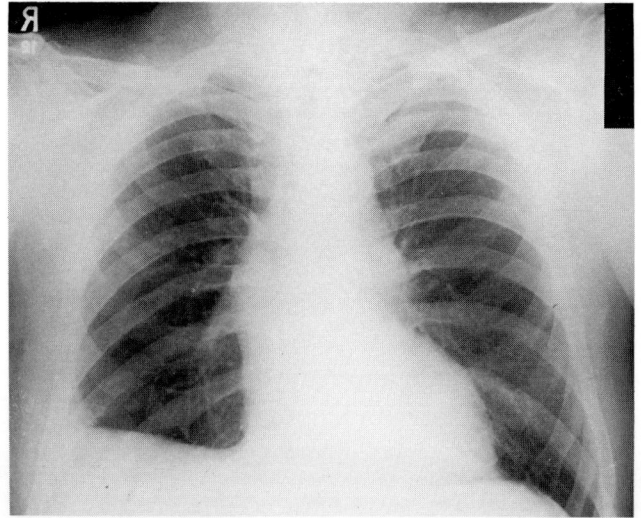

Figure 62a

Figure 62b

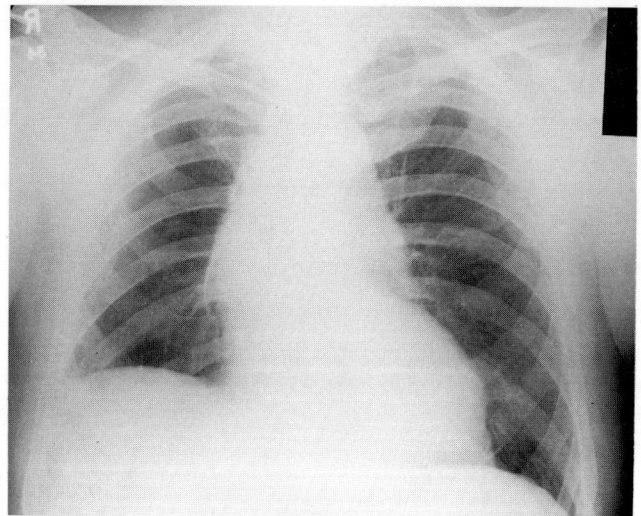

Case 62

A man of 58 years of age had been treated with radiotherapy for carcinoma of the bronchus. Figure 62a shows his chest x-ray near the start of treatment and 62b shows the x-ray six months later.

On both films there is elevation of the hemidiaphragm. In figure 62b the right lung is more radiolucent than the left.

To further evaluate the cause of this breathlessness ventilation/perfusion scanning, with emission CT of the perfusion study was undertaken. Computed tomography of the chest was also performed.

The planar images of the ventilation/perfusion scans show decrease in both ventilation and perfusion in the right lung. The emission CT showed profound decrease in

Figure 62c

Perfusion   Ventilation

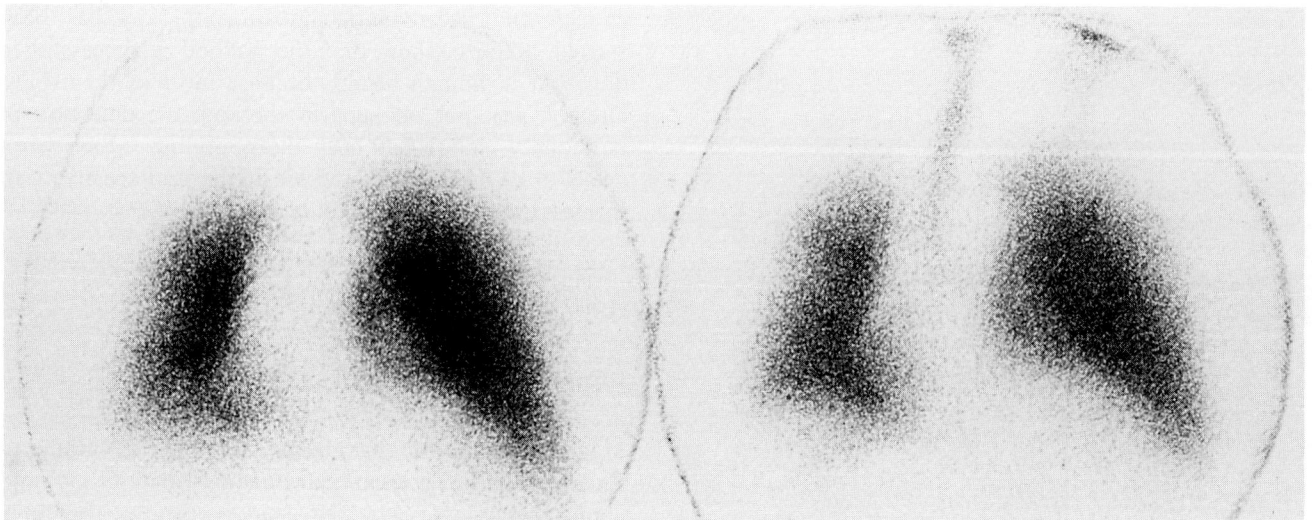

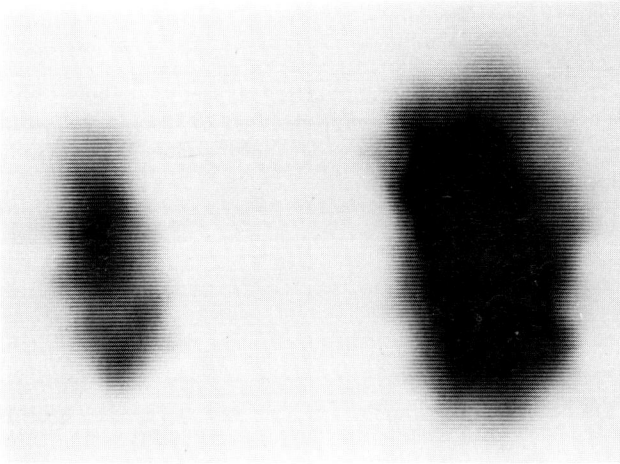

Figure 62d

perfusion in the right lung. CT showed decreased vascularity in the affected lung and paramediastinal fibrosis involving the right hilum. The fibrosis has a straight lateral edge and is very similar to that shown in Case 38.

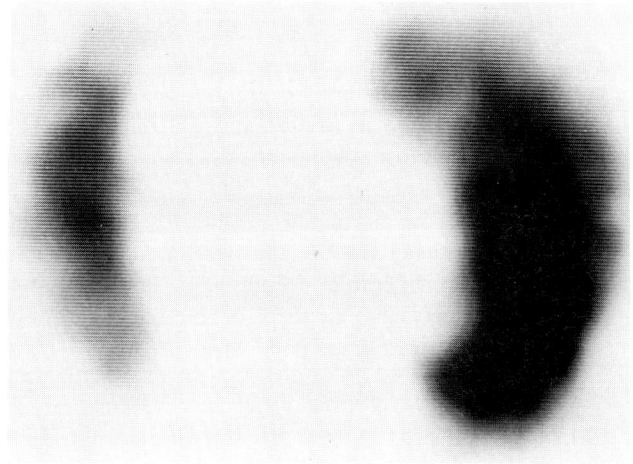

Figure 62e

Figure 62f

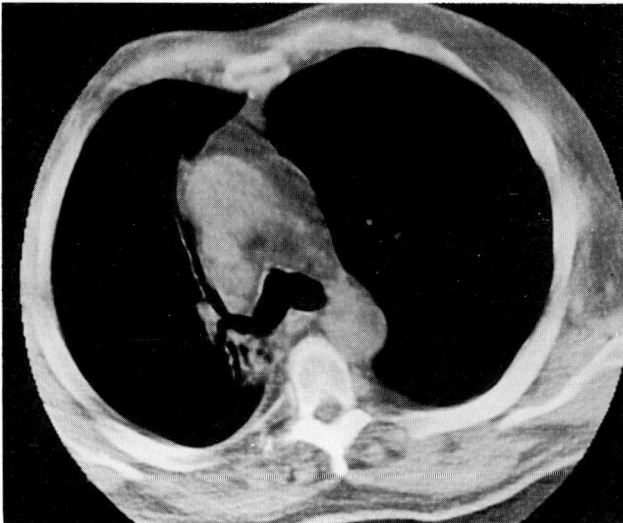

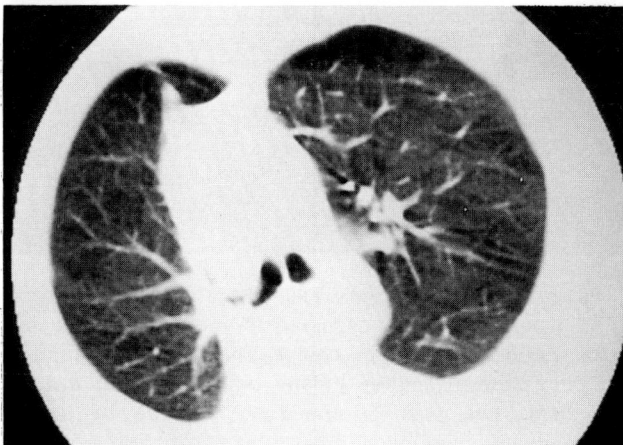

Figure 62g

The changes in vascularity of the right lung in Case 62 have mainly occurred as a result of the hilar fibrosis and this in turn resulted from irradiation.

If the second chest x-ray (fig. 62b) is re-examined, it is possible to see that there is paramediastinal fibrosis, and the vessels in the right lung have reduced in size compared with the left lung and indeed are smaller than on the previous film.

Radiation pneumonopathy and pulmonary vascular changes

Pulmonary changes following irradiation have been discussed in Chapter 7, page 61. Initially there is pneumonitis in the field of irradiation and this may or may not be followed by fibrosis.

The advent of transmission computed tomography (CT) and single photon emission computed tomography (SPECT) has made possible the detection and analysis of lesions that are not visible on the standard x-rays and ventilation/perfusion scans [56, 57].

Areas of decreased perfusion due to the exudative pneumonitis or due to fibrosis can be shown and any changes outside the radiation field can be documented.

Changes in pulmonary vascularity within the area of pneumonitis or fibrosis are inevitable. In addition changes in pulmonary vascularity outside the radiated field are fairly common if the hilar and mediastinum are involved. Mismatched defects may be seen but should not be confused with pulmonary emboli because the mismatch is one of degree rather than the subsegmental or segmental defects that are seen in pulmonary emboli. Initially the defects are confined to the area of the radiation field. It is seemingly only later that the rest of the lung may become avascular and at that stage the perfusion defect is usually matched with a ventilation defect.

In addition to the decreased vascularity that can be seen in some patients outside the irradiated field there may also be considerable decrease in lung volume, apparently greater than that to be accounted for simply by shrinkage of the irradiated part of the lung.

Case 63

A girl aged 22 presented with a previous history of Hodgkin's lymphoma and the following CT appearances.

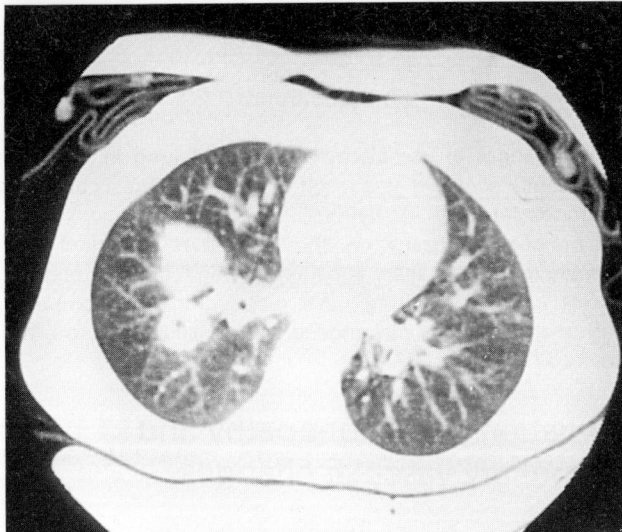

Figure 63a

Figure 63b

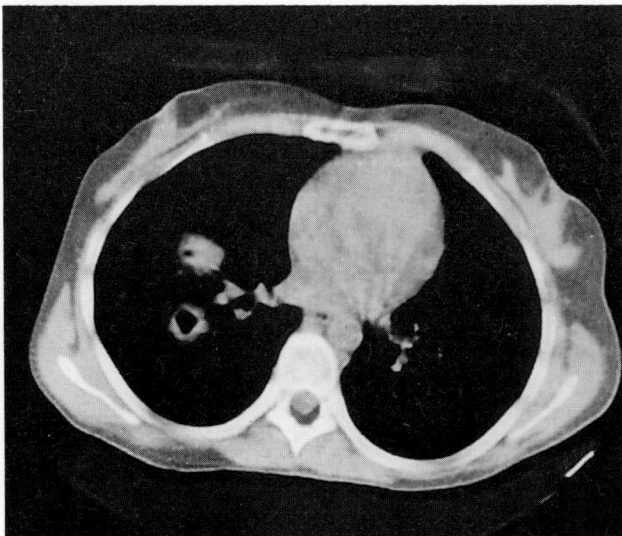

There were cavitating masses present in both hilar regions. Further radiotherapy resulted in disappearance of the opacities and CT scans 18 months later showed only slight residual abnormality.

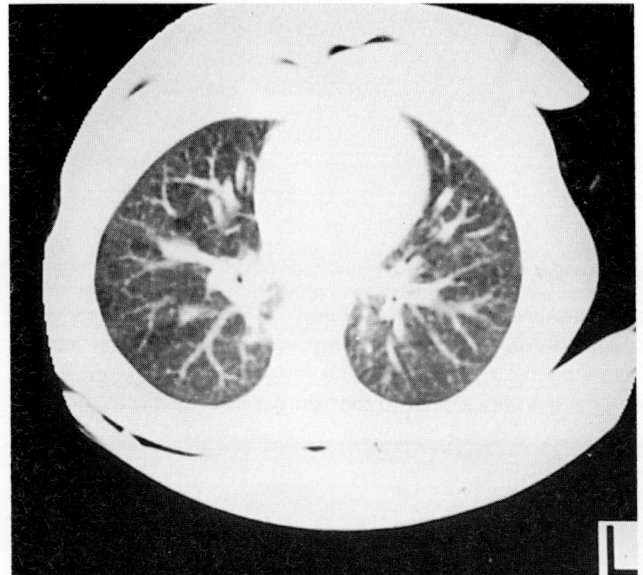

Figure 63c

Figure 63d

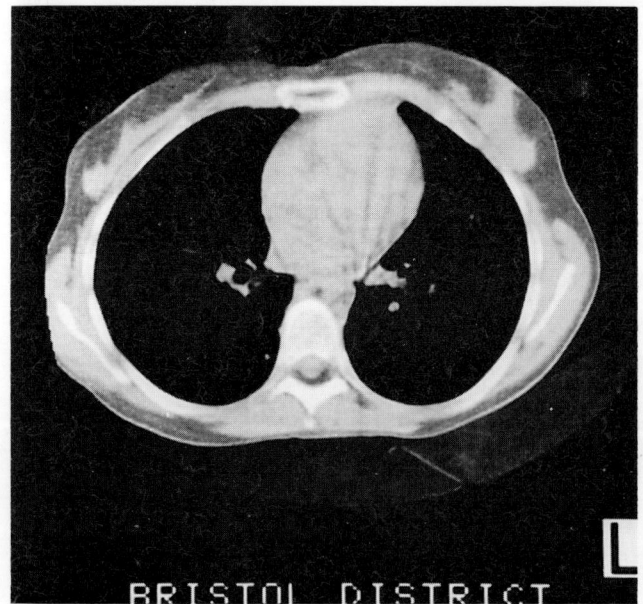

The patient, however, gradually became breathless and further investigation was necessary 21 months after the start of the second radiotherapy course. The chest radiograph at that time showed slightly greater opacification of the left lung field, this was presumed to be due to pleural thickening and pulmonary fibrosis.

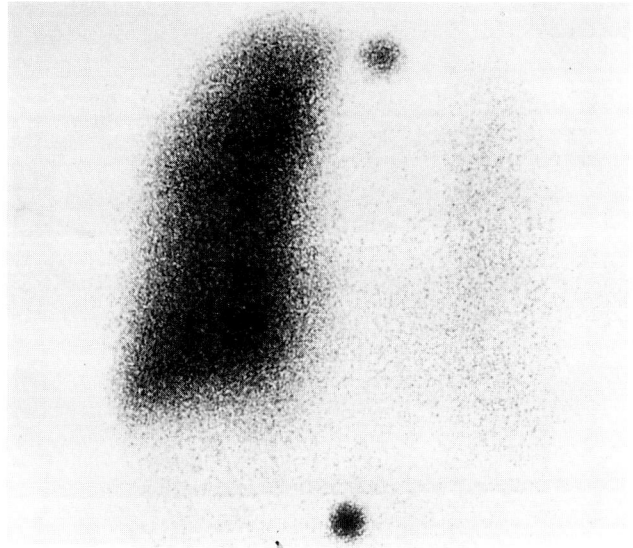

Figure 63g

Figure 63h

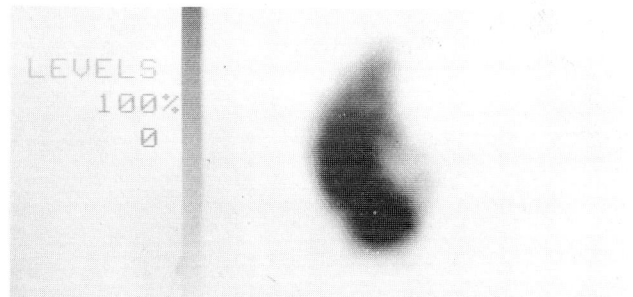

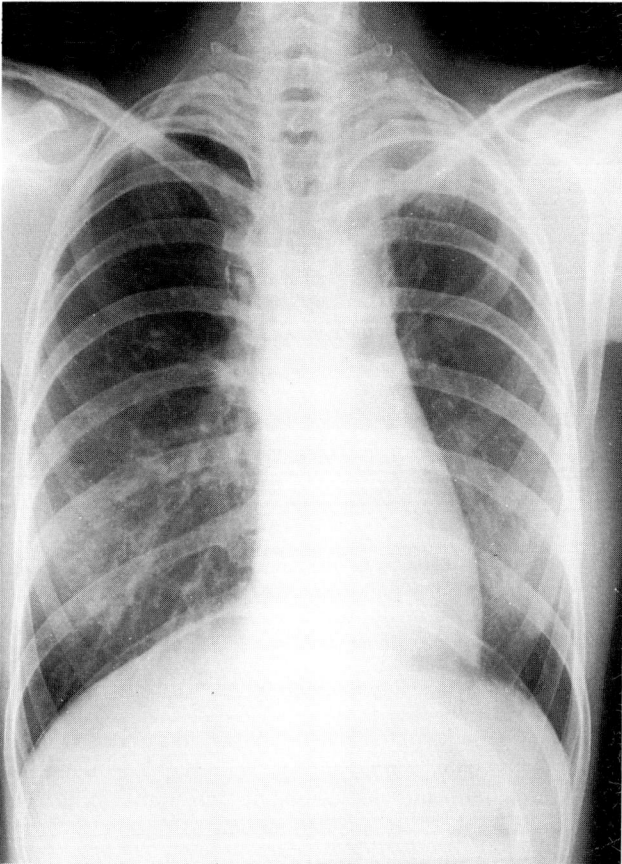

Figure 63e

On auscultation there was lack of air entry to the left lung. This was confirmed by ventilation/perfusion scanning. The ventilation/perfusion scans showed no ventilation

and only slight perfusion in the left lung. The emission CT showed no perfusion in the left lung fields. In figures 63i, 63j and 63k the transmission CT series over a period of 9 months is shown.

Figure 63f

Figure 63i One year after recurrence

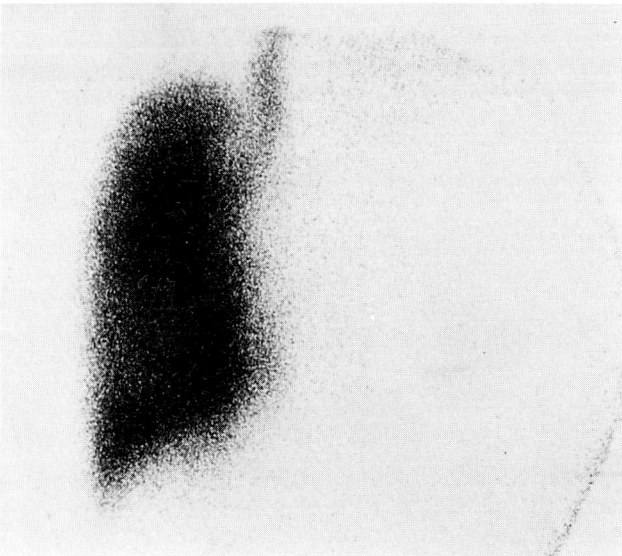

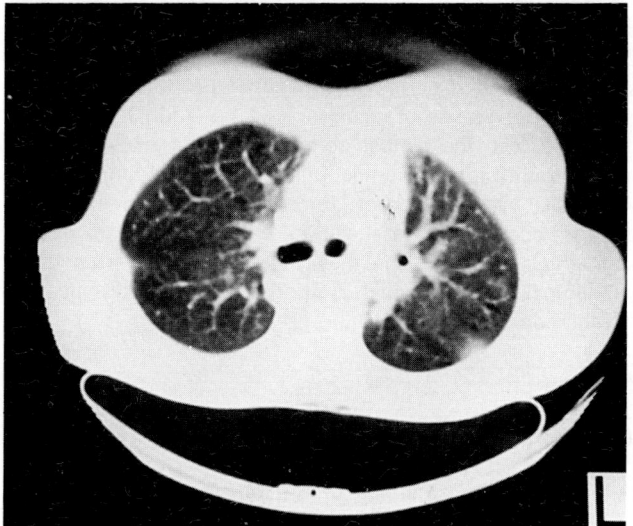

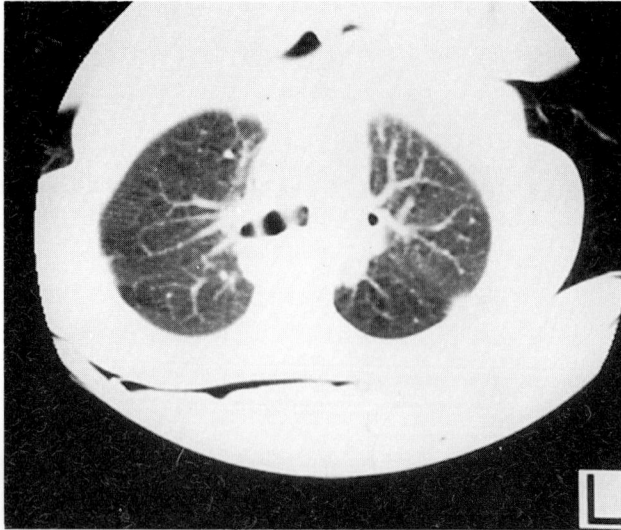

Figure 63j At 18 months

Figure 63k At 21 months

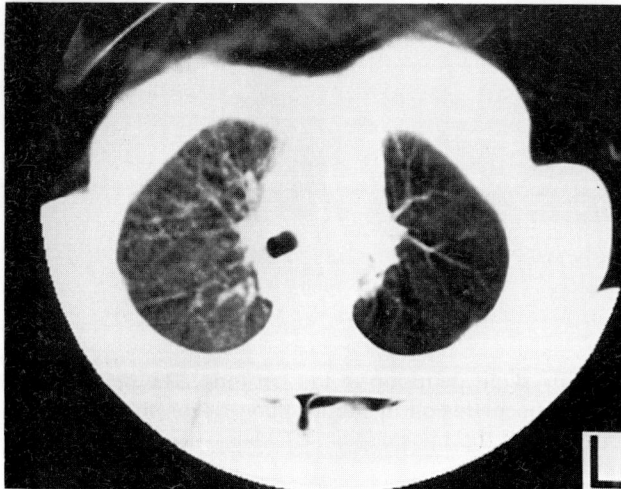

On careful analysis of the CT it is possible to see a decrease in size of pulmonary vessels with the left lung being markedly worse affected than the right. On the latest scan the left upper lobe bronchus is no longer visible. The shape of the fibrosis remained unchanged throughout and there is no evidence of recurrence of the Hodgkin's disease.

In this case the almost complete loss of perfusion was matched with loss of ventilation. Some of the diminution in vessel size had occurred at 18 months, but the most marked change occurred in association with obstruction of the segmental bronchi. This may have been exacerbated by subclinical infection which is another possible complication of radiation therapy.

Case 64

A patient with carcinoma of the breast was treated with radiotherapy. Her chest x-ray is shown in figure 64a.

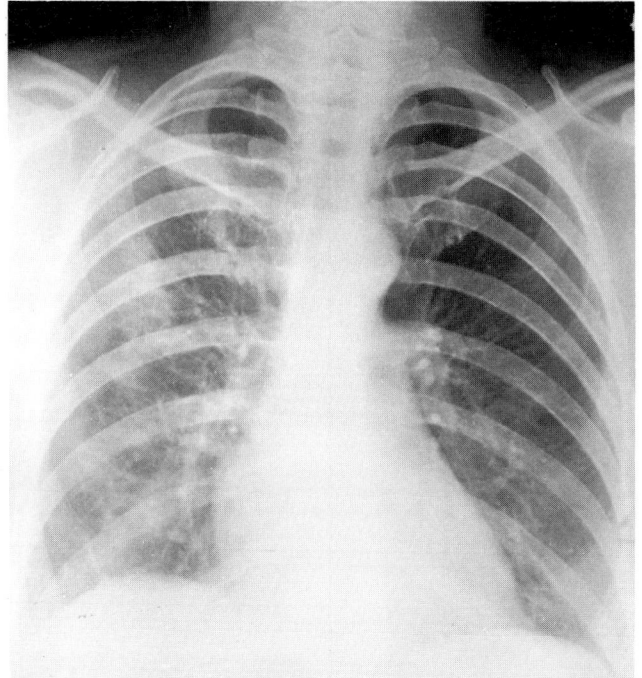

Figure 64a

There is slight opacification of the right lung field compared with the left.

Ventilation/perfusion scans are shown in figures 64b and 64c and the only abnormality is very slight reduction in both ventilation and perfusion of the right lung. The emission CT and CT scans are shown in figures 64d and 64e.

Figure 64b

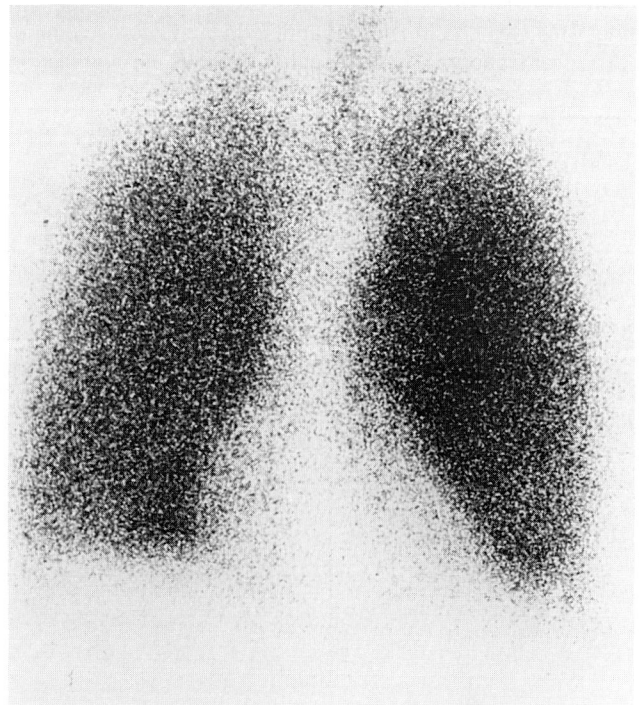

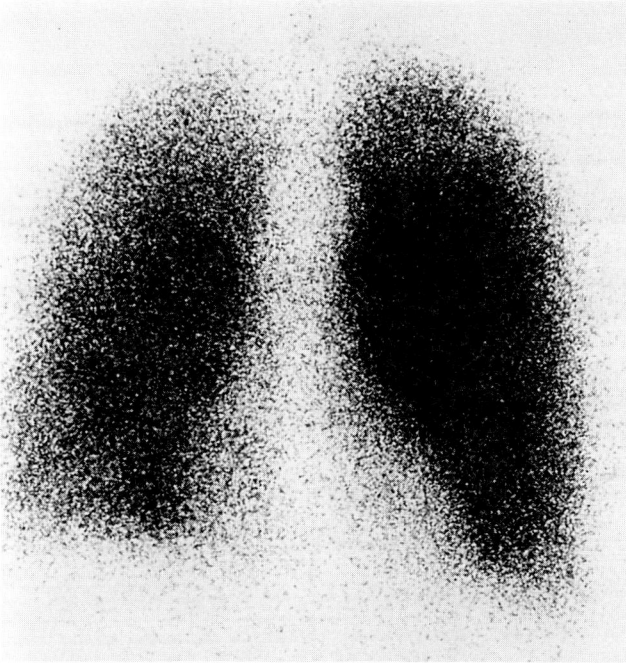

Figure 64c

Figure 64d

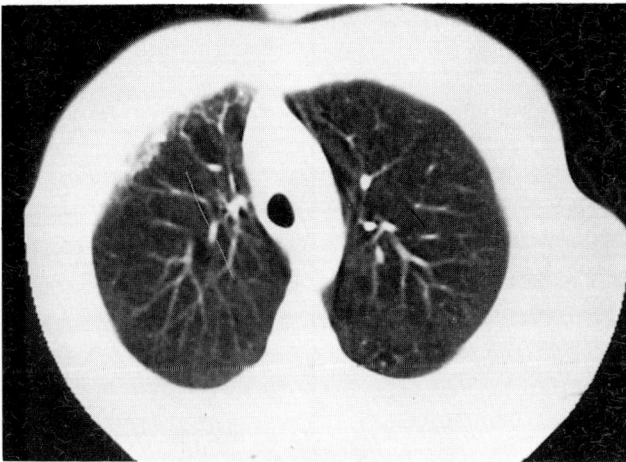

Figure 64e

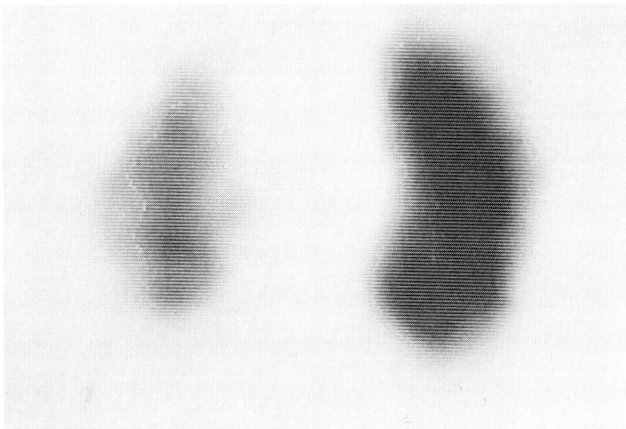

The emission CT showed considerable decrease in perfusion of the right lung. CT showed opacification of the right lung anteriorly but little change in the rest of the right lung. Emission CT is more sensitive than transmission CT in showing the vascular changes due to radiation. Emission CT is also considerably more sensitive than the planar ventilation/perfusion scan.

Summary: decreased density of the lung fields

Unequal density of one lung field compared with the other or patchy decreased density of the lung fields is a difficult sign to interpret on chest radiographs. Clinical presentation is important, since without relevant signs or symptoms an area of decreased density on a chest radiograph may not warrant further investigation. True decrease in density may result due to conditions such as emphysema, pneumothorax and pulmonary emboli. Unilateral radiolucency of the hemithorax may, however, also result from rotation of the patient or to loss of overlying soft tissues. It is always important to consider whether the area of radiolucency may be the normal area and the opposite lung denser due to a pathological condition such as consolidation or pleural effusion. In addition to the usual inspiration PA and lateral films an expiration PA film may be of value in showing air-trapping due to obstructive emphysema and in showing a small pneumothorax. High KV chest films may be particularly useful because the penetration of the mediastinum will enable lesions such as collapsed lobes to be seen.

Computed tomography is an investigation of considerable value in the investigation of patients with decreased lung density since the true density of the lungs can be seen without the confusion of overlying soft tissue and bones. Thus CT is a very sensitive method of demonstrating pulmonary emphysema, pneumothorax and most of the other causes of reduced lung density.

Pulmonary embolism can result in reduced lung density but is not the main presenting feature of that condition. More important symptoms and signs are pleuritic chest pain, haemoptysis and breathlessness. The main investigative modality for pulmonary embolism is scintigraphic ventilation/perfusion scanning. This is probably best performed using technetium-labelled albumin and inhalation of krypton gas. A chest radiograph should always be performed on the same day, since the presence or absence of pulmonary abnormalities on the chest x-ray may considerably alter interpretation of the scans. Pulmonary angiography may be required in patients with suspected pulmonary embolism if the ventilation/perfusion scans are equivocal or if the possibility of surgical intervention is being seriously considered.

Any form of damage to the pulmonary vessels can result in reduced lung density and thus mediastinal fibrosis or hilar fibrosis due either to infection (such as histoplasmosis) or due to radiation therapy may result in pulmonary radiolucency.

10 Elevation of the diaphragm

The diaphragm may be elevated because it is pushed up, pulled up, or paralysed. It may appear to be elevated due to a number of conditions that create a false impression as to the position of the diaphragm.

With true elevation of the diaphragm plain films of the chest may reveal the cause. The pulmonary causes of diaphragmatic elevation have mainly been dealt with in the preceding chapters (fibrosis, collapse, carcinoma etc). They will not be further discussed in this chapter.

Table 15 Elevation of the diaphragm

1	Pulled up	Pulmonary collapse, fibrosis, infarction, film on expiration
2	Pushed up	Ascites, subdiaphragmatic mass or abscess, intestinal distension
3	Paralysed	Carcinoma of the bronchus, phrenic nerve palsy, avulsion or crush, eventration
4	Simulated	Subpulmonary effusion, ruptured diaphragm, diaphragmatic hernia

Subdiaphragmatic masses, organomegaly, ascites, distension of the bowel and subphrenic abscess may push the diaphragm up. Investigations that assist in demonstrating these conditions start with plain films of the abdomen, including erect and supine films and coned views at the level of the diaphragm. Ultrasound of the abdomen will demonstrate some of the conditions that push the diaphragm upwards. If a subphrenic abscess is present, ultrasound may show a loculated cystic area between the diaphragm and liver. Other investigations that may assist in the demonstration of a subphrenic abscess include computed tomography, colloid scanning of the liver, gallium scanning and labelled white cell scanning.

If the hemidiaphragm is paralysed, paradoxical movement on respiration can be shown by fluoroscopy or real-time ultrasound. Thus, on inspiration the affected diaphragm may move upwards. Fluoroscopy is often difficult to interpret but coned views of the diaphragm in full inspiration and expiration may assist.

In eventration of the diaphragm, part or all of the hemidiaphragm is deficient in musculature. Pathologically an eventrated diaphragm consists of a thin membranous sheet attached peripherally to normal muscle at points of origin from the rib cage [58]. Partial eventration is most common in the anteromedial portion of the right hemidiaphragm. When the right hemidiaphragm is 'elevated' due to eventration, sonographic features include demonstration of a normal liver beneath the diaphragm, thinning of the cupola and, on real-time scanning, paradoxical movement.

In a recent paper [59], a selected series of 22 patients with right-sided diaphragmatic humps and juxtadiaphragmatic masses were examined by real-time and static grey scale ultrasound. Ultrasonography provided a useful adjunct to conventional chest x-rays by accurately defining the extent and contents of the humps and masses. The diagnoses made included localized eventration, loculated effusion, subphrenic and hepatic abscesses. Also clearly shown were hydatid and pericardial cysts, an aortic aneurysm, a fat pad and hepatic metastatic deposits. In all cases the ultrasound provided a reliable and accurate diagnosis. Khan and Gould [59] concluded that ultrasound should be regarded as the examination of choice for scanning diaphragmatic humps and juxtadiaphragmatic masses.

Case 65

A 50 year old man had undergone an oesophagogastrectomy and splenectomy. He had a stormy post-operative period with a right-sided pneumonia that was slowly clearing when he was discharged home. He was readmitted with a two-day history of recurrent rigors and

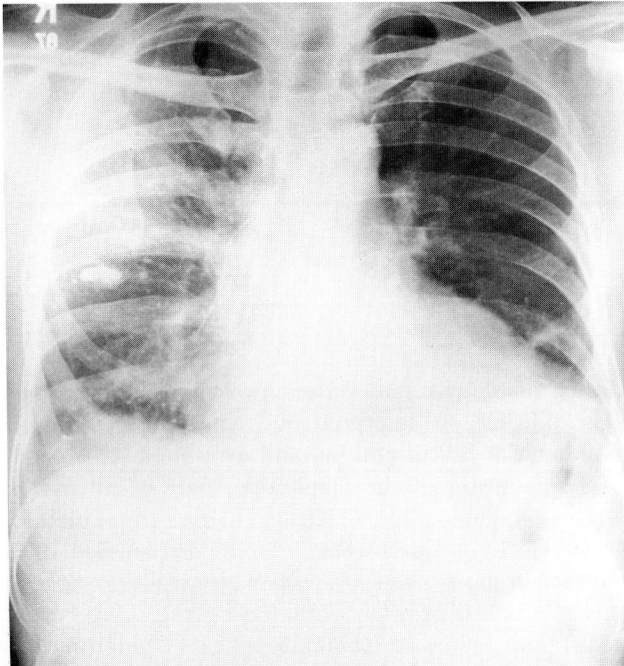

Figure 65a

pain in the left upper quadrant and loin. His chest x-ray is shown.

There is patchy opacification in the right lung field due to the resolving pneumonia. (In fact it was much improved compared with the previous films!) A calcified opacity is also present in the right mid-zone.

There is subsegmental collapse in the left lower zone and elevation of the left hemidiaphragm. Ultrasound was done of the left upper quadrant of the abdomen.

Figure 65b

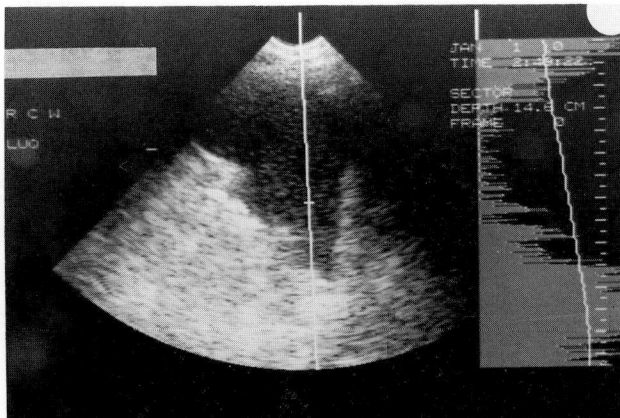

The ultrasound shows a mass of low echogenicity in the splenic bed. The appearances could have been due to haematoma or abscess but with the signs and symptoms the latter was far more likely.

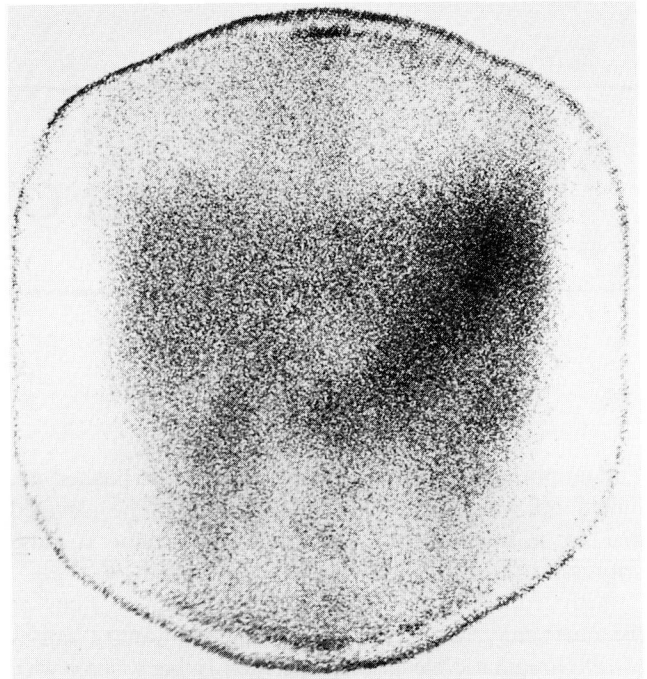

Figure 65c

Gallium scanning (fig. 65c) showed increased uptake in the hypochondrium.

The pattern was similar in shape to bowel but on later scans the area of increased uptake was unchanged in shape

Figure 65d

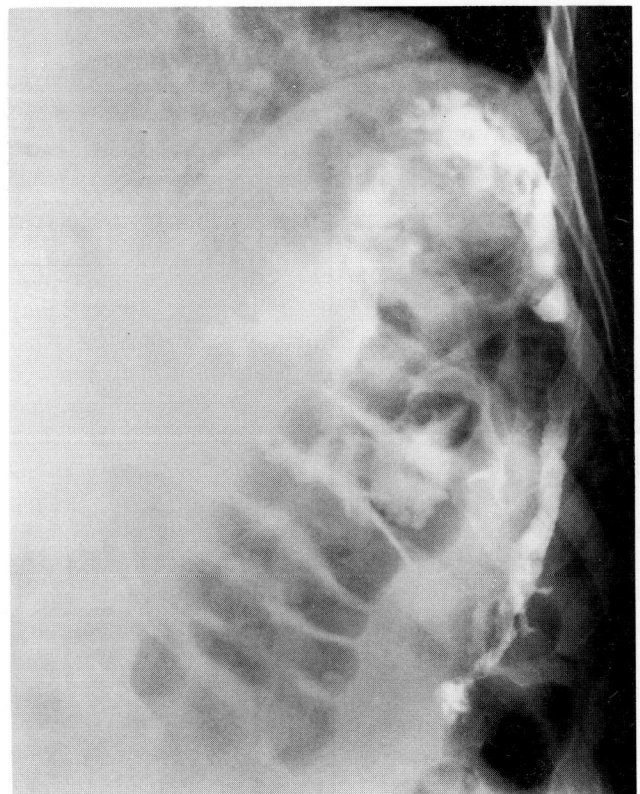

or site and was relatively more obvious compared with the background uptake. These were features of an abscess.

The abscess subsequently 'pointed' over an old drain site in the left upper quadrant. A sinogram is shown in figure 65d. Contrast medium is shown in the splenic bed and left paracolic gutter. The abscess thus involved the subphrenic and paracolic areas.

Some conditions may mimic the appearances of a raised hemidiaphragm. Perhaps the most common of these is subpulmonary effusion. Pleural fluid lying above the diaphragm but below the lung will appear opaque on chest x-ray and on an erect film may take the same shape as the diaphragm. The superior surface of the effusion may then be mistaken for the top of the hemidiaphragm. On careful analysis of the chest x-ray, if a patient has a subpulmonary effusion, there may be two signs to help distinguish the appearance from a raised hemidiaphragm: (1) The apparent dome of the hemidiaphragm may be more laterally placed than usual, (2) there is usually slight blunting of the costophrenic angle. Differentiation of effusion from elevation of the diaphragm can be made by three methods:

1 Films of the chest with the patient lying on his side (lateral decubitus films).
2 Ultrasound.
3 Computed tomography.

If subpulmonary effusion is suspected, it is most simple to perform lateral decubitus films. The problem of differentiation between pleural effusion and other pleural abnormalities is discussed in Chapter 11.

A life-threatening condition that may be easily and catastrophically forgotten is that of rupture of the diaphragm. This should be considered in any case of severe chest or abdominal trauma. The condition is of great importance because of the complication of hernial bleeding or strangulation.

If the hemidiaphragm has been torn but herniation of the bowel has not occurred, the only available radiological signs may be the presence of an associated pneumoperitoneum or pneumothorax [60]. There may be signs of associated intra-abdominal trauma such as rupture of the liver or spleen. If herniation of gut has occurred, the features on the chest radiograph may be non-specific but include:

1 Abnormal pattern obscuring the lung base due directly to the herniated bowel. This may give rise to a wrong diagnosis such as subphrenic abscess or traumatic pneumatocele.

2 Haemothorax or haemopneumothorax.
3 Herniation of the stomach and collapse of the left lung may mimic pneumothorax.

Barium studies may be helpful by showing herniation of gut and ultrasound or CT may show herniation of omentum, liver or other viscera.

Case 66

A man aged 55 presented with a long history of aortic stenosis with recent worsening of his shortness of breath. The chest x-ray is shown.

Figure 66a

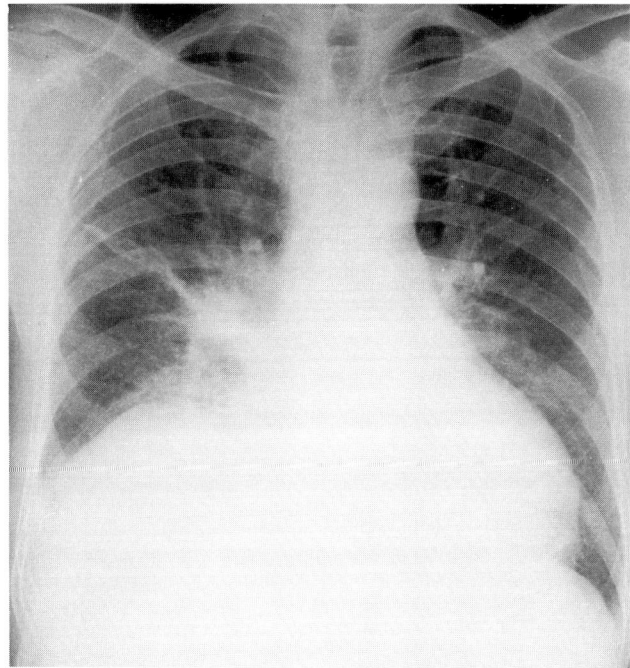

PA chest films and lateral show an apparently raised right hemidiaphragm and right hilar mass. A penetrated film (fig. 66c) two weeks later shows the heart is still enlarged, septal lines are present due to failure. The hilar mass and elevation of the right hemidiaphragm are still present. Bronchoscopy was performed at this stage and no abnormality was detected. CT scan was undertaken.

CT scan at the anatomical level of T6 (fig. 66d) shows a large right-sided pleural effusion tracking up to the posterior wall of the bronchus intermedius. CT scan at the level of T8 (fig. 60e) again shows the large effusion and shows calcific aortic stenosis. The pleural effusion was

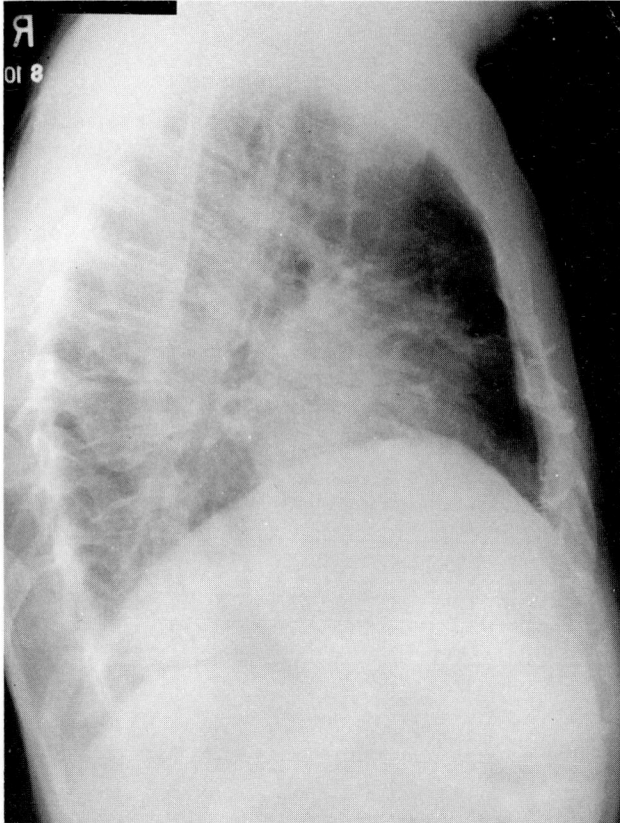

Figure 66b

Figure 66c

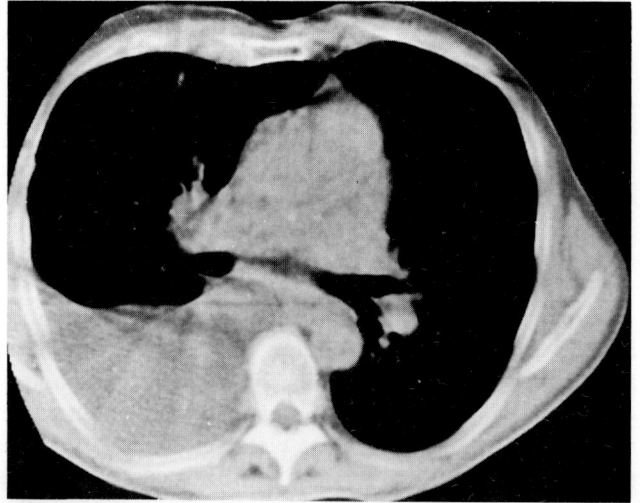

Figure 66d

Figure 66e

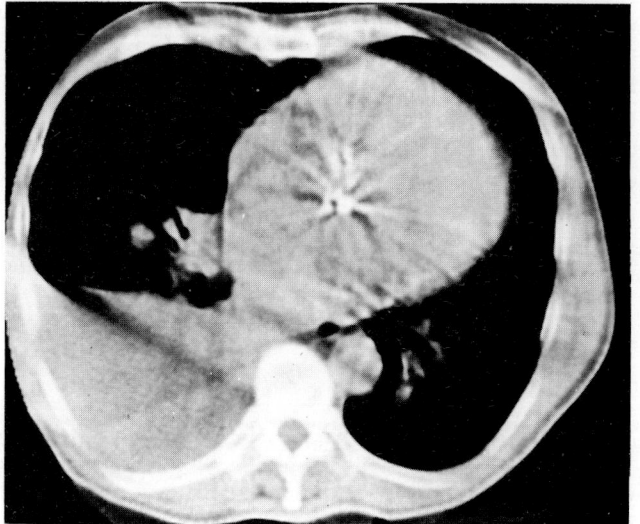

Figure 66f

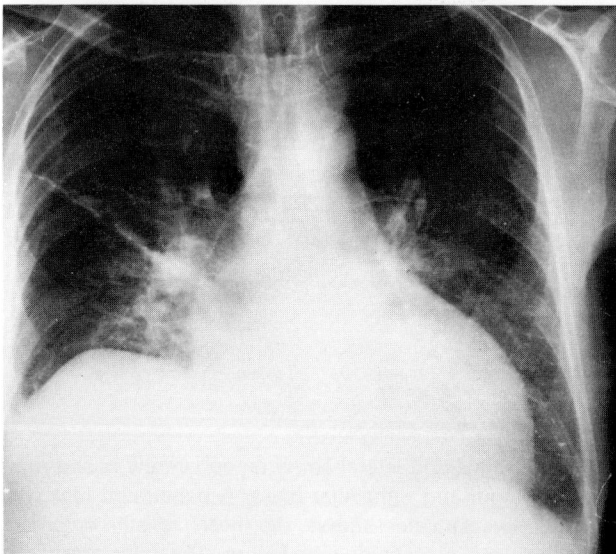

taken to be the cause of the apparently raised hemidiaphragm and was in a subpulmonary position when the patient was erect. The effusion was tapped. No malignant cells were found. The patient underwent valve replacement. A post-surgery film is shown in figure 66f, at which time there has been almost complete resolution of the pleural effusion and the hilar mass has completely disappeared.

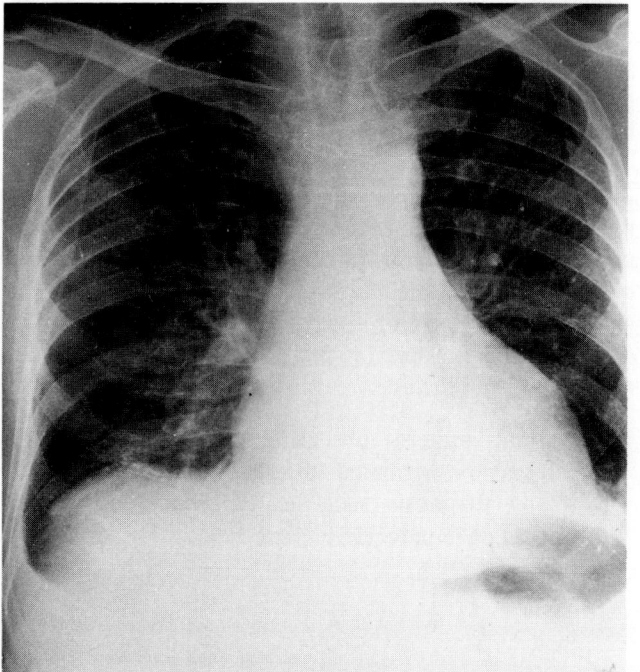

Case 67

A man aged 63 presented with a history of aortic stenosis of a moderate degree and recent worsening of dyspnoea. The chest x-ray shows appearances very similar to the last example.

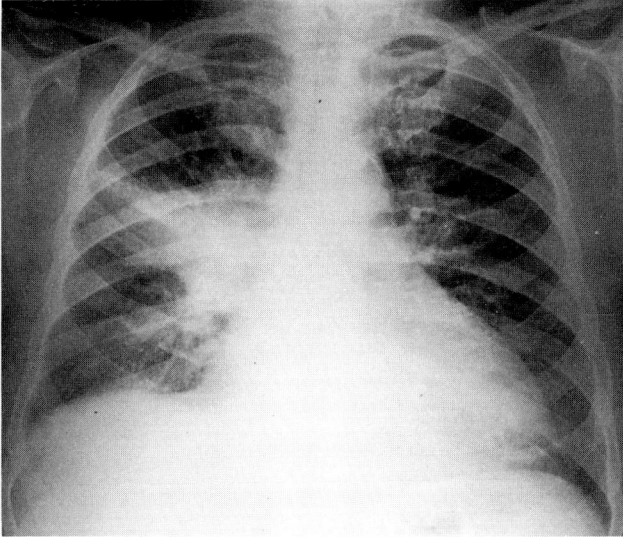

Figure 67a

Figure 67b

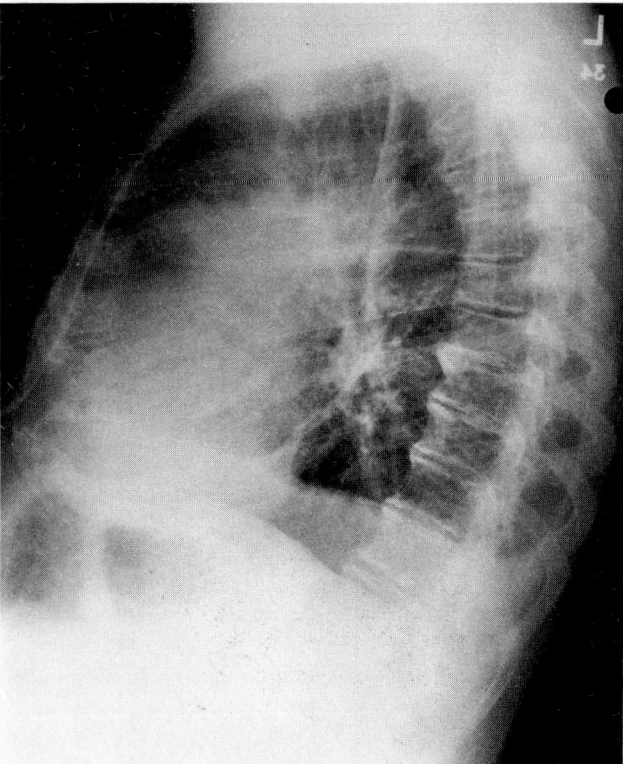

On the PA film there is slight elevation of the right hemidiaphragm and a right hilar mass. These appearances are confirmed on the lateral film. A lateral decubitus film was undertaken.

There is a large pleural effusion tracking up the chest wall and into the horizontal fissure. The hilar mass has not disappeared, however. Bronchoscopy was undertaken and showed a bronchial carcinoma at the right hilum.

Figure 67c Lateral decubitus film

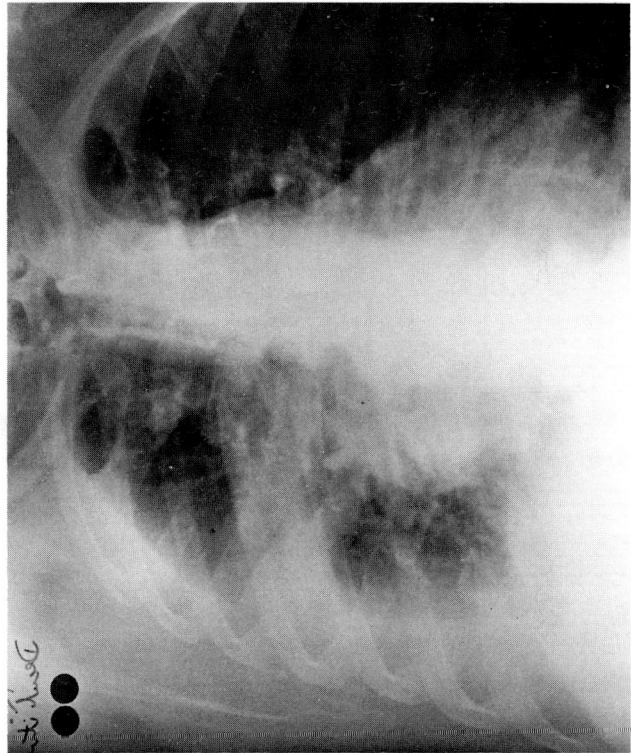

Case 68

A woman aged 47 had recently undergone cholecystectomy. She had grumbling pyrexia post-operation.

The chest x-ray showed blunting of the costophrenic angles bilaterally and the right hemidiaphragm appeared elevated. Ultrasound was undertaken in order to look for a subphrenic abscess. Figures 68b and 68c show the ultrasound of the right hemidiaphragm with an explanatory line drawing and figures 68d and 68e the left hemidiaphragm.

The ultrasound scans were performed with the patient lying supine. They beautifully demonstrated bilateral pleural effusions but no subphrenic abscess was detected.

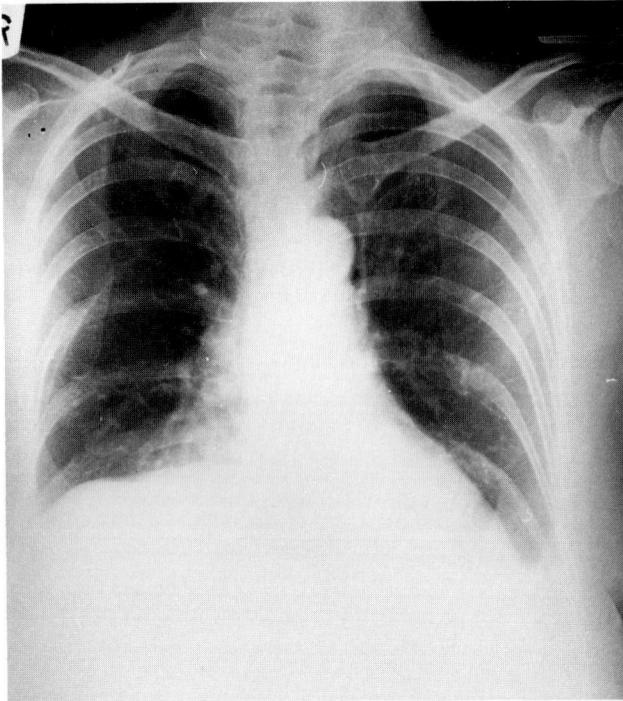

Figure 68a

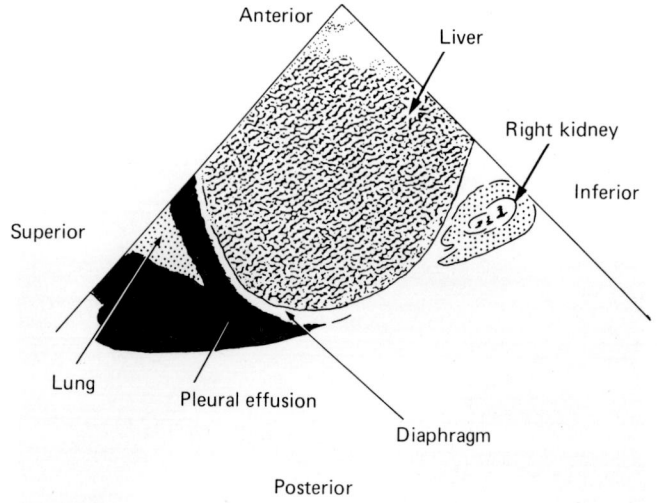

Figure 68b

Figure 68c

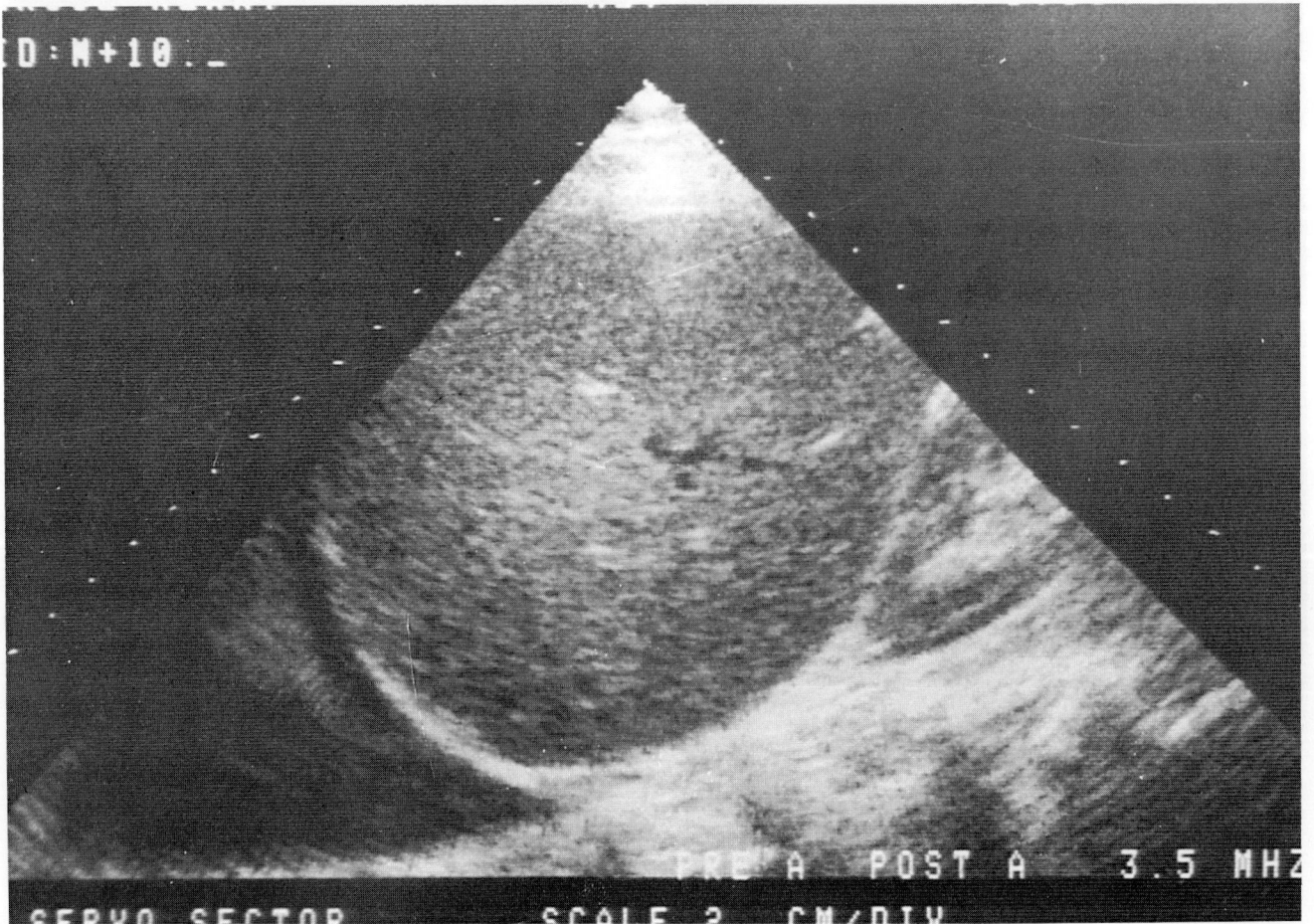

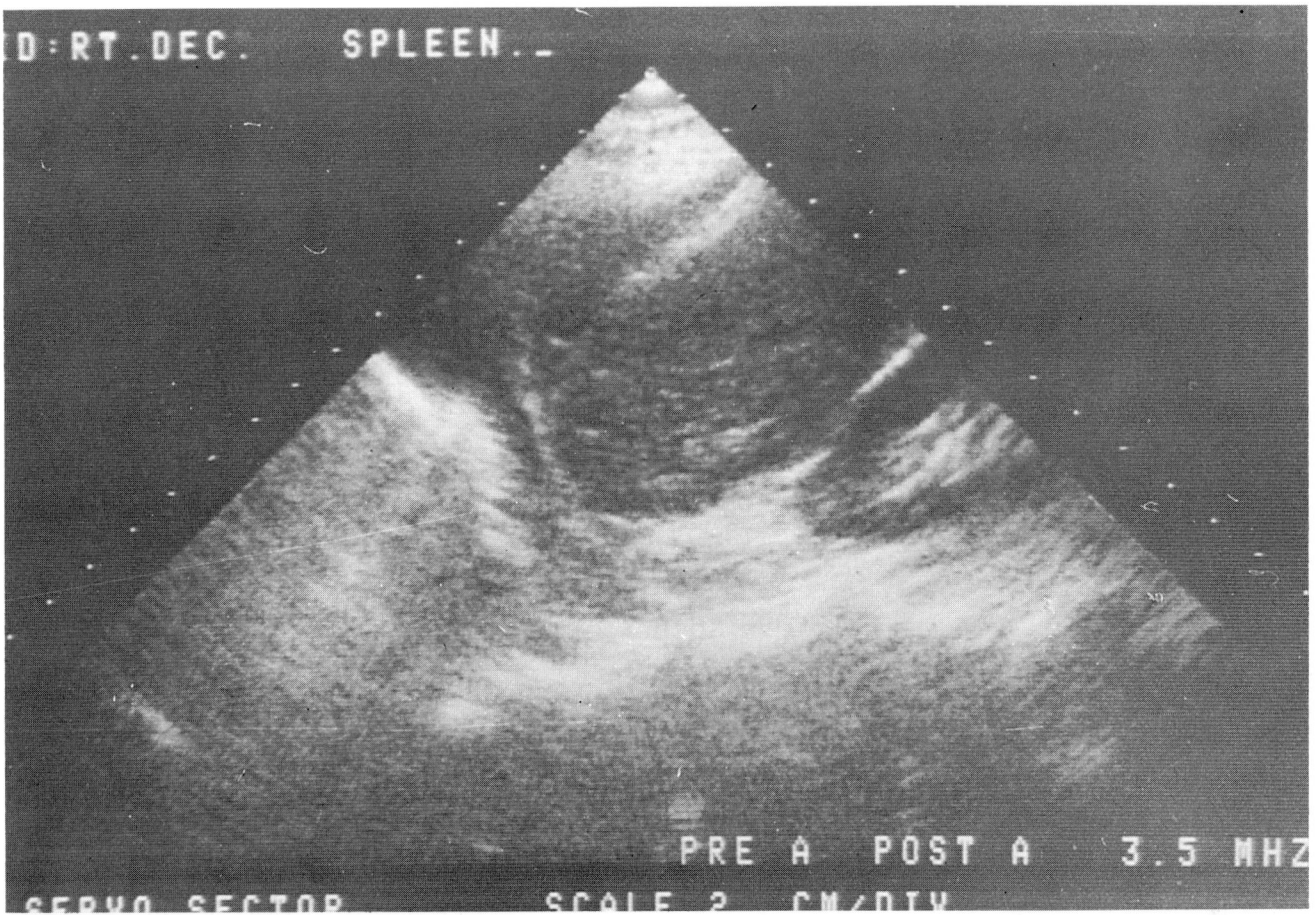

Figure 68d

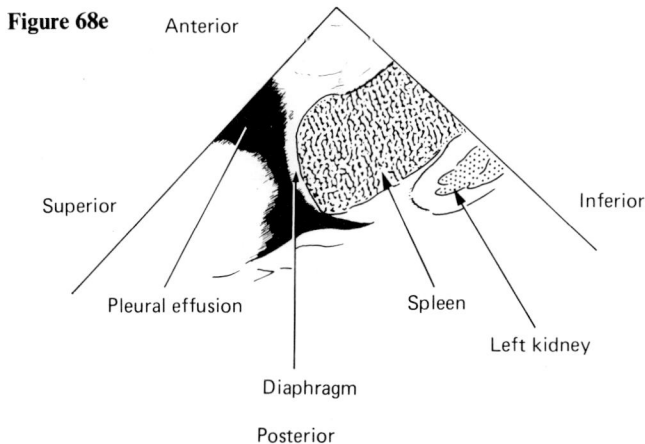

Figure 68e

The patient subsequently underwent laparotomy which confirmed the ultrasound findings that no subphrenic abscess was present. (Oh ye of little faith! Matthew 8:26).

The last three cases demonstrate how it is possible to simulate signs by different conditions. Subpulmonary effusions were demonstrated in all three cases and this is a much more common site for effusion than has previously been recognized. In each case the appearances on the plain film were suggestive of a raised hemidiaphragm and, if suspected at all, only a small pleural effusion was thought to be present.

In the first case there was no mass at the right hilum, the appearances being due to an encysted effusion. Bronchoscopy had been negative. In the second case the appearances of the hilum were almost identical but bronchoscopy revealed a carcinoma. If a patient has a persistent hilar mass, bronchoscopy is mandatory unless a complete explanation is forthcoming. (See also Chapter 12.)

A pleural effusion may present in association with ascites in a number of conditions. In such circumstances the fluid may be clearly demonstrated by ultrasound or by computed tomography.

Case 69

In the figures ascites and pleural effusion are demonstrated by CT and the diaphragm is seen sandwiched between the two collections of fluid.

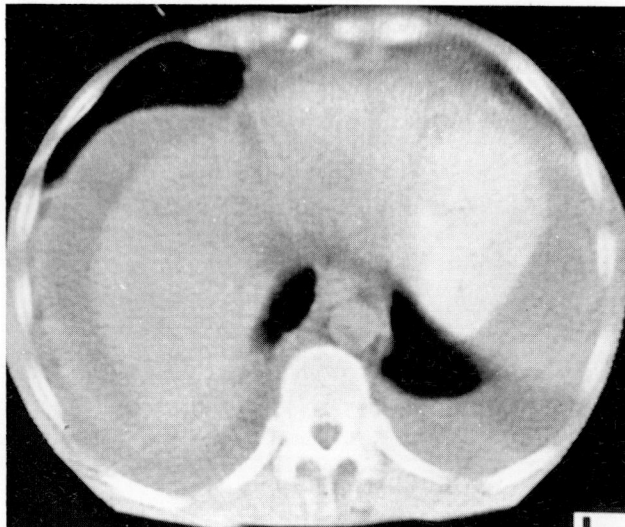

Figure 69a

Figure 69b

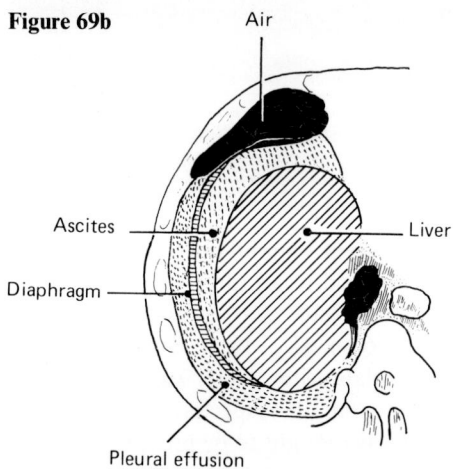

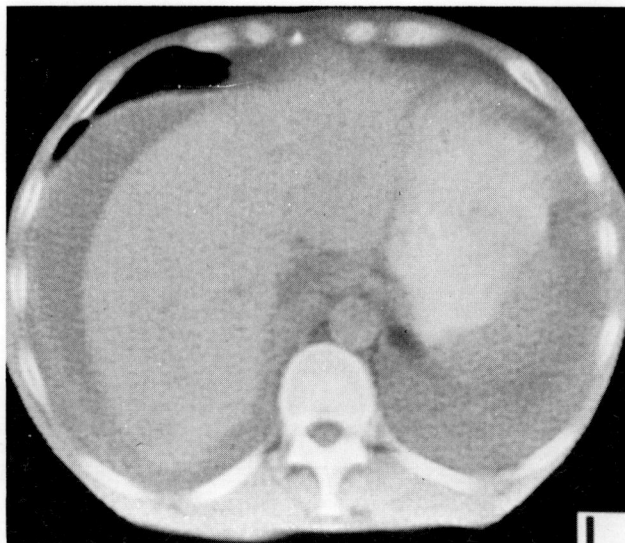

Figure 69c

Figure 69d

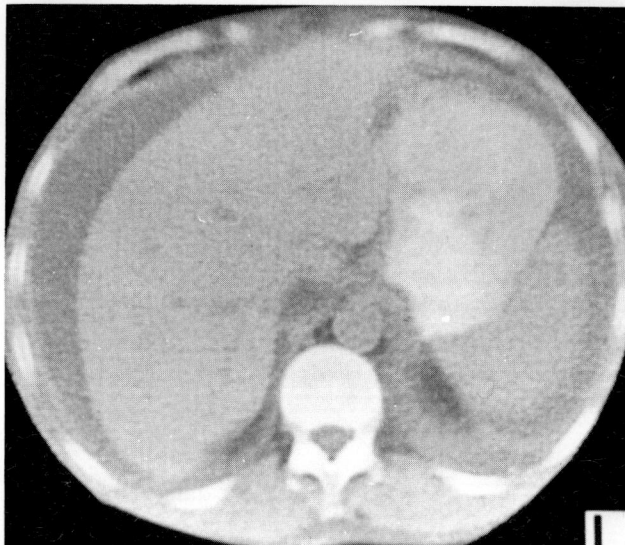

Summary elevation of the diaphragm

The diaphragm may be elevated because it is pulled up by pulmonary abnormality, pushed up by subdiaphragmatic lesions or because it is paralysed. Elevation of the hemidiaphragm may be simulated by subpulmonary effusion, ruptured diaphragm or diaphragmatic hernia.

The pulmonary abnormalities that may cause elevation of the hemidiaphragm have been discussed in previous chapters but include pulmonary collapse, fibrosis and infarction. Subdiaphragmatic abnormalities pushing the diaphragm up, including ascites and subdiaphragmatic masses or abscesses, can be well demonstrated either by ultrasound or CT. Paralysis of the hemidiaphragm can be demonstrated by fluoroscopic screening but ultrasound is another investigation that can be of value, particularly on the right side where the liver can be used as a convenient 'window' for visualizing the diaphragm. Ultrasound may also be useful in showing subpulmonary effusions that simulate a raised hemidiaphragm. Lateral decubitus films and CT may also be used to this end.

11 | Pleural and chest wall lesions

Abnormalities of the pleura and chest wall are often difficult to assess on plain chest radiography. Gross pleural abnormality is usually obvious on chest x-ray but even when there is a large pleural opacity, it may be difficult to distinguish between pleural effusion, empyema, pleural fibrosis and neoplasia.

Films taken of the patient lying on his side using a horizontal beam can be very helpful. Such a radiograph is usually called a 'lateral decubitus' film and the side on which the patient is lying denotes which decubitus film has been taken. Both lateral decubitus films may be needed. This technique is an easy but accurate method of showing a small pleural effusion or a pneumothorax. (See Case 67.)

Ultrasound

Ultrasonography of the chest has proved successful in the evaluation of pleural fluid and pleural masses [61–67]. Ultrasound can demonstrate that a pleural opacity is due to fluid but it is not possible to differentiate between transudation and exudation in the early stages, since both are anechoic and the margin of the lung is well defined. However, by sequential evaluation, it is possible to show changes in inflammatory exudates suggesting fibrosis and thickening of the pleura. Thus, empyema can be identified, being seen as a complex pleural mass containing areas of relatively increased and decreased echogenicity, alternating with thick, coarse-appearing, irregular septa, with no clear demarcation between pulmonary and pleural components [66]. Fibrothorax is a less aggressive result of inflammatory exudation and can be identified as an opacity originating within the pleura with dense fibrosis as an echoic rind around the lung and a trabeculated encysted effusion within. This may progress to become an organized fibrous opacity with a more homogeneous echogenic pattern.

Table 16 Pleural lesions

1 **Transudate**
   (a) cardiac failure
   (b) renal failure
   (c) hypoproteinaemia
   (d) over-transfusion
   (e) fibroma of ovary

2 **Exudate**
   (a) pneumonia
   (b) tuberculosis
   (c) carcinoma of bronchus
   (d) subphrenic abscess, pancreatitis
   (e) pulmonary embolus

3 **Haemorrhage**
   (a) trauma
   (b) infarction
   (c) carcinoma of bronchus

4 **Chyle**
   (a) thoracic duct obstruction (malignancy)
   (b) filariasis
   (c) lymphomatosis
   (d) surgery
   (e) trauma

5 **Pleural plaques and masses**
   (a) asbestos exposure
   (b) haemorrhage
   (c) infection
   (d) rib fracture
   (e) radiation
   (f) scleroderma
   (g) pleural malignancy
   (h) mesothelioma
   (i) adenocarcinoma secondaries
   (j) primary carcinoma of bronchus
   (k) extension from other malignant tumours, e.g. thymoma

Note: In some cases there is a combination of causes of the pleural opacification, e.g. pleural metastases and effusion.

Real-time ultrasound can be useful when draining pleural effusions. Lipscomb, Flower and Hadfield [67] assessed the contribution of ultrasound in the diagnosis and management of patients with pleural disease. The ultrasound was performed with the patients sitting and most examinations were performed at the bedside. In 48 per cent of patients ultrasound was helpful either in clarifying the diagnosis or by aiding aspiration and biopsy. The overall accuracy combining radiology and ultrasound was higher than either modality alone and they concluded that ultrasound should be used more widely in pleural disease to complement plain chest radiography (see also Case 68).

Case 70

A man aged 51 presented with cough and purulent sputum and fever. His symptoms cleared with antibiotics but his chest x-rays are shown in figures 70a and 70b.

Figure 70a

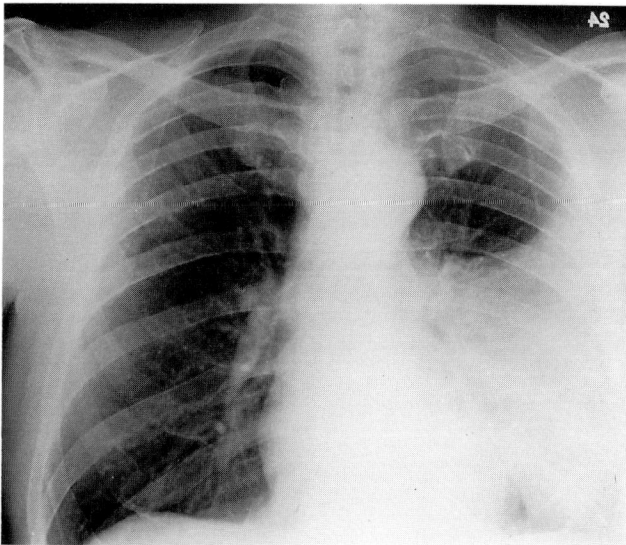

There is opacification of the left mid and lower zones. The lateral film shows that it is anteriorly positioned. Ultrasound at that time showed an area of low echogenicity, i.e. fluid. A needle was introduced into the opacity and a small amount of fluid containing altered blood was withdrawn. On analysis this grew nothing and no malignant cells were demonstrated. CT was next performed and a repeat ultrasound.

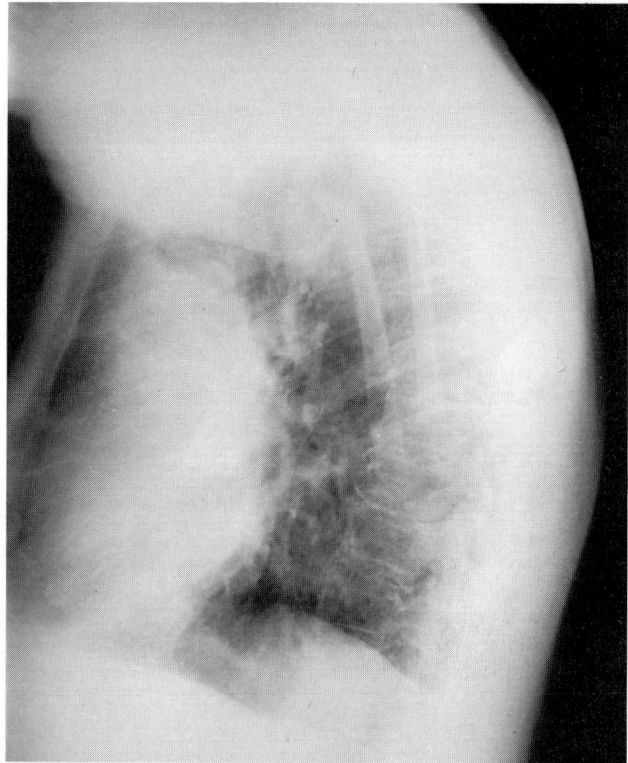

Figure 70b

Figure 70c

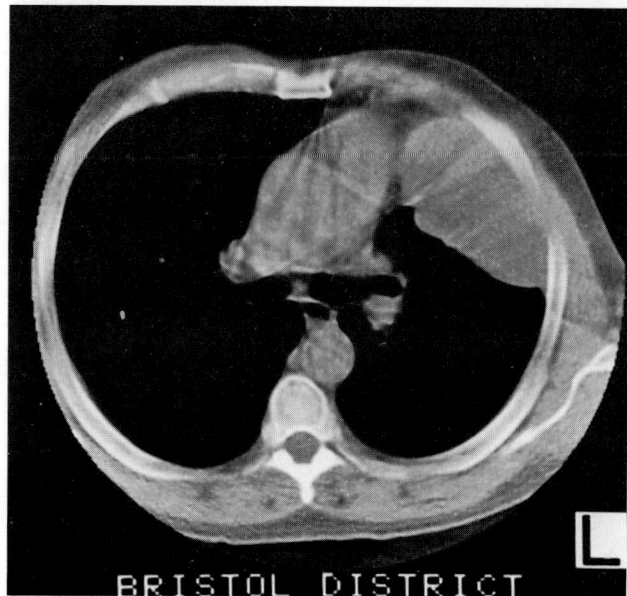

CT showed the lesion to be pleural and it had a well demarcated edge. Ultrasound showed septa running throughout the encysted fluid. The appearances were those of fibrous reaction in an inflammatory effusion (fibrothorax) [66].

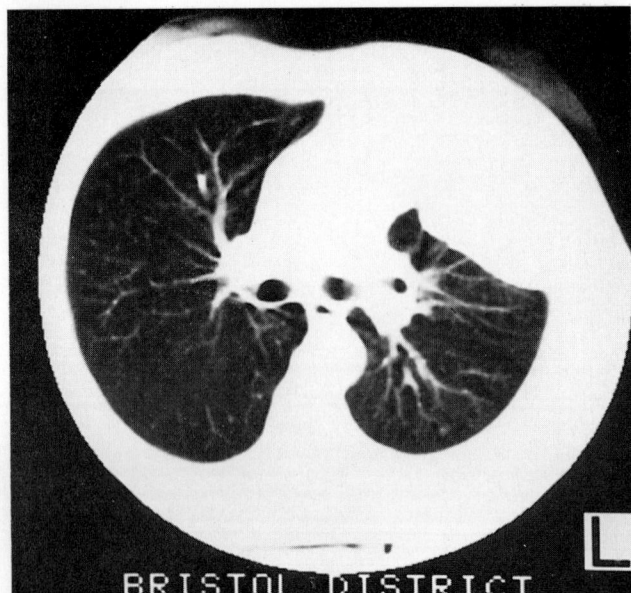

Figure 70d

Figure 70e

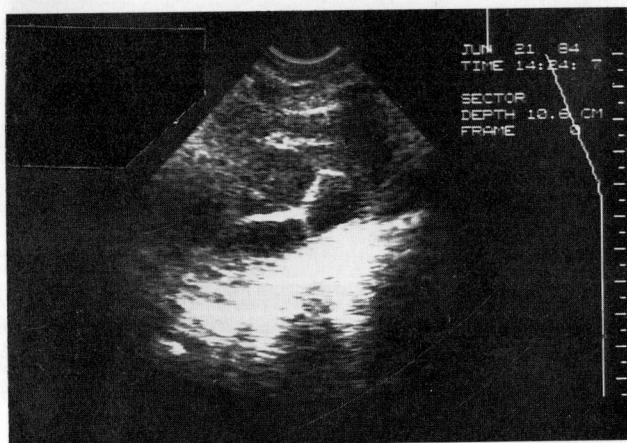

Computed tomography

Computed tomography is probably the best imaging technique for the investigation of the pleura because:

1 CT will reveal minimal abnormalities not seen on plain radiography:
   (a) small pleural plaques
   (b) calcification
   (c) small effusion
   (d) small pneumothorax

2 CT can be used to differentiate between pulmonary, pleural and chest wall lesions.

3 By turning the patient from supine to prone and by careful analysis of the density of structures, it is possible to distinguish between fluid and solid pleural opacities. This is considerably complemented by the use of ultrasound as described earlier.

4 CT is of great value when the radiograph is obscured by pleural thickening. CT enables the underlying lung to be studied. (See Case 27.)

Contrast medium is not usually required when CT is performed to examine the pleura. It may, however, assist in the differentiation between a cyst and a solid mass, demonstrating areas of necrosis within a mass or in identifying a hypervascular abscess wall. Occasionally the insertion of a little air into the pleural cavity when performing CT permits further information regarding the site and nature of a pleural mass to be obtained.

Case 71

A 76 year old lady with maturity onset diabetes was found to have considerable abnormalities on her chest x-ray with no obvious cause. No previous films were available. Over a period of some months she had developed increasing right-sided chest pain.

The chest x-ray showed loss of volume in the right hemithorax and pleural opacification.

Figure 71a

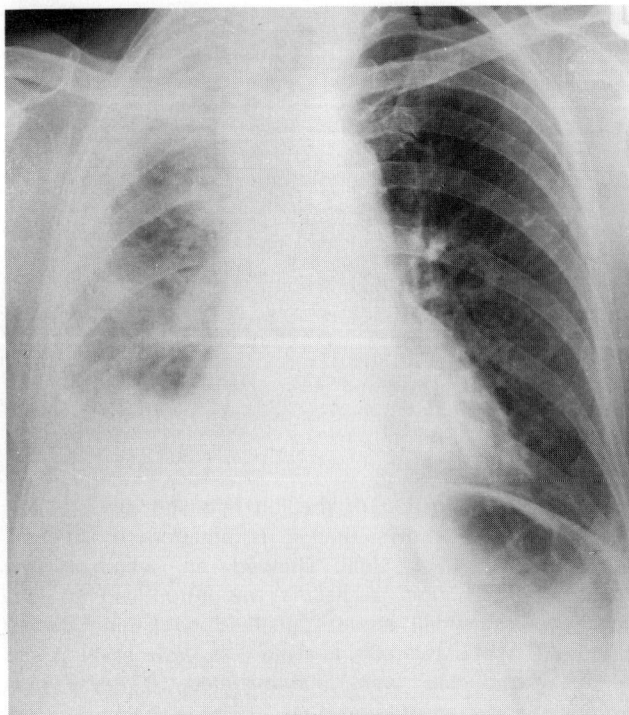

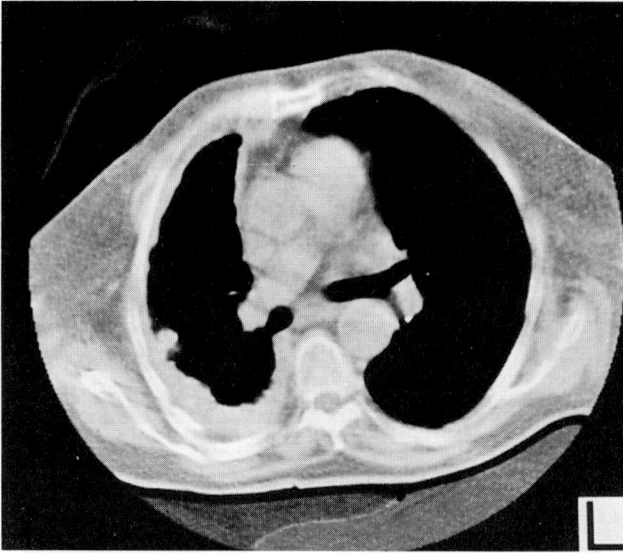

Figure 71b

CT scans showed lobulated pleural opacification which was of soft tissue density, circumferential and did not shift when the patient was scanned in the prone position (fig. 71c). The features were considered to represent pleural malignancy—possibly a mesothelioma—although there was no history of asbestos exposure.

Figure 71c

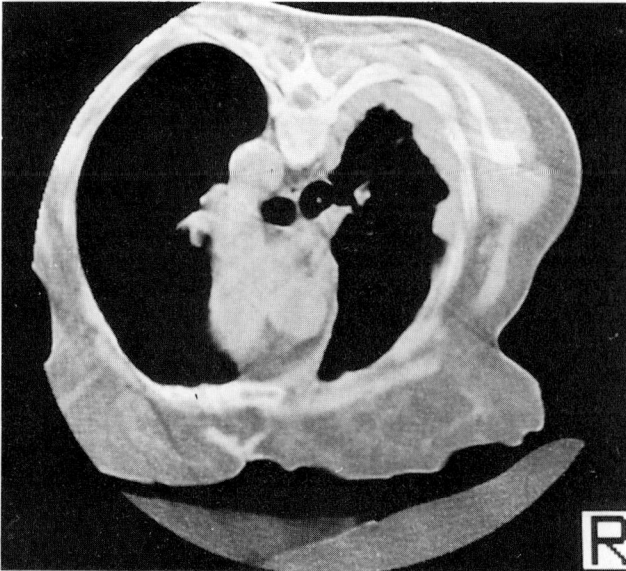

To help with further management a percutaneous needle biopsy of the pleura was performed under local anaesthetic. This showed adenocarcinoma.

As discussed previously (Chapter 8), the features of adenocarcinoma involving the pleura and mesothelioma can be impossible to distinguish radiologically.

Biopsy

Fluoroscopy, ultrasound and CT are all of assistance when biopsy of a pleural mass is contemplated. With pleural masses biopsy can be undertaken using a larger cutting needle than is the case for intrapulmonary lesions since the risk of pneumothorax is much less. Thus it may be possible to obtain a tissue core for histology as well as smears for cytology.

If needle biopsy is not successful, it is sensible to consider 'thoracoscopy'. This is a technique that is gaining popularity in Great Britain. Either a rigid or a flexible endoscope is passed through a small incision into the pleural cavity. Under direct vision it is then possible to biopsy areas of pleural thickening or masses. This technique may be more difficult to undertake if there have been repeated attempts at pleural biopsy or tapping of effusion.

Thoracotomy is considered by some to be the best method of obtaining a pleural biopsy. Certainly thoracotomy will enable the largest possible specimen to be obtained but there may be considerable morbidity.

The best method of biopsy will vary from patient to patient depending on factors such as the size of lesion, the severity of symptoms and the general condition of the patient.

Case 72

A woman aged 69 presented with severe chest pain and a tender swelling on the anterior chest wall.

Figure 72a

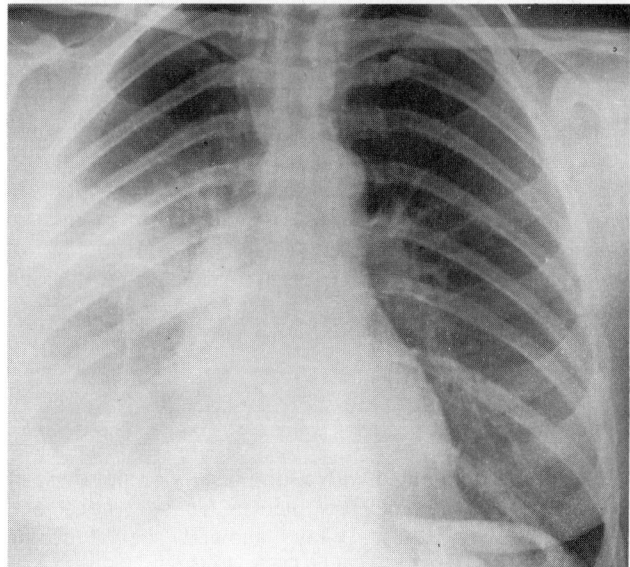

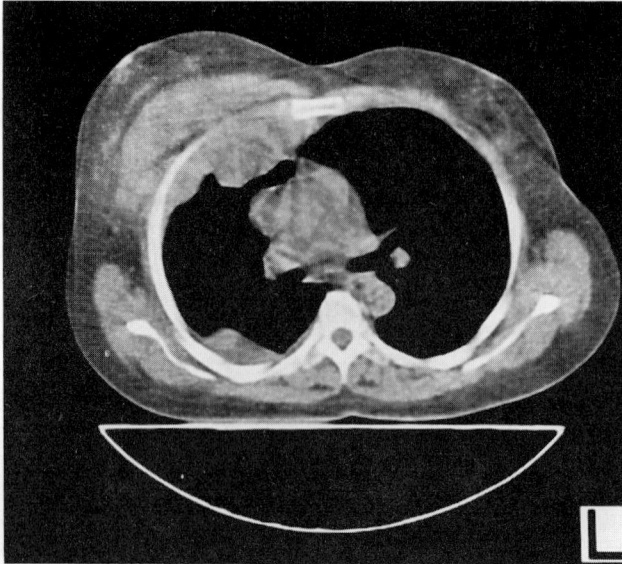

Figure 72b

Figure 72c

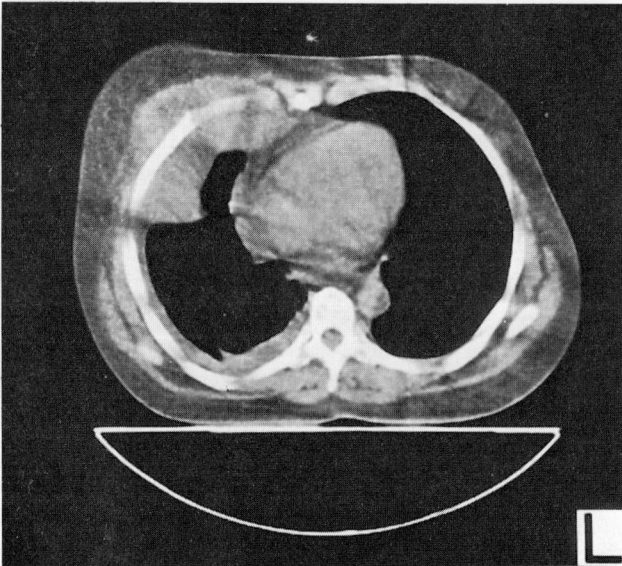

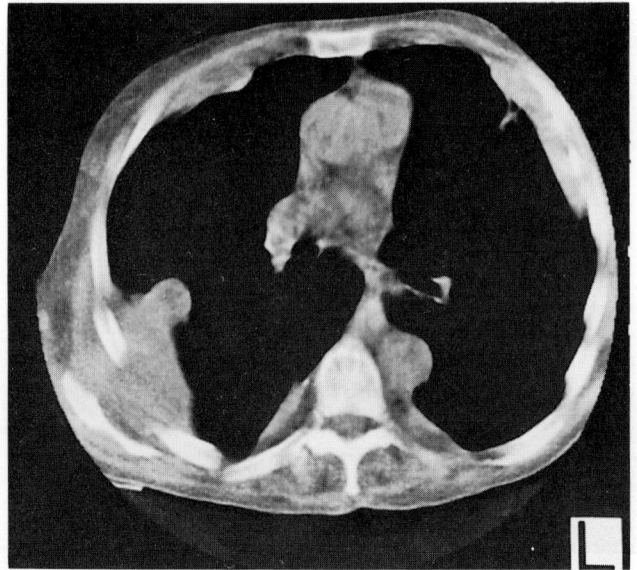

Figure 73a

Figure 73b

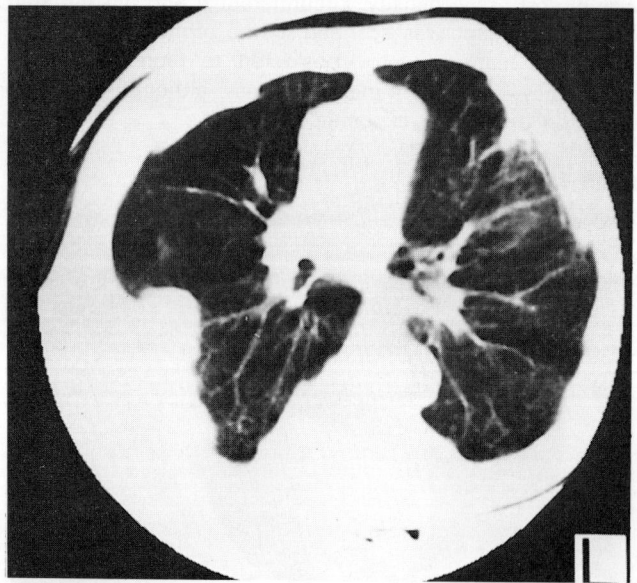

The chest x-ray showed opacification in the right mid and lower zone. CT showed circumferential nodular pleural thickening with extension anteriorly through the chest wall into the subcutaneous tissues. Histological diagnosis of mesothelioma was obtained. There was no history of asbestos exposure and no pleural thickening in the left lung.

Case 73

A dock worker presented with a long history or shortness of breath and a short history of pain in his right chest and right shoulder. Chest x-ray showed hazy pleural opacification in both lung fields. CT is shown.

CT showed pleural plaques bilaterally some of which had fat between the chest wall and the plaque and were calcified between the plaque and the lung tissue. Further pleural fibrosis and pulmonary fibrosis were present. A large mass was present in the right posterolateral region extending through the chest wall and invading behind the scapula. A diagnosis of mesothelioma was made histologically.

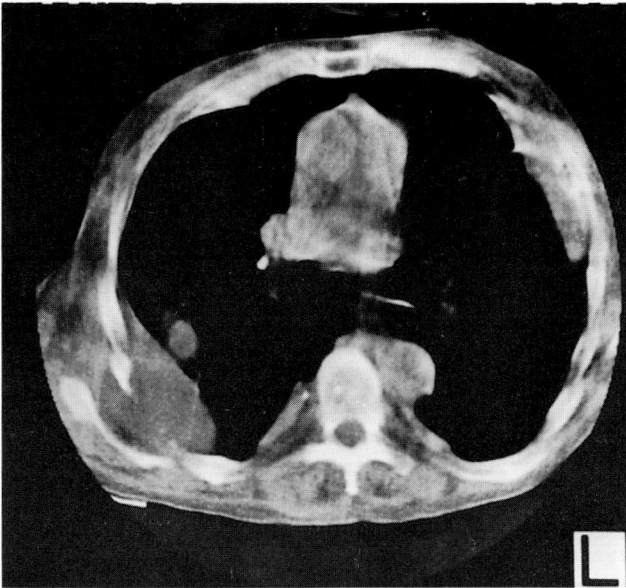

Figure 73c

Figure 73d

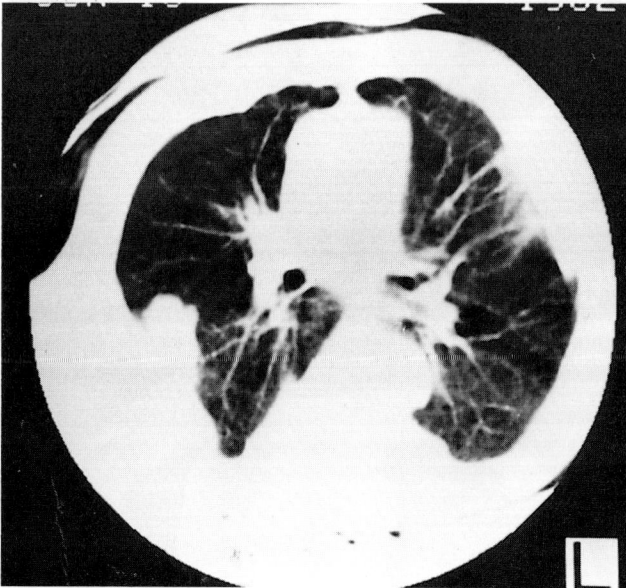

The investigation of asbestos exposure

Asbestos exposure can result in a number of thoracic manifestations. The most important of these include pulmonary fibrosis, pleural plaques and calcification, pleural mesothelioma and carcinoma of the bronchus.

The pleural and pulmonary lesions can be difficult to assess from the plain chest films and further information can be obtained by respiratory function studies and by computed tomography. If there is pulmonary fibrosis, this may result in impaired gas transfer and decreased lung volume.

Features of asbestos exposure shown by CT include:

1 Pleural plaques (often with typical features of layers of fat, fibrosis and calcification).

2 Pulmonary opacification and distortion of vessels due to fibrosis and a sub-pleural line of fibrosis [7].

3 Pleural masses and pulmonary masses due to carcinoma or mesothelioma.

Case 74

A patient with long-term exposure to asbestos presented with the following chest x-ray and CT appearances.

There are multiple calcified pleural plaques in both lung fields. The calcification over the hemidiaphragm which is arrowed is a characteristic appearance of asbestos exposure but does not occur in the majority of the patients.

Figure 74a

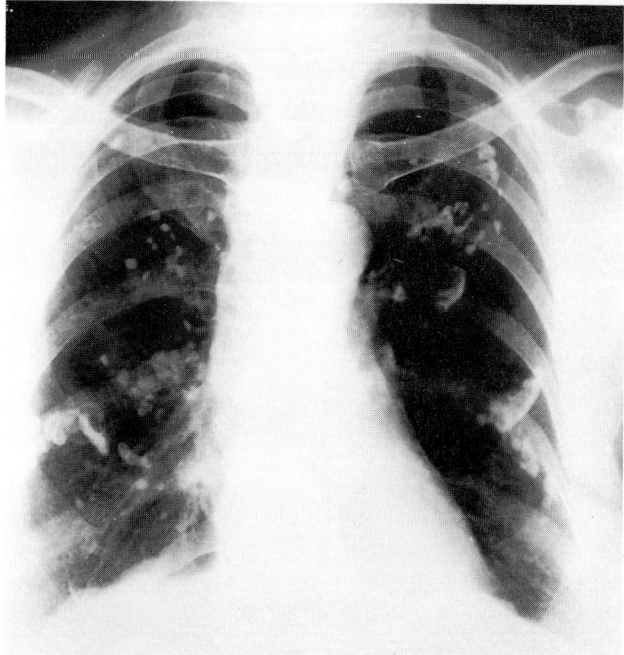

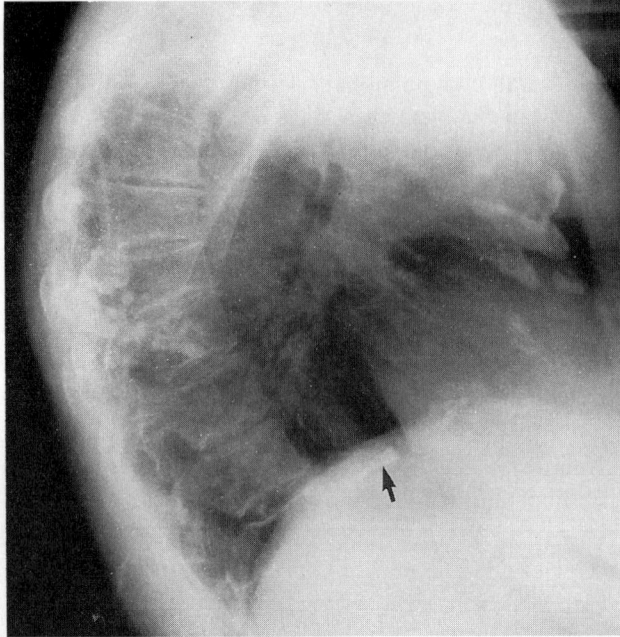

Figure 74b

Figure 74c

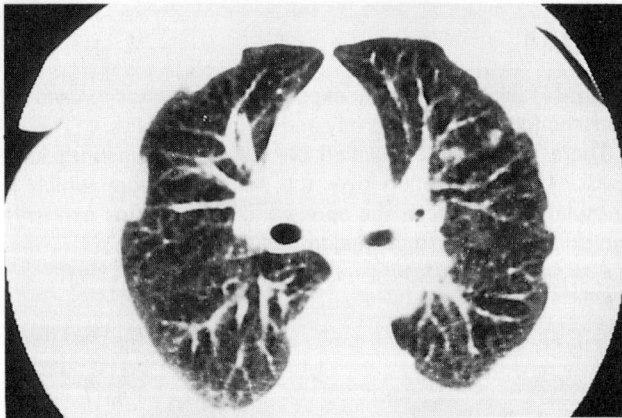

Figure 74d

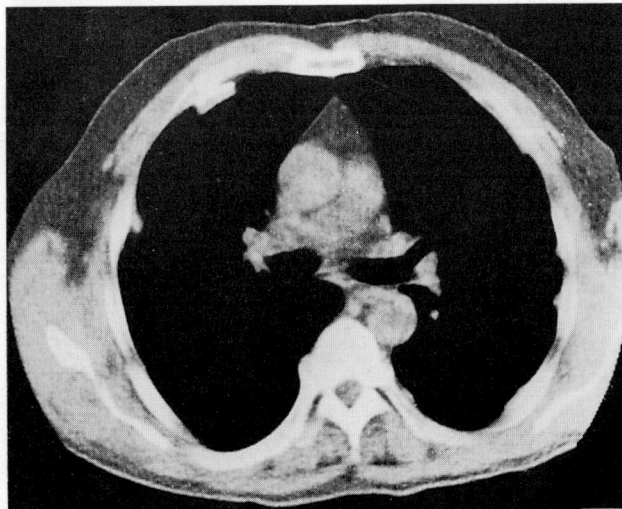

Two further examples of the pulmonary and pleural changes due to asbestos exposure are shown.

Cases 75 and 76

In each of these cases there are multiple pleural plaques. In addition there is a subpleural line which in Case 76, figure 76b has been arrowed. This subpleural line probably represents pulmonary fibrosis. In Case 75 there is distortion of vessels and considerable pulmonary fibrosis.

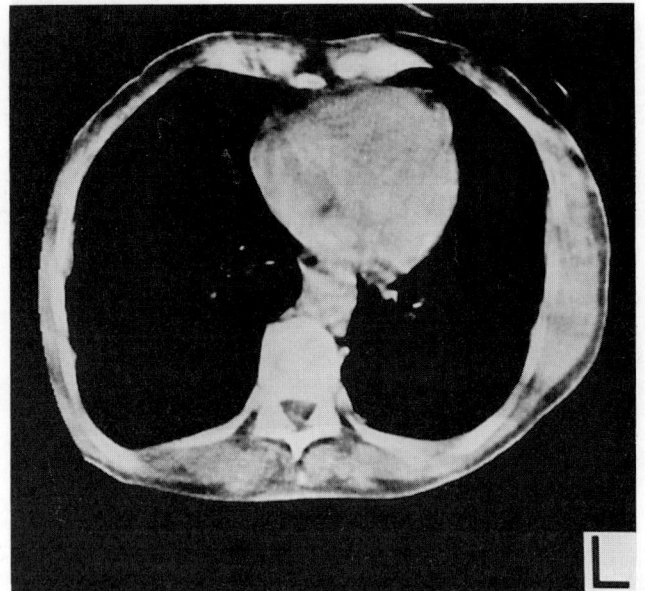

Figure 75a

Figure 75b

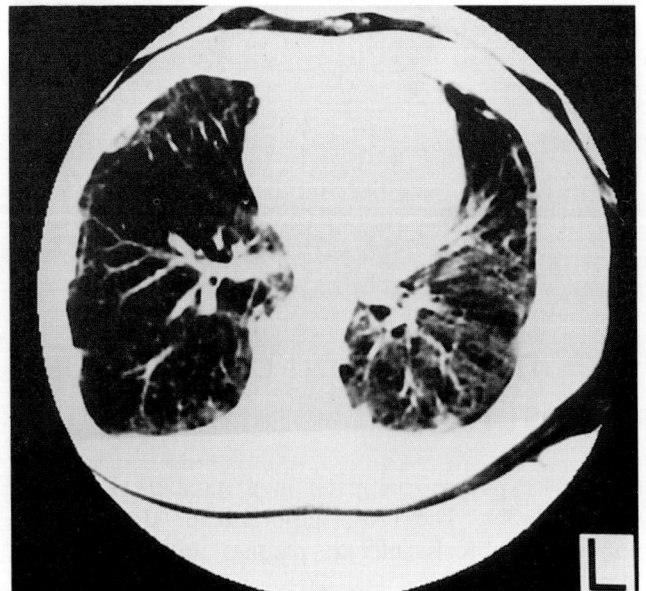

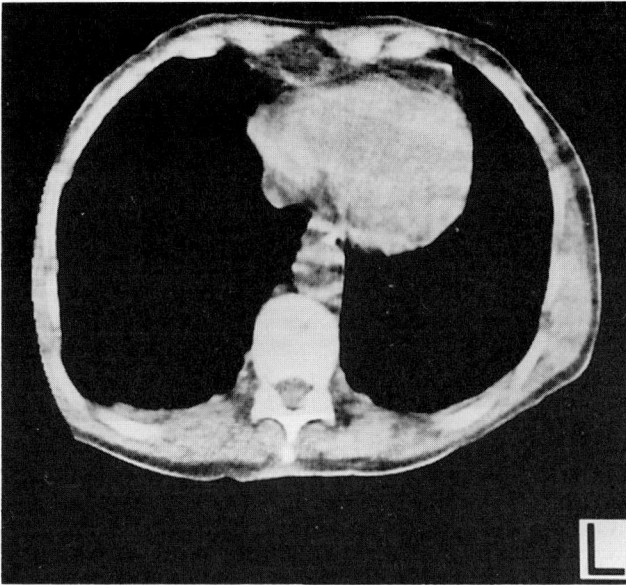

Figure 75c

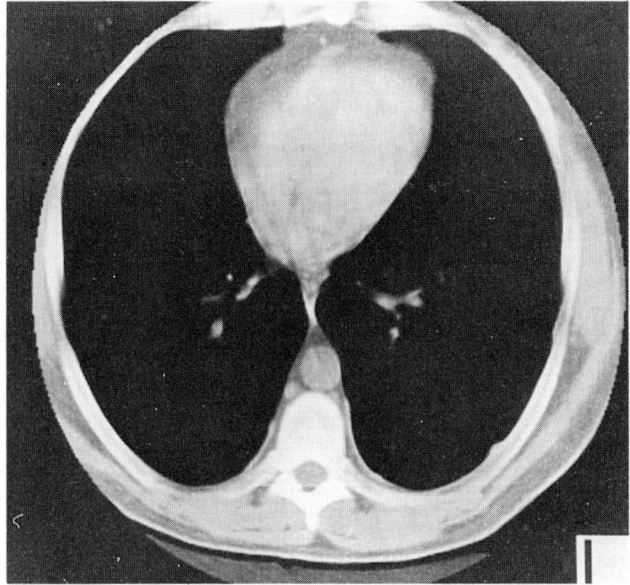

Figure 76a

Figure 75d

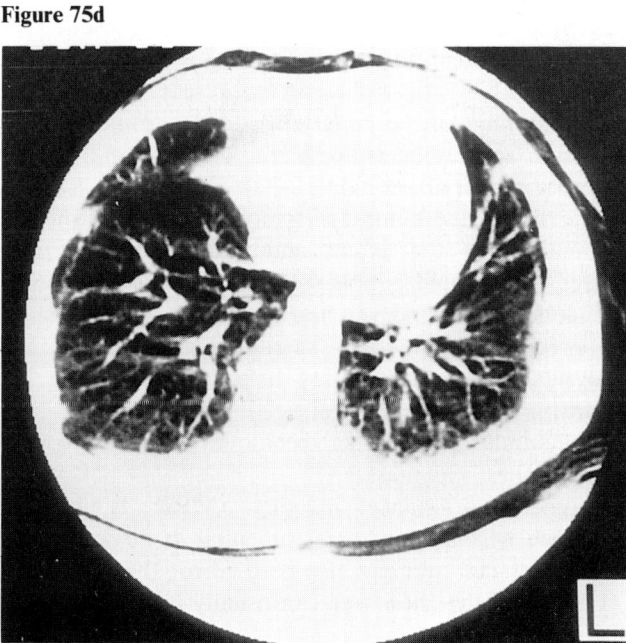

Figure 76b

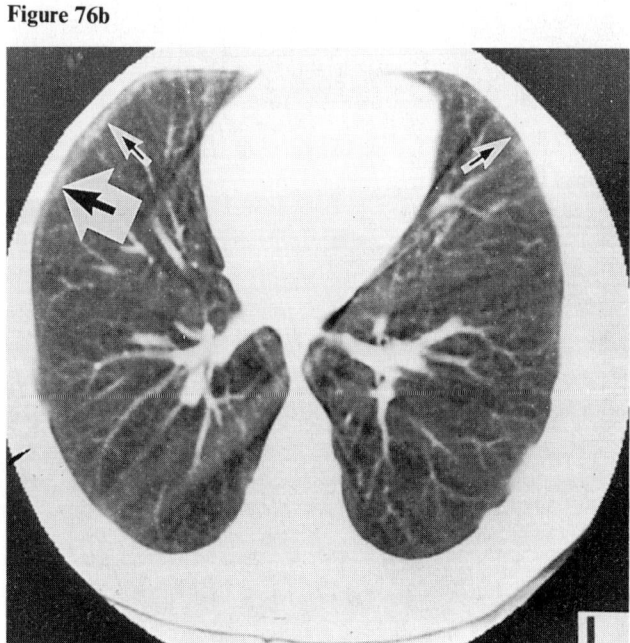

Case 77

A 32 year old man with a history of teratoma had the following CT scans.

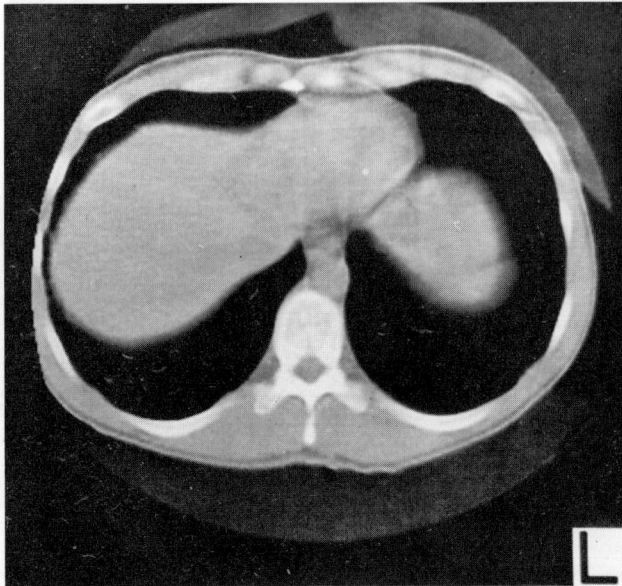

Figure 77a

Figure 77b

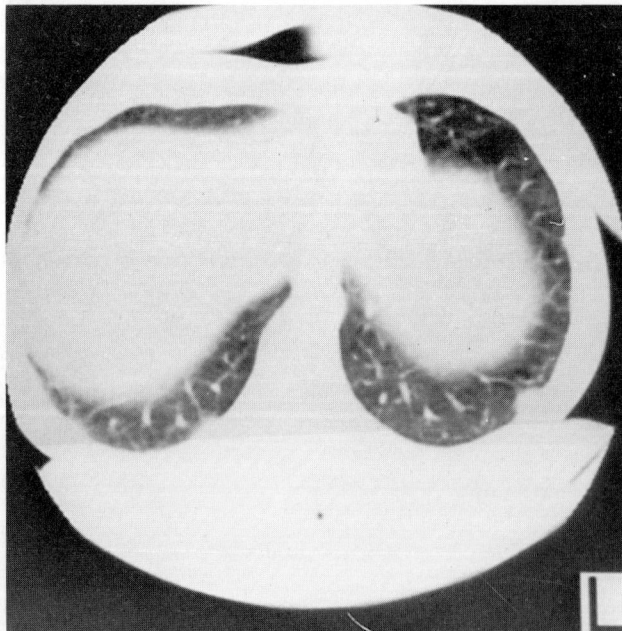

There are small bilateral pleural opacities. These are similar in appearance to pleural plaques, although there is no evidence of calcification or fat beneath the lesions. In addition to these pleural opacities the CT scans of the upper and mid thorax showed multiple pulmonary metastases. These lesions represented metastatic deposits from the teratoma.

This case demonstrates the fact that any one sign shown radiologically can be due to a variety of causes. It is only when several signs can be pieced together like a jigsaw to make up a complete picture that the results can be pathognomonic of any particular diagnosis. See also Case 102, Chapter 13.

Chest wall lesions

Chest wall lesions may involve the ribs, intercostal structures or overlying soft tissues. Common chest wall lesions include soft tissue tumours (such as lipoma), secondary deposits in ribs, and neurofibroma. All such lesions may result in opacities visible on plain chest films. Examination of the patient will often reveal a swelling at the site of a chest wall mass and oblique or tangential films may help in distinguishing whether or not there is involvement of ribs and any intrathoracic extension. If a lytic rib lesion is present, scintigraphic bone scanning can be undertaken to determine whether the lesion actively takes up the radioisotope and if there are other similar abnormalities.

Ultrasound and computed tomography are also useful in determining the extent and nature of chest wall masses. Ultrasound is able to distinguish between solid, semi-solid, cystic and vascular structures. CT will show the precise anatomy and surrounding structures and analysis of the density may help in determining the nature of the lesion. Thermography and transillumination are other techniques that can be used to assess chest wall masses.

Magnetic resonance imaging (MRI) is a new technique which shows great potential in distinguishing between tissues, and can also be used for the chest wall.

Lesions of the chest wall can usually be biopsied with ease either by needle biopsy or excision.

Case 78 (*Courtesy of Dr Grayson of Derriford Hospital*)

Peter, aged 18, presented with left subcostal pain. A retroperitoneal mass was found at operation arising from an intercostal nerve. Further investigation included a chest x-ray and CT scan.

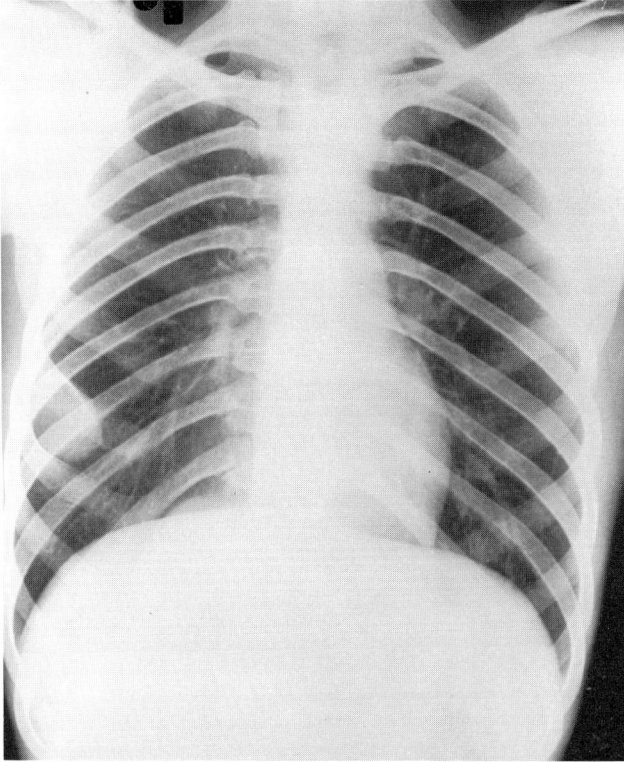

Figure 78a

On the chest radiograph, there are two opacities in the right hemithorax, one adjacent to the right lateral chest wall and one just visible situated in the right cardiophrenic angle. The opacity adjacent to the chest wall has a well-defined medial border but the lateral margins merge with the chest wall and cannot be clearly distinguished. This is a sign of a pleurally based or chest wall lesion rather than an intrapulmonary mass. On the CT scans, the lower lesion is situated in the posterior costophrenic recess involving the crus of the diaphragm and extending from the intervertebral foramen at the T10 level. The laterally placed lesion can be seen to lie in the chest wall and to bulge into the chest

Figure 78b

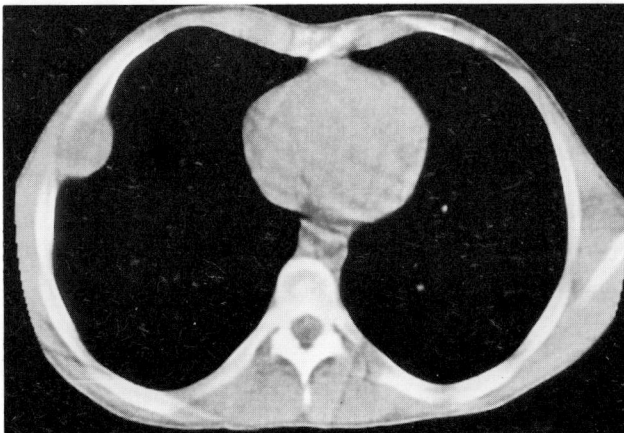

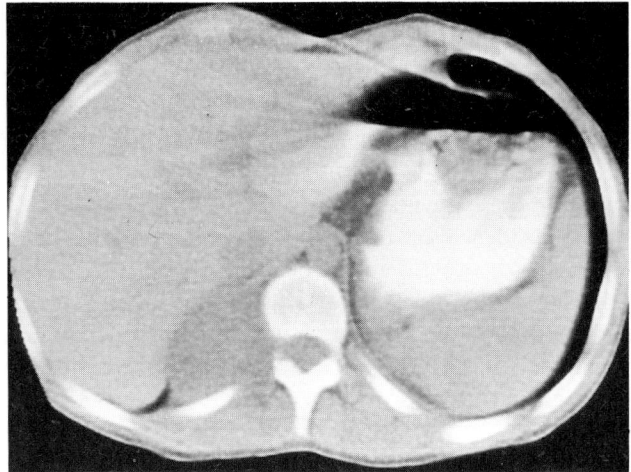

Figure 78c

rather than arise from it. The appearance of masses in these sites is consistent with multiple neurofibromata.

A spinal radiculogram was performed to assess whether there was any evidence of intraspinal extension, even though there were no neurological symptoms or signs. This revealed an intradural extramedullary filling defect at the T9-T10 level posteriorly and slightly to the right.

Neurofibromatosis, van Recklinghausen's disease (eponymously described in 1882 by the Professor of Pathology in Strasbourg) is inherited as a Mendelian dominant and is characterized by both skin and neural lesions.

The skin lesions include a diffuse increased pigmentation, café-au-lait spots, generalized freckling and cutaneous tumours. The neural component of the disease involves peripheral, spinal and cranial nerves which may be diffusely or nodularly thickened. Tumours of the neurilemmal sheaths of the peripheral nerves or nerve roots may occur. The spinal nerve tumours may grow inwards through the intervertebral foramen or outwards producing a paraspinal mass and the classical dumb-bell tumour.

Up to 50 per cent of people with neurofibromatosis have intracranial tumours. Bilateral acoustic neuromas are said to be pathognomonic of the disease. Other tumours include optic nerve gliomas, optic nerve sheath meningiomas, pontine gliomas and intracranial meningiomas [68].

There are other manifestations of the disease which may be seen radiologically. In the chest these include narrow deformed ribs known as 'ribbon ribs' and posterior mediastinal neural or intercostal tumours. The latter may cause inferior rib notching. There is also a higher incidence of anterior thoracic meningocele in this condition. Other abnormalities may affect the skull, spine and limbs.

One-third of the cases of neurofibromatosis are found incidentally on routine examination with no patient symptomatology, one-third are seen seeking medical advice regarding the cosmetic aspects of the disease and one-third present with neurological symptoms.

The incidence of malignant sarcomatous change is reported as between 5 and 12 per cent.

Treatment is directed towards lesions which enlarge and may therefore be undergoing sarcomatous change. Treatment is also required for spinal decompression when there are neurological signs related to a nerve tumour.

Case 79

A man aged 57, a heavy smoker with a past history of haemoptysis, had a plain chest radiograph on which a rounded mass was seen superimposed on the heart shadow (*arrowed*). This could not be identified on the lateral film.

Figure 79a

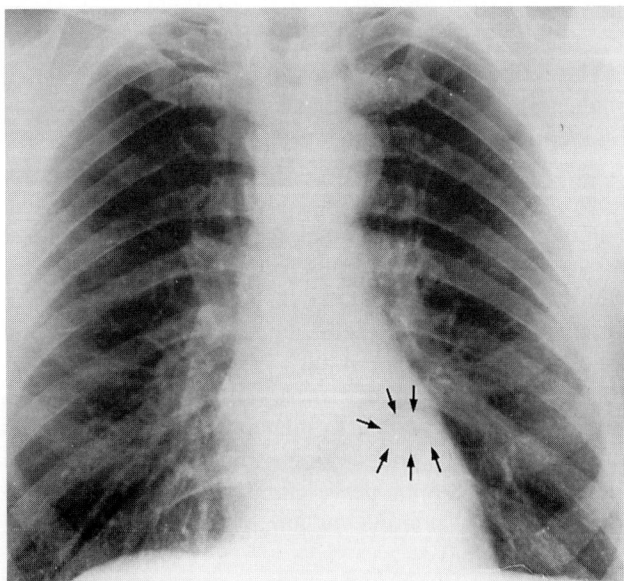

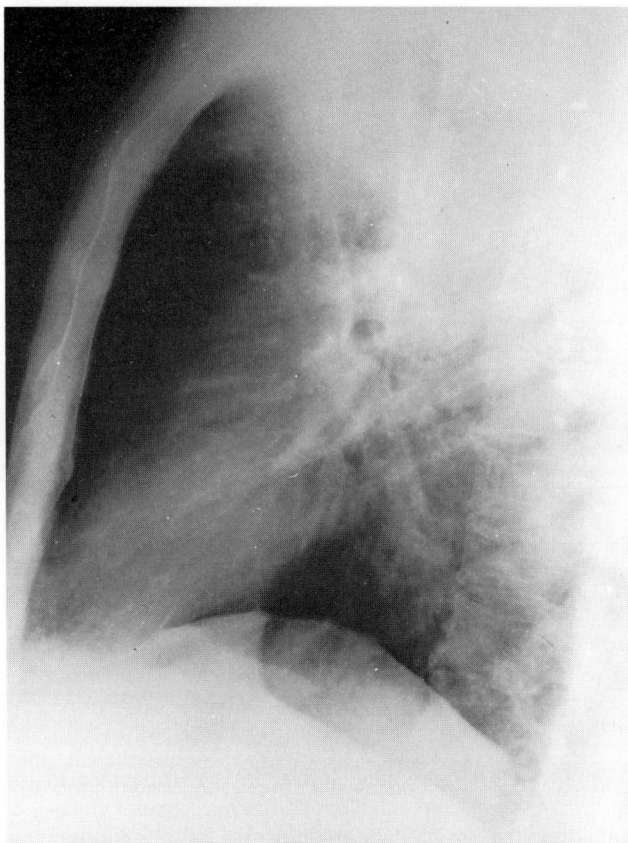

Figure 79b

Figure 79c

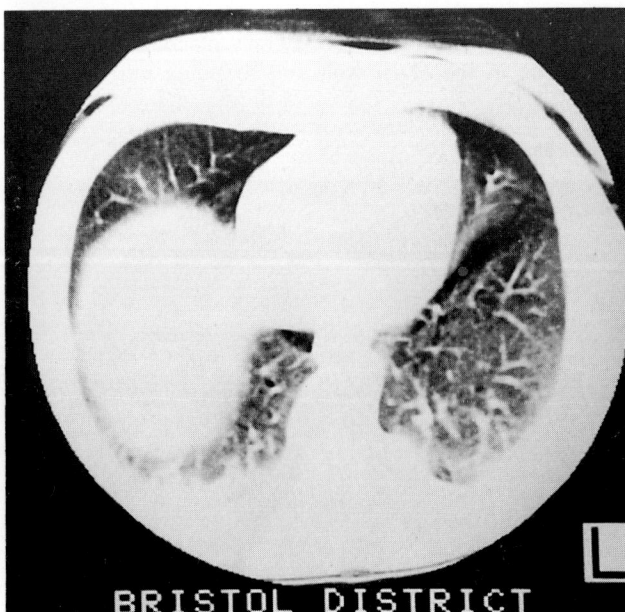

Hilar tomography failed to show the opacity. CT was performed (figs. 79c and 79d). This showed no abnormality in the left lung field but there was expansion of the head of a left rib. Conclusion: benign cartilage tumour of the head of a rib.

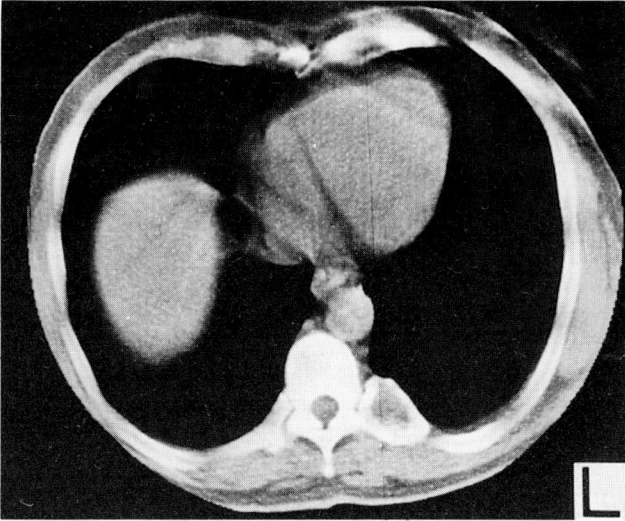

Figure 79d

Case 80

A patient had the following appearances on a chest x-ray.

There is a large mass projected over the left hemithorax and the left border of the heart. The lower margins are seen well but the upper margin is incomplete. If there is an incomplete upper border, it is important to consider whether or not the lesion is outside the chest. The patient should be physically examined. In this case the oblique view showed a pedunculated lipoma of the chest wall. If the patient is examined carefully, chest wall lesions such as lipoma and fibroma should be easily detected by inspection.

Figure 80a

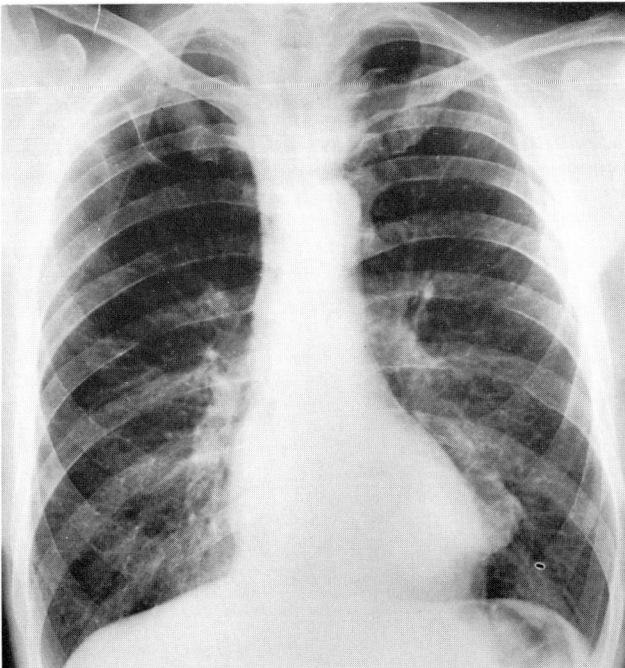

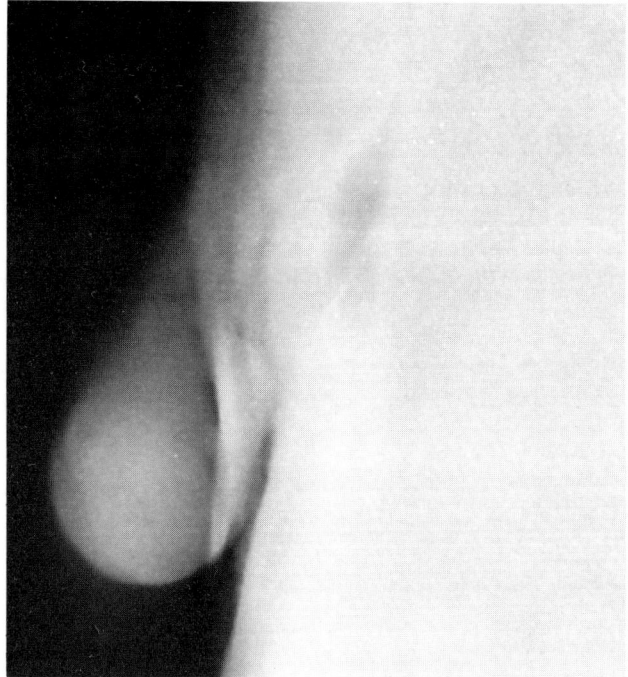

Figure 80b

Case 81

Magnetic resonance images of the chest from an Elscint machine showing a mass in the posterior chest wall with parameters of fat. Conclusion: lipoma. Good differentiation of muscle, fat, great vessels and bone are seen but the lung fields are only poorly visualized with magnetic resonance due to the low density of tissue and the intrinsic lack of protons from which to obtain images.

Figure 81

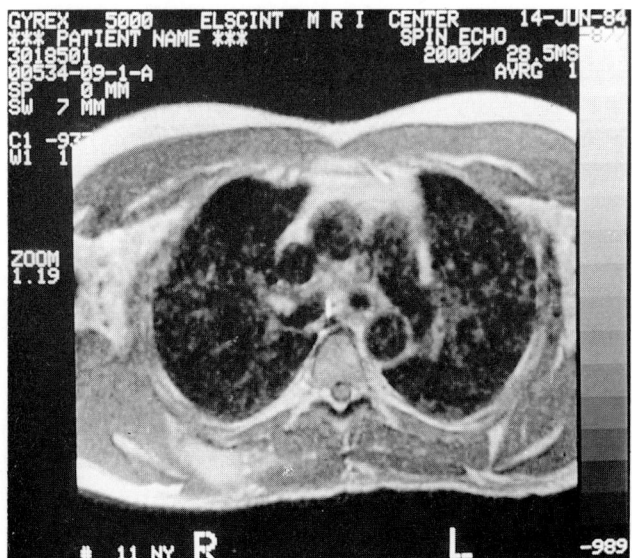

Case 82

Magnetic resonance imaging of the chest wall showing a view of a woman's chest after mastectomy for carcinoma of the breast and subsequent implantation of a silicon prosthesis. (TR = 2000, MST = 28 ms, Elscint.)

Figure 82

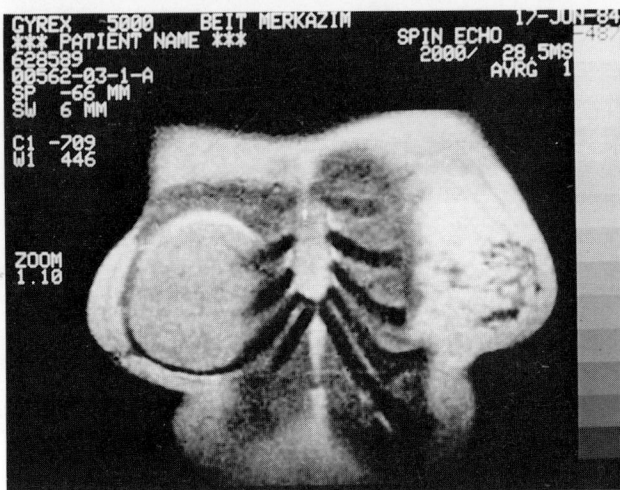

Summary: pleural and chest wall lesions

Whilst gross pleural abnormality is usually obvious on chest x-ray, subtle abnormalities may not be visible on plain chest radiography. In addition it may be difficult to distinguish between pleural and pulmonary lesions.

Investigations that can be of assistance include lateral decubitus films, ultrasound and computed tomography. Ultrasound will reveal whether an abnormality is of a solid nature or fluid. It can therefore be particularly helpful in assessing pleural effusion.

Computed tomography is the best imaging technique for the investigation of the pleura and is able to reveal minimal abnormalities not seen on plain radiography and to differentiate between pulmonary, pleural and chest wall lesions.

Biopsy of pleural lesions can be performed by percutaneous needle biopsy, by thoracoscopy (endoscopic examination of the pleural cavity) or by open biopsy.

Chest wall lesions are usually palpable on physical examination. Ultrasound and CT may again be useful in determination of the exact extent, site and consistency of the mass. Newer techniques such as magnetic resonance may have a role in the investigation of chest wall and pleural lesions.

12 Hilar enlargement

When prominence of the hila is detected on a chest radiograph a number of questions are posed. The first problem is to decide whether the enlargement is in fact at the hilum or is anterior or posterior to the hilum. Enlargement of the hila can be simulated by masses anterior or posterior to the hilum and these can, of course, be due to any of the causes of a pulmonary mass. Close inspection of the PA film is, of course, vital and, if the hilar vessels can be seen through the shadow of the opacity, it is clear that the mass is not actually at the hilum, but superimposed by projection. This can sometimes be decided from the lateral film, but often tomography is necessary. If the exact site of the lesion is not known, then it may be useful to perform lateral tomography first, followed by AP tomography. An alternative form of tomography is computed tomography and this is being used more commonly as the facility becomes available.

The next important question is whether or not the abnormality is a mass or whether it is an enlarged vascular structure, for example, the pulmonary arteries. This can also be determined by tomography, although for definitive differentiation, CT, angiography or digital vascular imaging may be necessary.

It is important to determine whether there is bilateral or unilateral hilar enlargement since this will profoundly affect the choice of diagnostic tests. If the mass is unilateral in a British adult, by far the most common cause is bronchogenic carcinoma but worldwide, tuberculosis is probably more common (see also Case 25). If the latter is likely, a Heaf test or a Mantoux are indicated. Sputum should be sent for culture and microscopy performed. Acid-fast bacilli should be looked for and cytology undertaken for malignant cells. If these tests are negative and the hilar mass is still present, bronchoscopy is almost mandatory.

Computed tomography is undertaken in many centres as a staging procedure for carcinoma of the bronchus. It will show whether or not there is enlargement of hilar or mediastinal lymph nodes. If the nodes are very large and seen to invade mediastinal structures, it is possible to infer, with considerable certainty, that the lymph nodes are involved with metastatic spread. If, however, the nodes are only slightly enlarged (say 1.5 to 2.5 cm) they may be large due to reactive changes. Thus a biopsy of the mediastinal or hilar nodes may be necessary and the demonstration of enlarged nodes, particularly in the hilum, does not necessarily imply that the carcinoma is inoperable. Staging of bronchial carcinoma is discussed in greater detail in Chapter 2 and mediastinal lymph nodes are discussed in Chapter 13.

Table 17   Hilar enlargement

Unilateral hilar enlargement
Common causes

1   Carcinoma of the bronchus (primary carcinoma or metastatic node enlargement)
2   Tuberculosis (in USA also fungal especially histoplasmosis and coccidioidomycosis)
3   Post-stenotic dilatation of the left pulmonary artery in pulmonary valvular stenosis
4   Simulated, i.e. pulmonary mass adjacent to, or superimposed on, the hilum

Bilateral hilar enlargement
Common causes

1   Sarcoidosis
2   Lymphoma and leukaemia
3   Bilateral pulmonary artery enlargement (pulmonary hypertension and shunts)
4   (Left heart failure)

Less common causes of unilateral or bilateral hilar enlargement

1   Pneumoconiosis (e.g. silicosis, berylliosis)
2   Viral disease (e.g. infectious mononucleosis)
3   Brucellosis

Note: Most of the causes of unilateral hilar enlargement can also less commonly cause bilateral enlargement (and vice versa).

Case 83

A man of 72 presented with a knobbly mass at the lower pole of the right hilum.

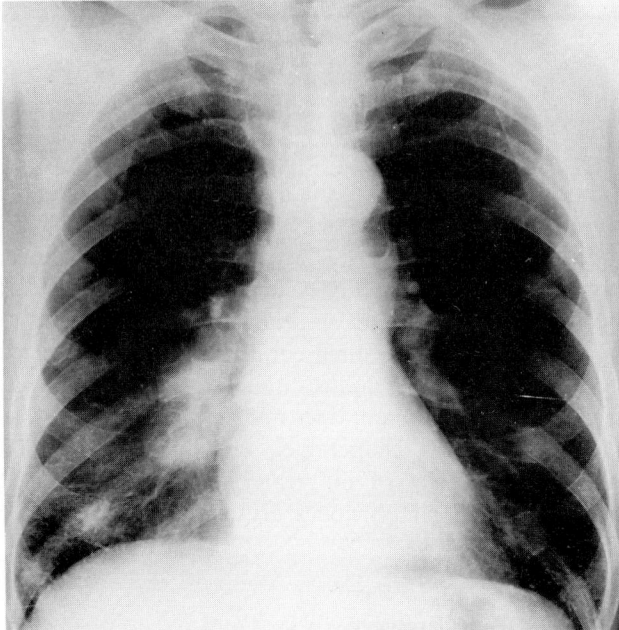

Figure 83a

Figure 83b

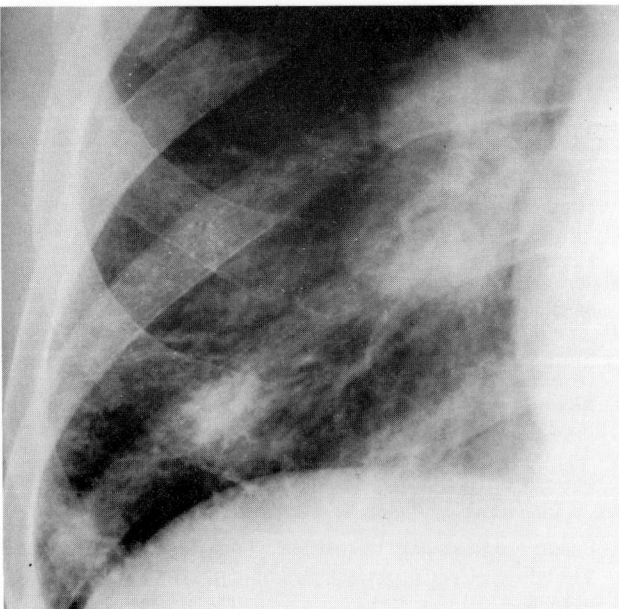

The chest x-ray also shows patchy opacification lateral to the mass and a few septal lines. Further investigation included computed tomography.

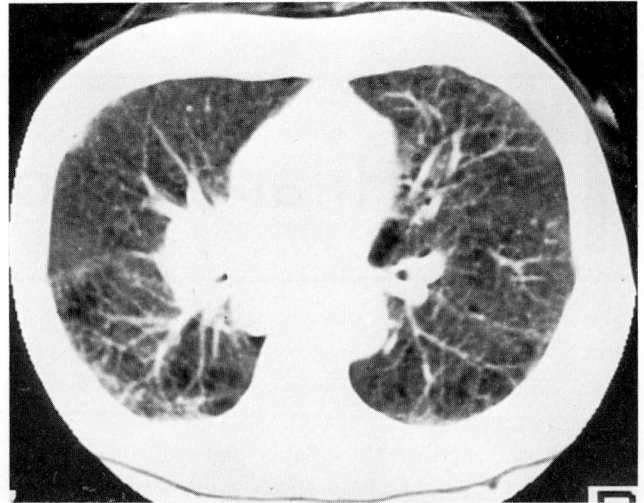

Figure 83c

The CT shows a number of abnormalities. There are marked changes of pulmonary emphysema in both lung fields.

There is a large mass at the inferior part of the right hilum obliterating the space between the basal pulmonary artery and the inferior pulmonary vein. Lateral and inferior to the mass there is consolidation and collapse of the right lower

Figure 83d

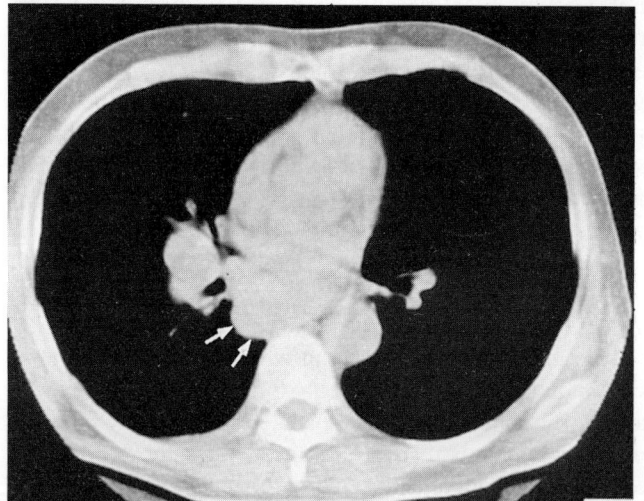

lobe, posterior and lateral basal segments. There is also interstitial oedema in these segments seen as linear opacities radiating from the hilum and thickening of the walls of bulla. There is a large bulging mass in the posterior mediastinum due to enlarged posterior mediastinal lymph nodes (*arrowed*). The mass can be seen as a convex bulge into the azygo-oesophageal recess of the right lung.

The appearances are those of a bronchogenic carcinoma with obstruction of bronchi, localized lymphangitis carcinomatosa and spread to the posterior mediastinal group of lymph nodes.

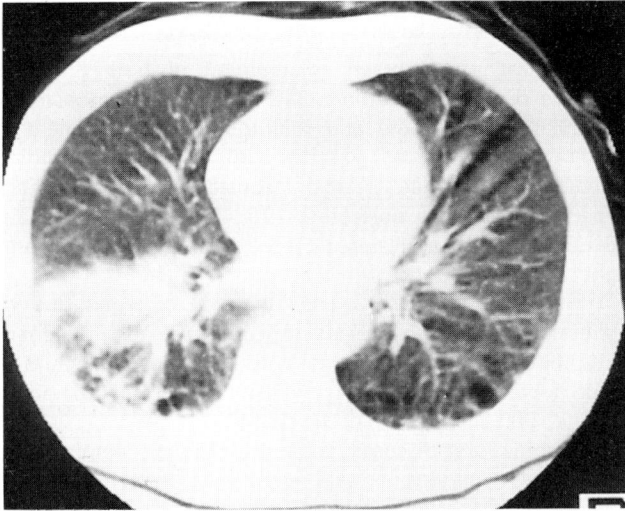

Figure 83e

Figure 83f

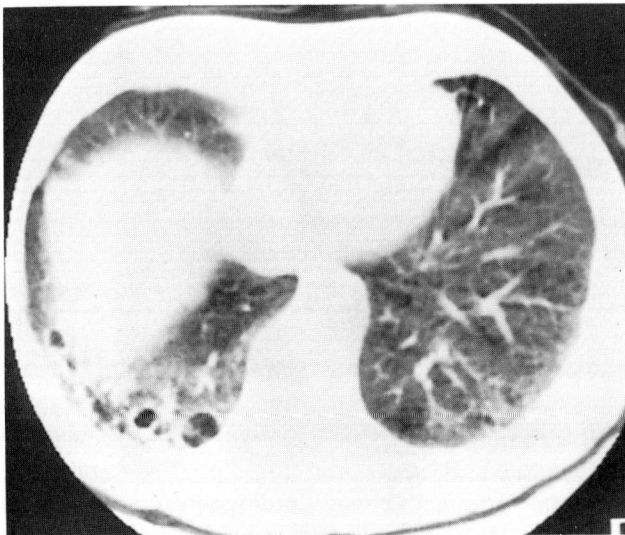

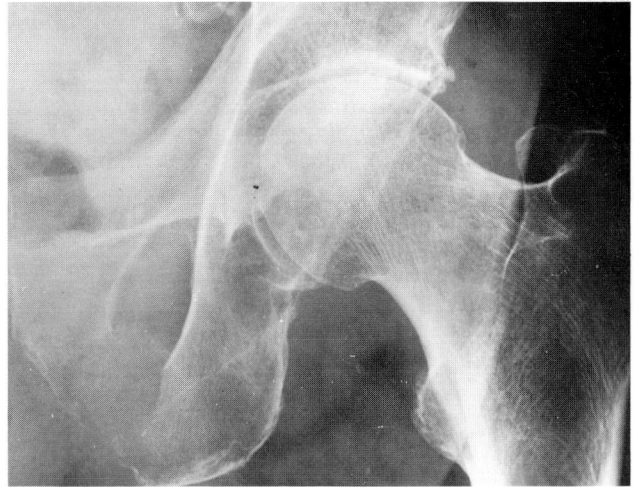

Figure 84a

The chest x-ray showed a mass in the left suprahilar region and enlargement of the left hilum. Sputum cytology was positive. Diagnosis: carcinoma of the bronchus.

Figure 84b

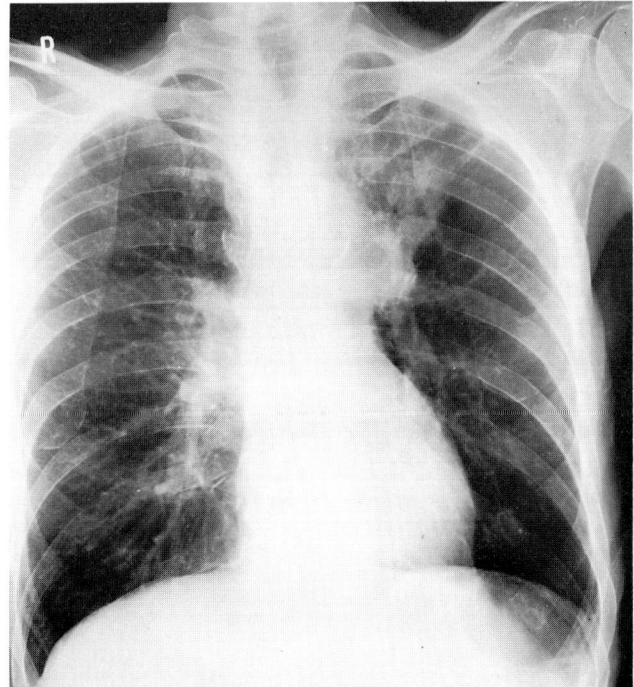

Case 84

A man aged 62 presented with a history of severe left hip pain. The hip radiograph is shown.

There is a radiolucent lesion is the ischium with ill-defined margins and destruction of the bony cortex. All of these features are those of an 'aggressive' lesion and a metastatic deposit is by far the most common cause in a man of this age. In men the most common primary malignancy giving rise to bony metastases is carcinoma of the bronchus whilst in women it is carcinoma of the breast.

Case 85

A woman aged 50 had undergone surgery for patent ductus anteriosus 20 years before and the PDA had only partially been closed. She now had attacks of paroxysmal tachycardia, collapsing pulse, a systolic murmur over the femoral vessels and pistol shot over the brachial artery.

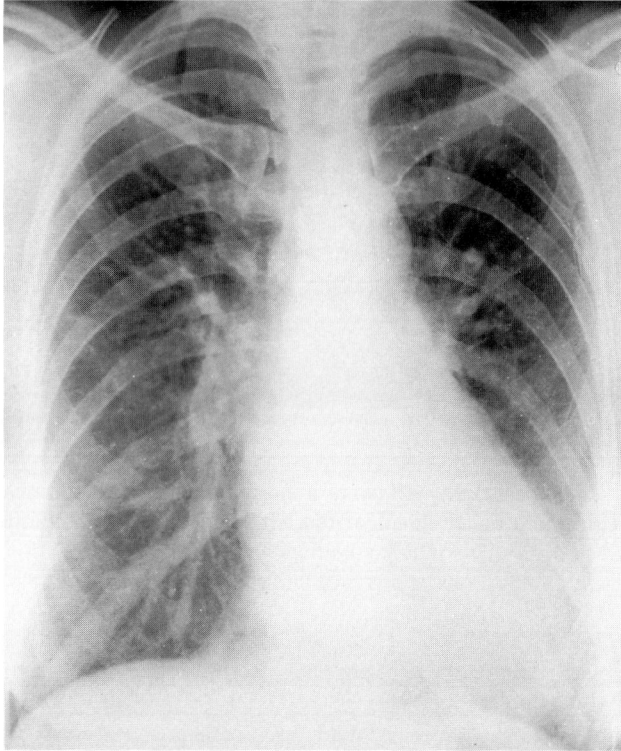

Figure 85a

Figure 85b

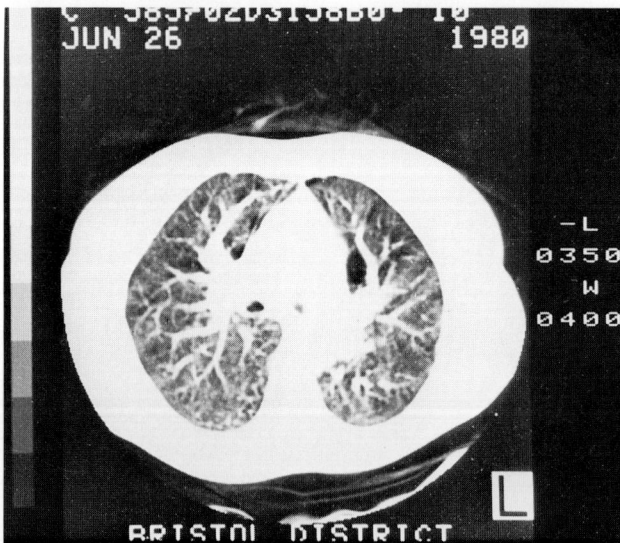

The chest x-ray is shown in figure 85a and CT in figure 85b.

The chest x-ray shows enlargement of both hila and probable pulmonary plethora. The CT clearly demonstrates the pulmonary plethora and that the hilar enlargement is bilateral and entirely vascular in origin. At cardiac catheterization there was considerable pulmonary hypertension with a pressure or 70/45 mmHg in the main pulmonary artery and step up of oxygen in both left and right pulmonary arteries indicative of a large shunt.

The main pulmonary arteries may be enlarged due to pulmonary arterial hypertension or increased pulmonary blood flow. Left to right shunts will initially cause increased blood flow and eventually can result in severe pulmonary hypertension and reversal of the shunt.

In chronic lung diseases, such as pulmonary emphysema, pulmonary hypertension can result due, probably, to the obliteration of the vascular bed and the consequent increased resistance to blood flow and due to the anoxia.

The importance of distinguishing enlarged vessels from enlarged lymph nodes must be stressed. If the hilar enlargement is vascular the next diagnostic tests will be directed at the cardiovascular system and include ECG, echocardiography and angiography.

If there is bilateral hilar lymph node enlargement, the list of common causes is fairly short and the main differentiation is between sarcoidosis and lymphoma. In sarcoidosis, the bronchopulmonary and right paratracheal nodes are the most commonly affected. The particular distribution in sarcoidosis often means that a clear line of air is seen between the medial part of the enlarged hilar nodes and the mediastinum. In lymphoma, the lymph node mass often affects nodes that are rarely affected in sarcoidosis. In particular the left paratracheal nodes and the subcarinal nodes are commonly affected. On chest radiographs and on CT of patients with lymphoma, the nodes are not discrete as they usually are in sarcoidosis. In lymphoma the mass may infiltrate around the vascular structures.

In sarcoidosis the Kveim test is usually positive. Gallium scans may be abnormal in active sarcoidosis, lymphoma and any form of inflammation. There is, however, a typical distribution in sarcoidosis involving hilar nodes, nasolacrimal and salivary glands.

Case 86

A patient presented with the following chest x-ray.

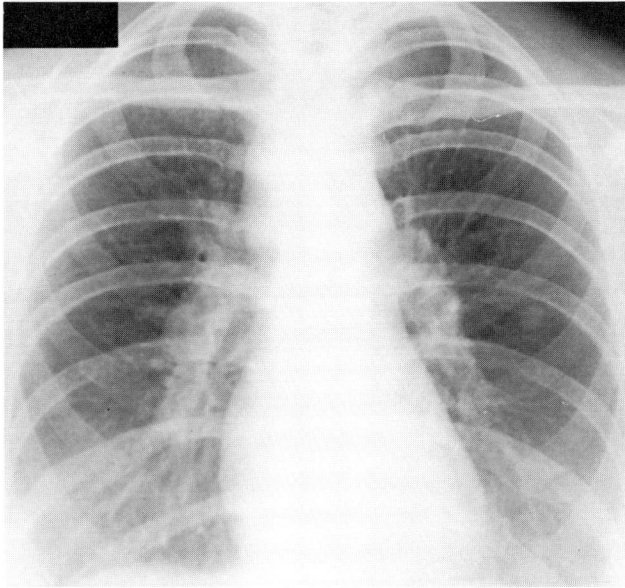

Figure 86a

There is bilateral hilar enlargement and right paratracheal lymph node enlargement.

Figure 86b

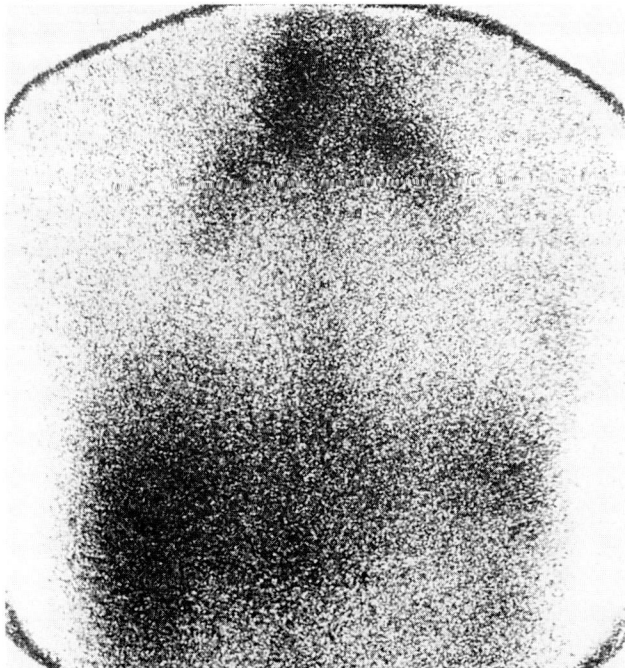

Gallium scans were performed and showed considerable uptake in the hilar and paratracheal nodes, nasolacrimal glands and salivary glands in a pattern typical for sarcoidosis.

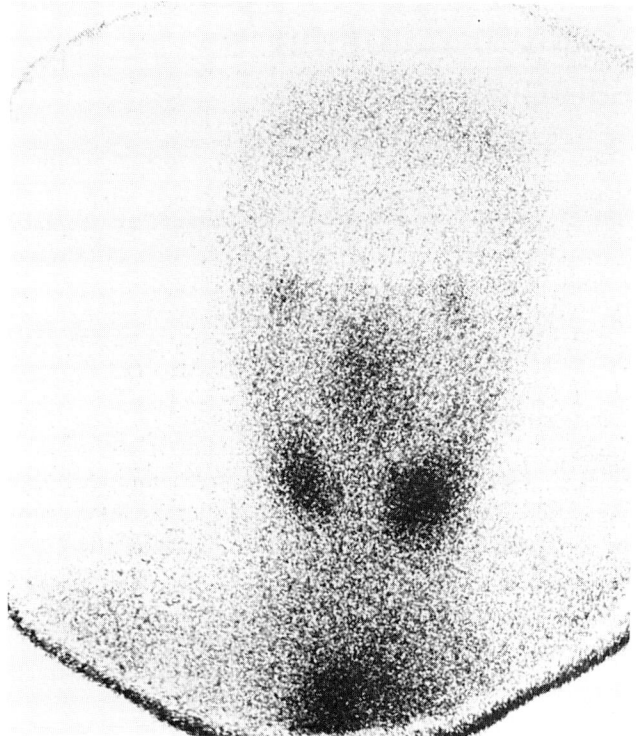

Figure 86c

Figure 86d

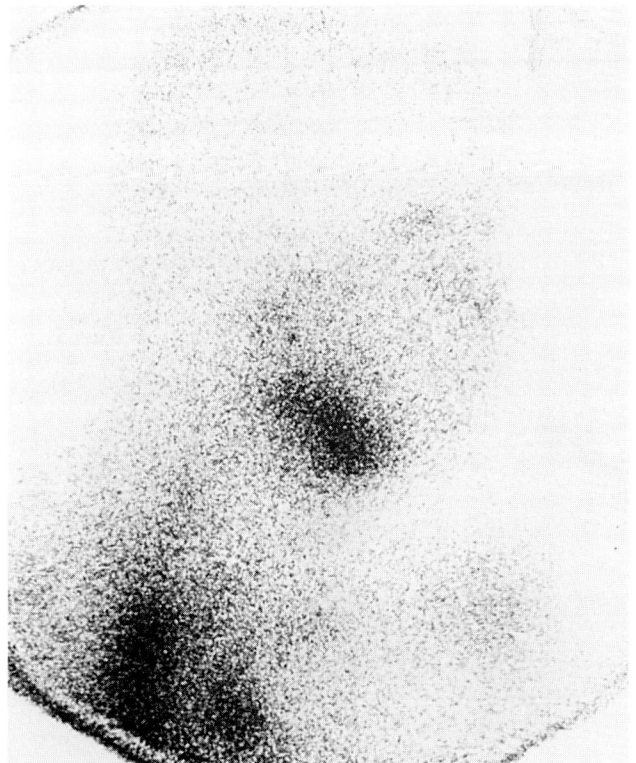

Gallium scanning in sarcoidosis

There are three main reasons for performing gallium scans in patients with sarcoidosis. The first is to distinguish areas of active and potentially treatable granulomatous reaction from inactive and untreatable fibrosis. This distinction may not always be easily made on plain chest radiographs and has already been discussed in Chapter 4, Case 18.

The second use of gallium scanning is to demonstrate the extent of disease activity. Sarcoidosis may affect a variety of extrathoracic sites including lymph nodes, spleen, liver, lacrimal and salivary glands, skin and upper respiratory tract mucosa. Gallium is concentrated by granuloma formation occurring at any of these sites [69, 70].

Thirdly, a characteristic pattern of gallium uptake may help support the diagnosis of sarcoidosis, although it is not yet certain whether the pattern can truly be considered as diagnostic.

Case 87

A lady aged 60 with a history of carcinoma of the breast had a bone scan showing worrying uptake in the thorax. Initially this was thought to be due to metastases in the ribs.

Figure 87a

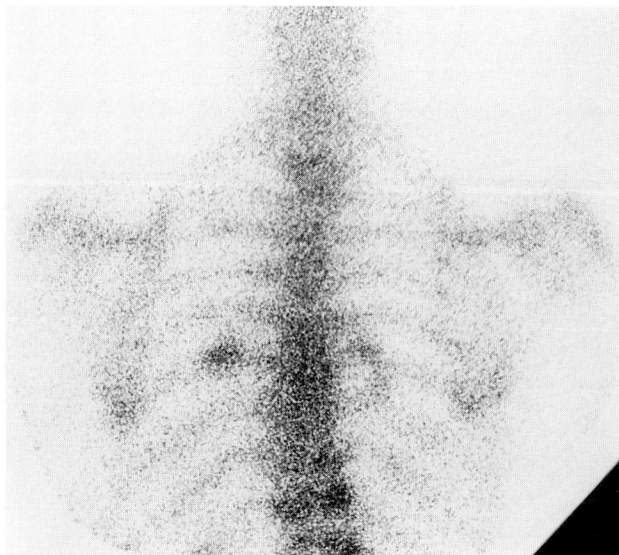

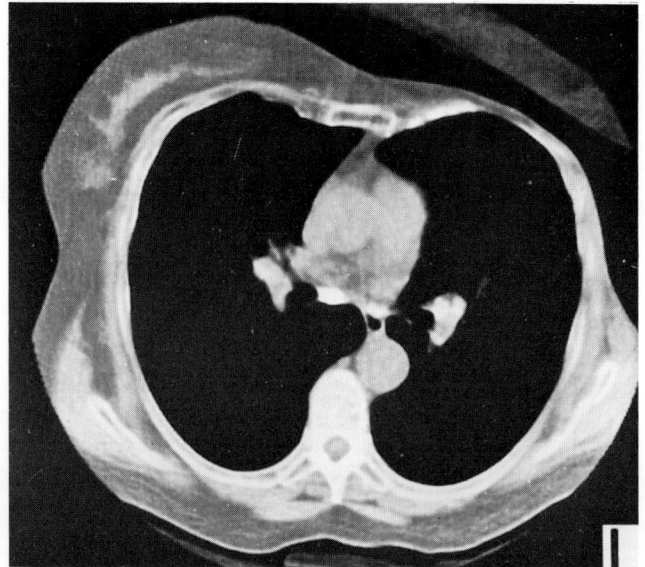

Figure 87b

Figure 87c

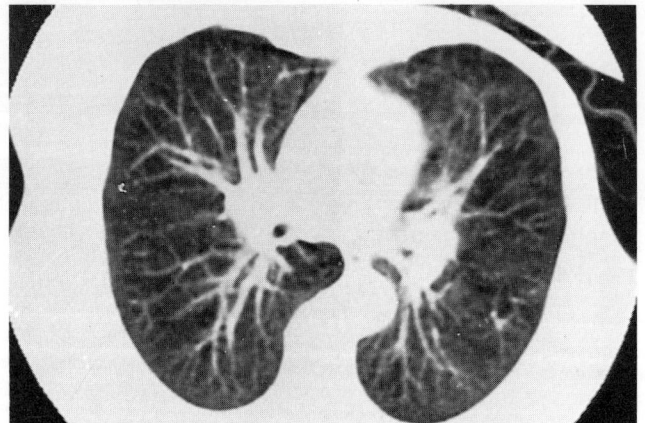

Figure 87d

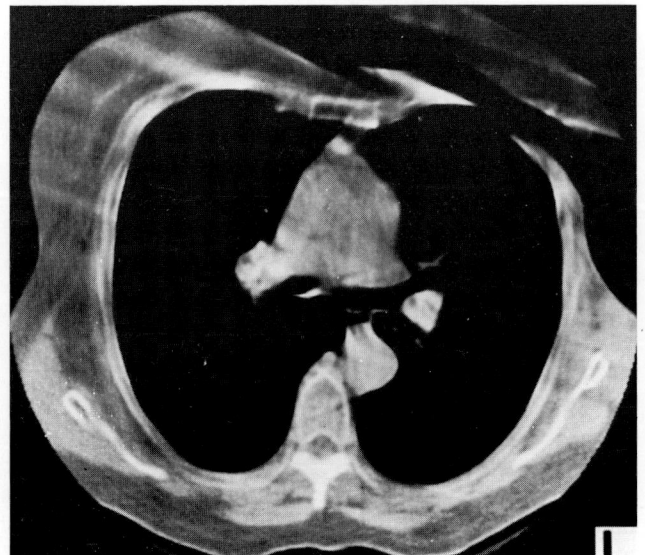

Figure 87e Emission CT

Emission CT of the bone scan showed the uptake to be in the centre of the chest and not related to bone. CT scans confirmed that the uptake was in calcified hilar and subcarinal glands.

The patient also had a previous history of pulmonary sarcoidosis and the calcified hilar nodes were the result of sarcoidosis.

Case 88

Chest x-ray showing gross widening of the mediastinum including and obliterating the hila. The appearances were due to Hodgkin's lymphoma and should be compared with the typical appearances of sarcoidosis seen in Case 86.

Figure 88

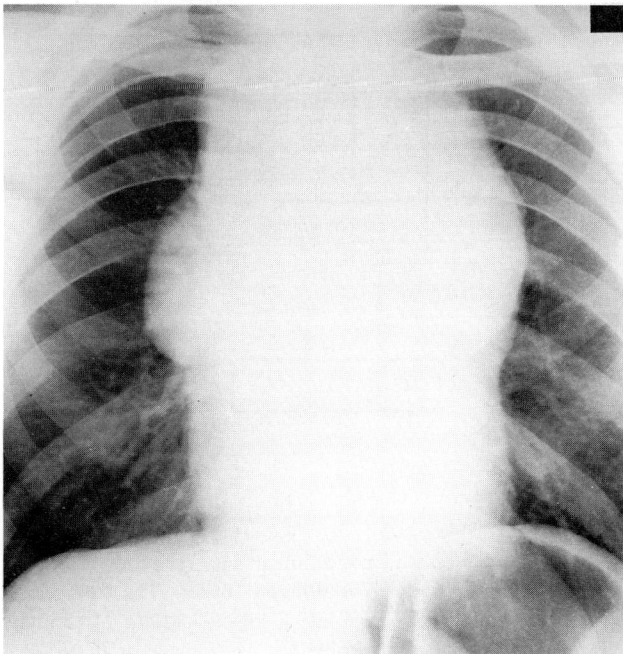

Summary: hilar enlargement

Apparent enlargement of the hila on chest radiography may be due either to an abnormality at the site of the hilum or to lesions in front of or behind the hilum. This problem can be resolved by lateral radiography or tomography. Next it is important to determine whether the abnormality is a mass or whether it is enlargement of a vascular structure and whether or not there are bilateral or unilateral lesions. For definitive differentiation CT, angiography or digital vascular imaging may be necessary. If there is a unilateral mass, by far the most common cause in an adult is bronchogenic carcinoma and the second most common is tuberculosis. Investigations should therefore be directed towards these and include microscopy and culture for acid-fast facilli and cytology for malignant cells. If the tests are negative, bronchoscopy is usually necessary.

If there is bilateral hilar lymph node enlargement, the main differentiation is between sarcoidosis and lymphoma. Investigations for these conditions would again include computed tomography but gallium scanning may also be useful and will show uptake in many of the conditions which cause lymph node enlargement. Biopsy may be necessary in order to determine the nature of hilar masses but whenever possible this should be performed by closed biopsy (e.g. transbronchial).

13 The mediastinal mass

A large number of imaging techniques can be used to assist in the diagnosis of a mediastinal mass.

A flow chart for diagnostic procedures of value in studying a mediastinal mass is shown below (Figure K).

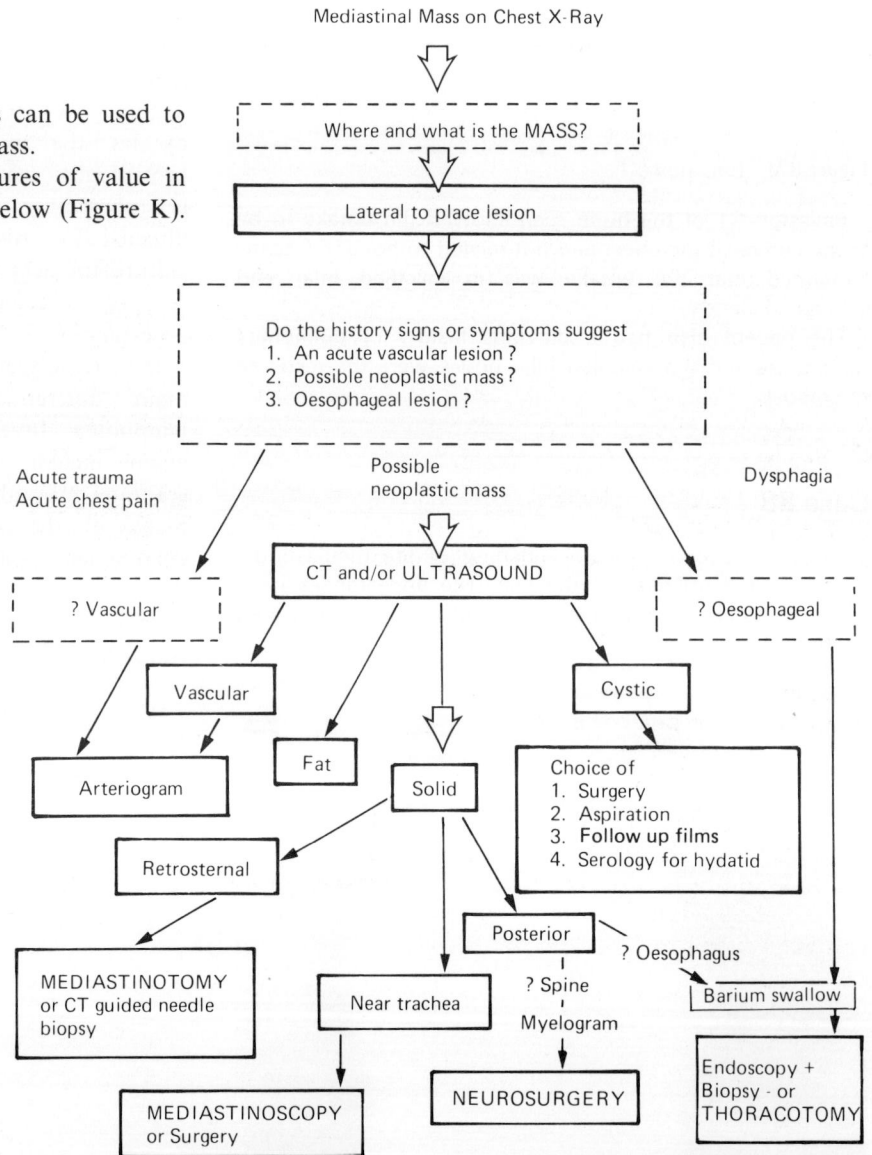

Mediastinal Mass on Chest X-Ray

Where and what is the MASS?

Lateral to place lesion

Do the history signs or symptoms suggest
1. An acute vascular lesion?
2. Possible neoplastic mass?
3. Oesophageal lesion?

Acute trauma
Acute chest pain

Possible neoplastic mass

Dysphagia

? Vascular

CT and/or ULTRASOUND

? Oesophageal

Vascular

Cystic

Arteriogram

Fat

Solid

Choice of
1. Surgery
2. Aspiration
3. **Follow up films**
4. Serology for hydatid

Retrosternal

Posterior

? Oesophagus

MEDIASTINOTOMY
or CT guided needle
biopsy

Near trachea

? Spine
Myelogram

Barium swallow

MEDIASTINOSCOPY
or Surgery

NEUROSURGERY

Endoscopy +
Biopsy - or
THORACOTOMY

Magnetic Resonance Imaging can be used to complement or replace CT or ULTRASOUND

Figure K Mediastinal mass on chest x-ray

Studying the flow chart.

Strict adherence to the flow chart is *not* recommended. At any stage of the investigation the diagnosis may become apparent and no further test may be required. In other cases with the knowledge of the clinical condition it may be prudent to perform the investigations in a different order. The flow chart should only be used to stimulate a logical pattern of thought with regard to a particular problem.

In most patients the mass is first detected by chest radiography, although in a few an abnormality of the mediastinum is shown initially by CT. The next investigation depends to a large extent on the clinical presentation and the site of the mass as judged by the chest PA film and lateral. If the presentation is the result of severe trauma, as in a road traffic accident, it may well be that the mediastinal mass is due to a haematoma indicative of injury to the large veins and possibly rupture of the aorta. In such cases there are often associated fractures and a pleural effusion (haemothorax). If traumatic rupture of the aorta is suspected, an arch aortogram should be undertaken as an emergency procedure.

Table 18 Table of causes of a mediastinal mass

Masses arising anywhere in the mediastinum
1. Lymphadenopathy (secondary carcinoma, lymphoma, sarcoidosis, tuberculosis)
2. Lipoma
3. Fibroma
4. Vascular origin: aneurysm, anomalous vessels, haematoma
5. Abscess

Superior mediastinum
1. Thyroid goitre
2. Pharyngeal pouch
3. Masses that arise anywhere in the mediastinum

Anterior mediastinum
1. Retrosternal thyroid
2. Thymoma and thymic cyst
3. Teratodermoid
4. Pericardial and pleuropericardial cyst
5. Morgagni hernia
6. Masses that arise anywhere in the mediastinum

Middle mediastinum
1. Cardiac abnormalities
2. Masses that arise anywhere in the mediastinum (especially lymphadenopathy and vascular abnormalities)
3. Bronchogenic cyst

Posterior mediastinum
1. Oesophageal abnormality (achalasia and carcinoma) and hiatus hernia
2. Aortic aneurysm and other masses that arise anywhere in the mediastinum
3. Neurogenic tumours (neurofibroma, ganglioneuroma, meningocele)
4. Spinal and paraspinal lesions
5. Bronchogenic and foregut cyst
6. Bochdalek hernia

Lesions 'simulating' a mediastinal mass
Pulmonary, pleural or chest wall masses abutting the mediastinum

Case 89

Alec W., aged 18 years, was involved in a serious road traffic accident. He was brought into the Casualty Department semiconscious and shocked. A radiograph of his chest is reproduced in figure 89a.

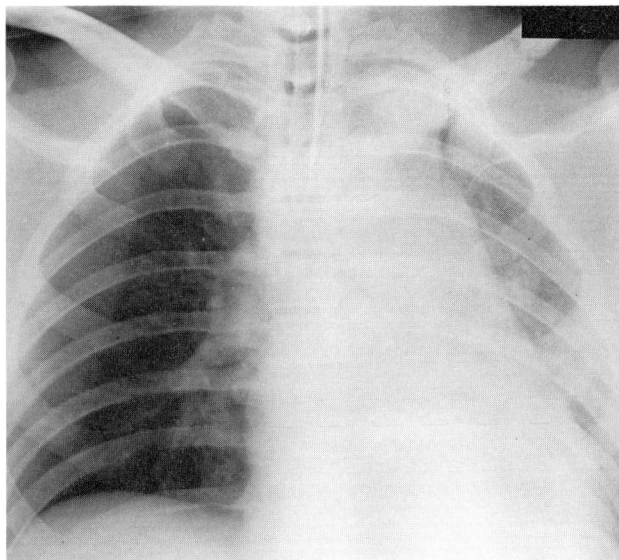

Figure 89a

The chest radiograph shows gross superior mediastinal widening, a left pleural effusion and the aortic arch is obscured. There is also a right-sided paraspinous mass and downward displacement of the left main bronchus.

The appearances are those of a mediastinal haematoma. Note also the fracture of the left clavicle.

An aortogram was performed.

Figure 89b is an arch aortogram subtraction film. There is a false aneurysm at the site of a tear of the lower thoracic aorta. There is also good visualization of the intimal flap.

This patient demonstrates the signs of mediastinal haematoma associated with a laceration of the lower thoracic aorta.

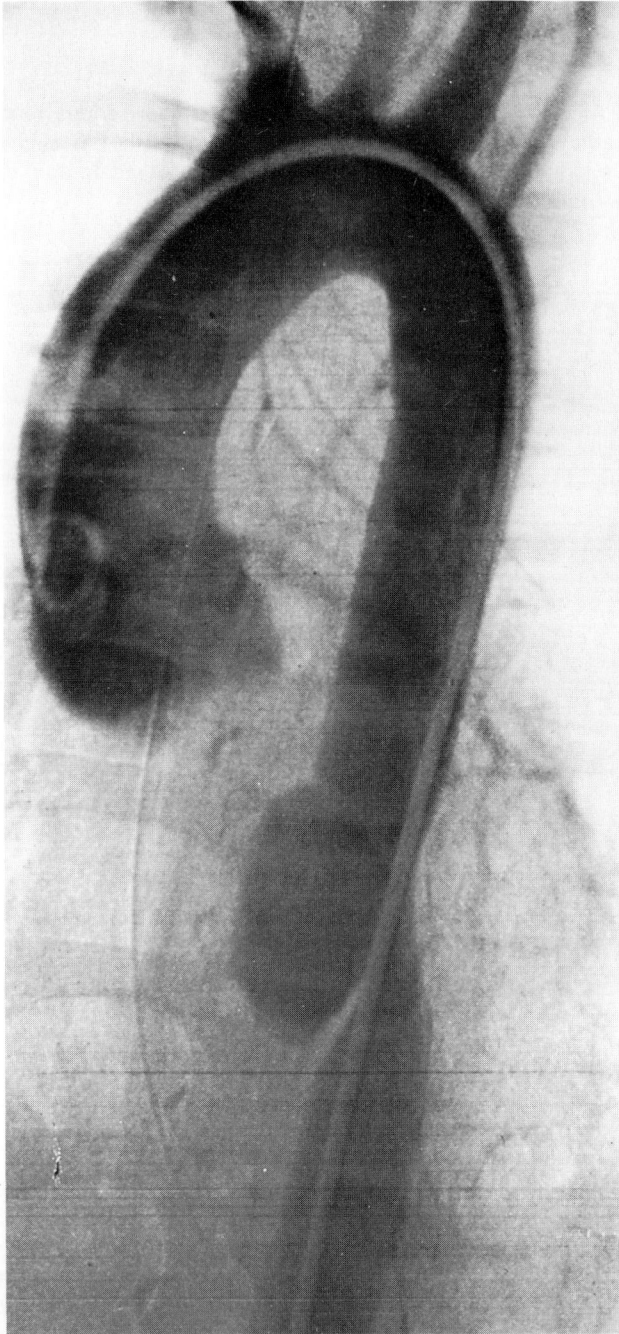

Figure 89b

The haematoma was gross in this case. Sometimes they are more subtle and may be hidden by the cardiac silhouette or manifest only as a shift of the trachea to the right. The commonest site for aortic injury is the isthmus. When a tear occurs, it tends to be subadventitial in young people, as opposed to submedial in older patients with atheromatous disease.

Some form of aortogram is essential to demonstrate the site of aortic injury or injuries and to exclude any associated vascular injuries especially the brachiocephalic trunk.

Aortography by the transfemoral root is quick, versatile and safe. In some centres aortography is performed by digital vascular imaging. By the use of digital subtraction it is possible to obtain pictures very much like figure 89b from an intravenous injection of contrast medium thus avoiding the necessity of arterial catheterization.

Alec went on to develop a paraplegia. This was the result of damage to the artery of Adamkiewicz which is the major supplying vessel of the dorsal and lumbar spine. It arises as the largest anterior radicular branch from one of the lower intercostal or upper lumbar (T8–L4) segmental arteries usually on the left.

Other complications that can arise from trauma to the aorta include catastrophic haemorrhage and renal failure. It must always be remembered that patients with this type of injury have received severe trauma and may well have head injury or other visceral damage such as ruptured spleen or liver.

Another interesting syndrome has been described following aortic trauma, described by Symbas 'The Post Traumatic Coarctation Syndrome' [71]. This comprises:

1 increased blood pressure and pulse amplitude in the upper extremity,

2 decreased blood pressure and pulse amplitude in the legs,

3 widened mediastinum on the chest film.

The exact aetiology of this condition is uncertain. A number of mechanisms have been suggested, including aortic compression by haematoma, occlusion by an intimal flap and reflux sympathetic aortic spasm. Whatever the mechanism there is characteristically a major intimal tear. The practical point is that the catheter is unlikely to pass from below and a transaxillary approach is indicated.

Case 90

David M. was not wearing his seat belt and was hence flung through his car windscreen when it ran into a bus. He was brought into the Casualty Department with lacerations to his head and face but became progressively shocked. After emergency resuscitation the following radiograph was performed (fig. 90a).

The chest film is similar to that of Case 89. Again there is widening of the mediastinum. There are, in this case, multiple fractured ribs on the right side. There is also a

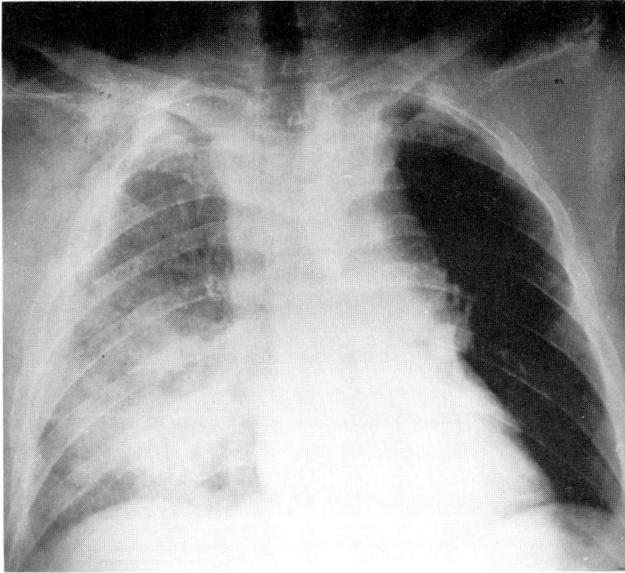

Figure 90a

Figure 90b

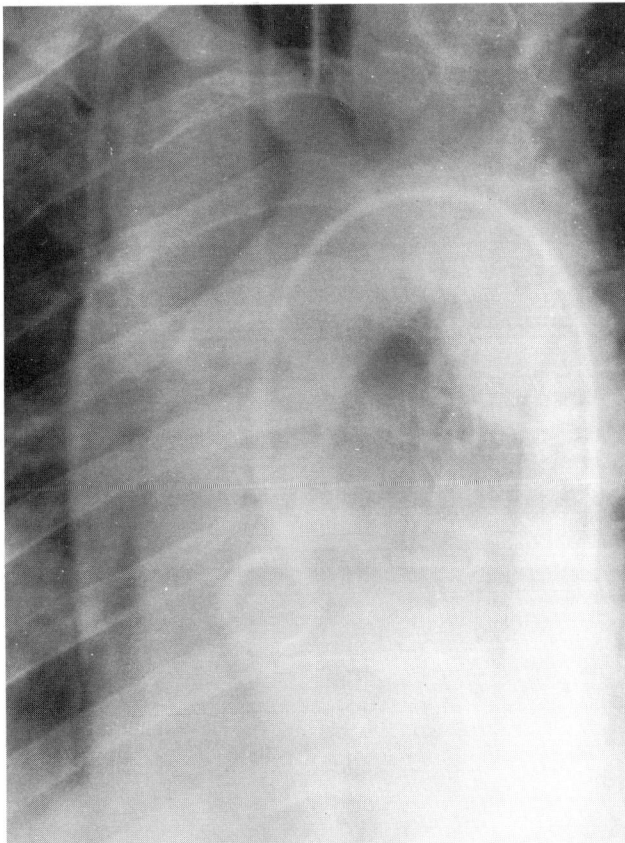

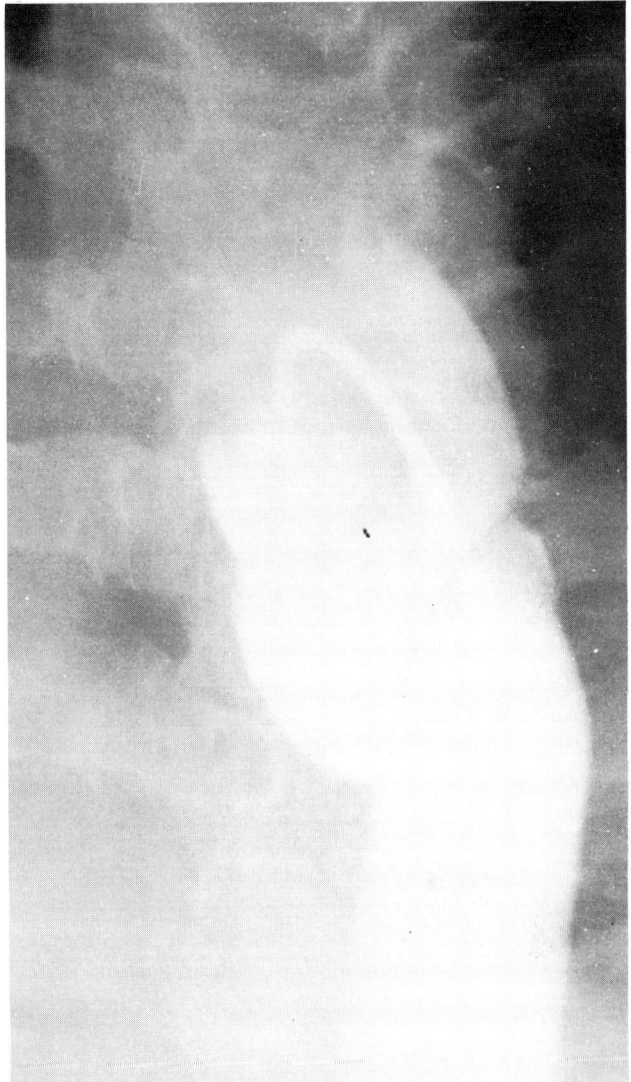

Figure 90c

right-sided pleural effusion and pulmonary opacification. The effusion is due to blood and the pulmonary opacification represents contusion (see also Case 24). An emergency aortogram was performed in order to demonstrate the site of aortic injury or injuries and to exclude any associated vascular injuries (e.g. brachiocephalic trunk).

The aortogram shows laceration of the aorta at the isthmus which is the commonest site of aortic injury occurring in 88 per cent of cases.

Rupture of the thoracic aorta is a very important condition to diagnose. Fifteen per cent of patients with laceration of the aorta by blunt trauma *do* survive long enough for the diagnosis to be made. If the diagnosis is missed, 90 per cent who survived the initial impact die within four months [72].

Points to consider in patients with chest trauma include:

1 There is an important association between fractures of the upper ribs and laceration of the aorta or great vessels.

2 Bilateral fractured ribs anteriorly may cause flail chest.

3 Fractures of the sternum may be associated with fractures of the thoracic spine.

4 Fractures of the lower ribs may be associated with ruptured spleen on the left or liver on the right.

Conditions such as pulmonary contusion, pneumothorax and ruptured diaphragm must also be considered. These subjects are covered in Chapters 5, 9 and 11.

Aortography is also undertaken as an emergency procedure if there are symptoms highly suggestive of dissecting aneurysm. Aortography may be indicated even if the mediastinum appears normal on chest radiography, since dissection can be present even if the chest x-ray looks virtually normal. However, in most cases of dissection of the aorta, there is widening of the mediastinum and in many cases there is a small left-sided pleural effusion. Computed tomography may be used with intravenous contrast medium, to show dissection and it appears that aortography and CT are complementary. In a few cases CT may demonstrate dissection that has been missed by aortography, but it can be debated whether or not this will change management significantly. Surgical management is usually indicated in cases involving the ascending aorta and causing significant aortic regurgitation.

Ultrasound has also been used to show aortic aneurysm. Using real-time ultrasound it is sometimes possible to see an intimal flap with dissection of the aorta, and by Doppler the flow in the true lumen and false lumen can be measured. Aortic regurgitation is important in dissection, since this will determine whether the patient is managed surgically or medically. Doppler can also be used to show aortic regurgitation elegantly. If dissection and regurgitation are demonstrated by ultrasound, it is still necessary to proceed to angiography since the surgeon will require to know the position and state of the coronary arteries. The combination of real-time ultrasound and Doppler will also show the abnormal flow in aberrant vessels and shunts—this will be covered in a forthcoming book on cardiovascular imaging.

It remains to be seen whether or not magnetic resonance imaging will find a place in the investigation of aortic aneurysm and dissection, but MRI is certainly capable of displaying the aorta and great vessels and of showing differences in flow and can demonstrate the coronary arteries.

Case 91

This is a normal example. Rapid sequential scanning on the IGE 9800 following intravenous injection of contrast medium.

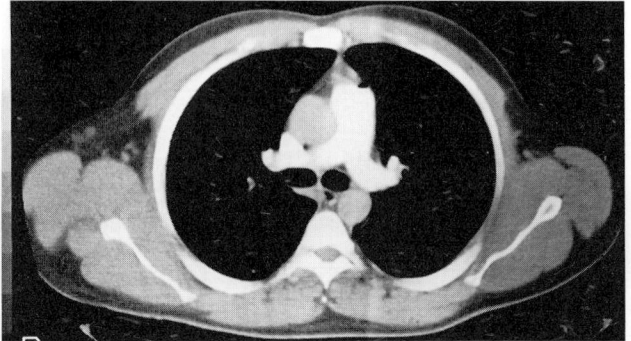

Figure 91a

Figure 91b

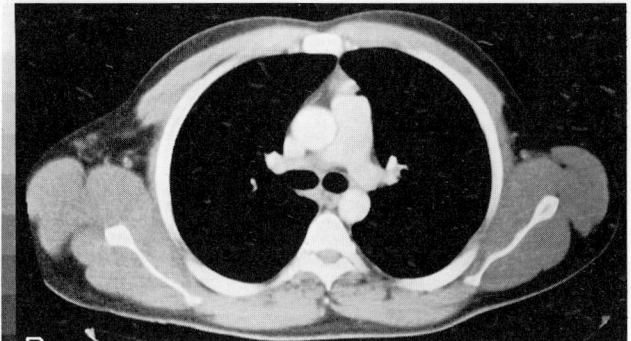

Figure 91c

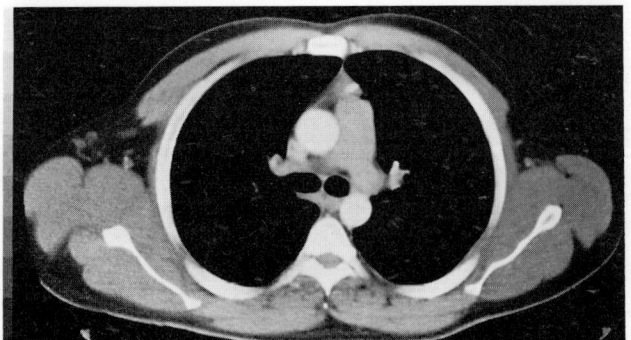

Initially the superior vena cava and pulmonary arteries and veins are opacified. In scan b all the major mediastinal vessels are opacified and in c the ascending and descending aorta contain contrast medium.

Case 92 (*Courtesy of Dr Thin-Thin Aye*)

The patient presented with acute onset of severe chest pain radiating to the back, weak femoral pulses and the following chest radiograph.

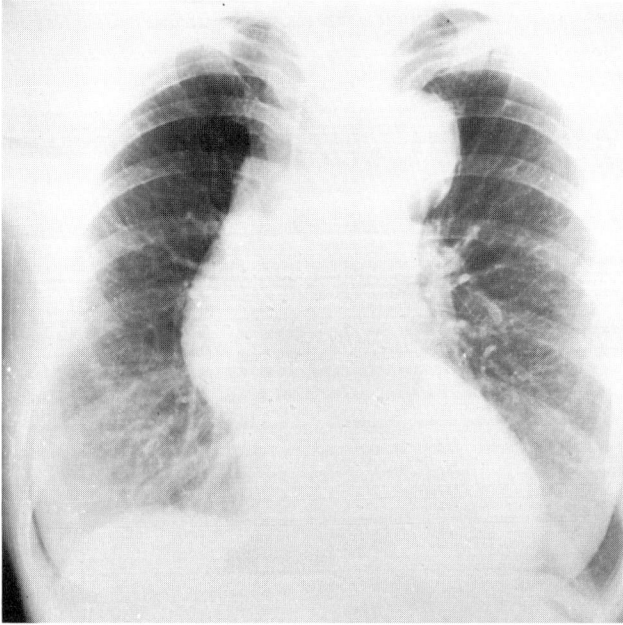

Figure 92a

Figure 92b

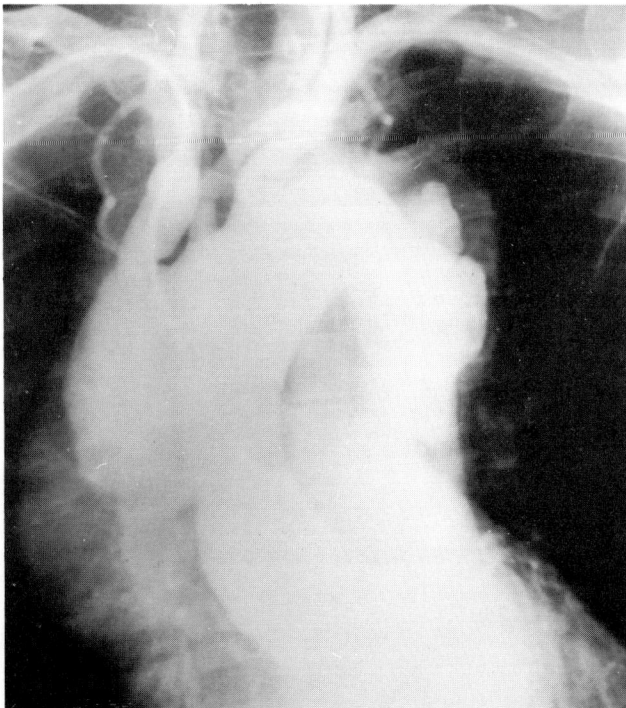

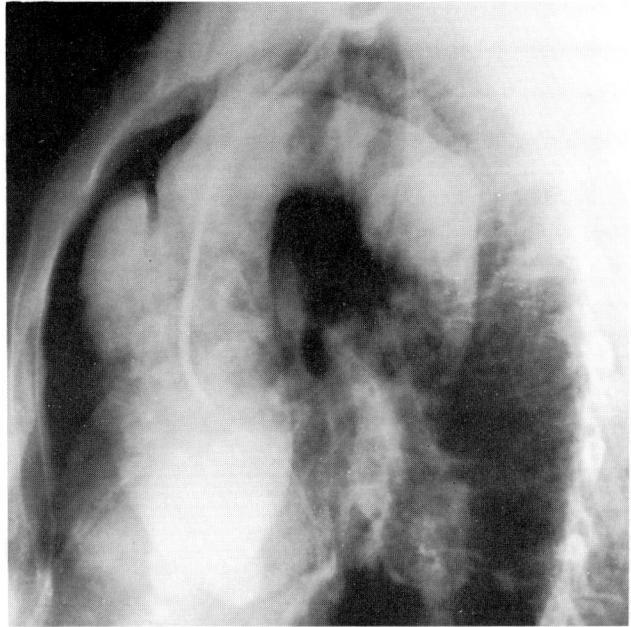

Figure 92c

The heart size is normal but there is marked enlargement of the ascending aorta and aortic knuckle. Aortography was performed via the right axillary artery.

There is widening of the ascending aorta and an intimal flap. These are the features of a dissecting aneurysm. The arch of the aorta is also involved and the brachiocephalic artery is dilated.

Computed tomography with an intravenous bolus injection of contrast medium shows the aortic aneurysm with the false lumen unopacified by contrast medium whilst the true lumen is opacified. Note also how the azygos vein is distended and contains contrast medium as a result of back flow from the partially obstructed superior vena cava.

Figure 92d

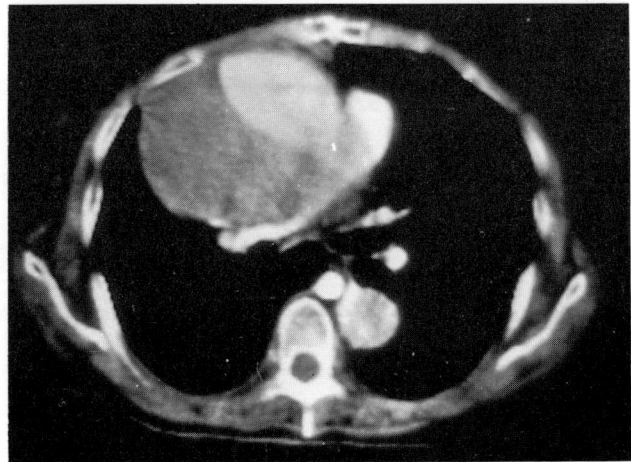

Case 93: Magnetic resonance imaging (normal example)

The aorta and pulmonary arteries are very clearly seen and can be distinguished with ease from other mediastinal contents. The chambers of the heart and the cardiac walls and septa can be identified in different phases of the cardiac cycle.

Figure 93   Multi-format display of gated heart images in axial and sagittal views (TR = 409 ms,   TE = 28 ms) (*Courtesy of Elscint*)

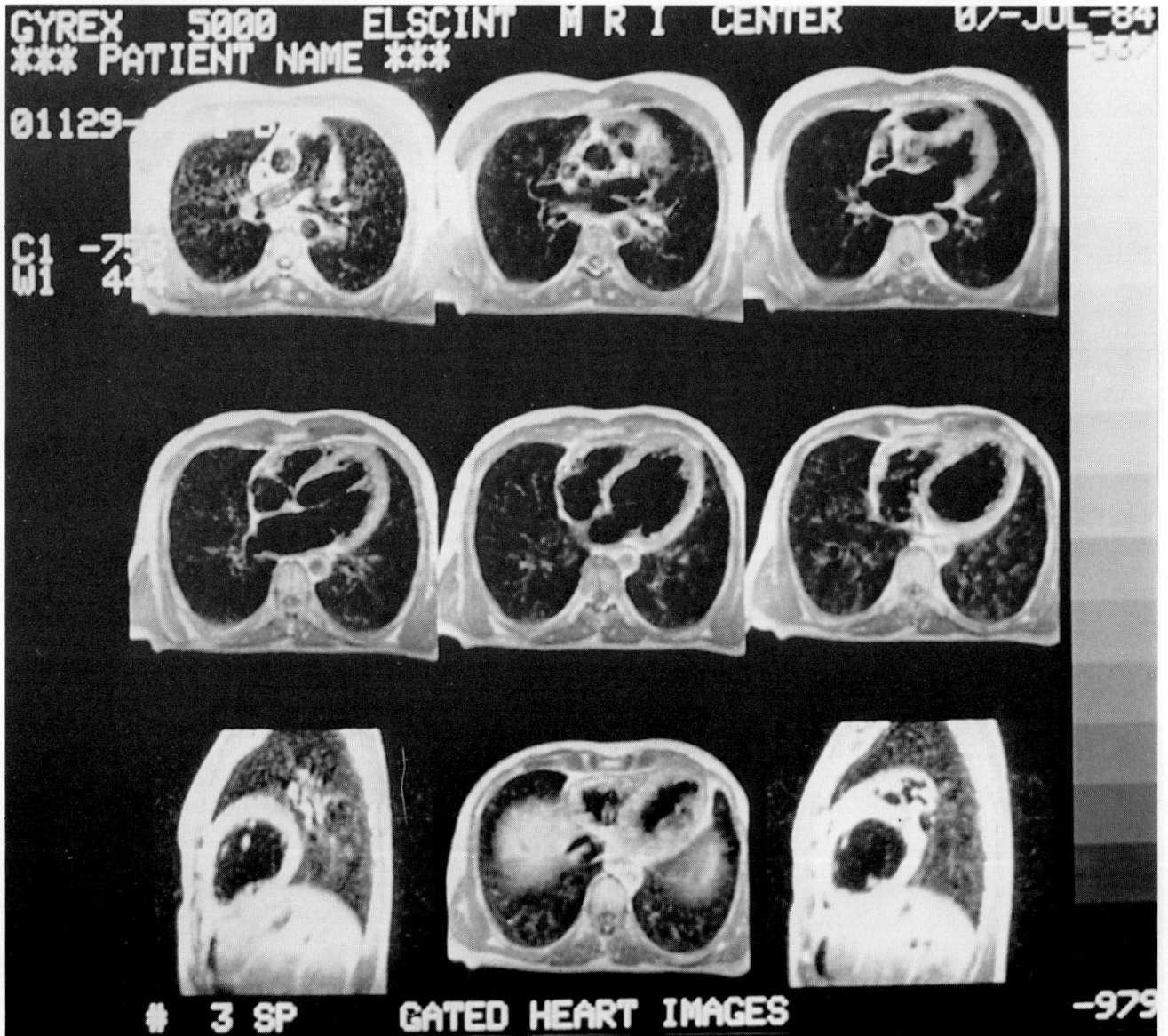

In other situations when a patient presents with a mediastinal mass it is as well to consider the various different structures that may give rise to masses in the particular site. In all parts of the mediastinum it is possible for masses to be vascular (aneurysms of various types), cystic or solid. Neoplastic masses can arise from many of the structures present including thymus and thyroid, the bronchi and trachea, the oesophagus and the nerve plexi. These will arise respectively in the anterior, the middle and the posterior compartments of the mediastinum. Solid masses that can arise anywhere in the mediastinum include lymphadenopathies, lipoma and fibroma. The commonest causes of lymphadenopathy are secondary carcinoma, tuberculosis, lymphoma and sarcoidosis.

A pulmonary mass, such as carcinoma of the bronchus, may arise in the periphery of the lung adjacent to the mediastinum and be indistinguishable from a mediastinal mass on the plain radiographs.

Superior mediastinum

In the superior mediastinum and neck the most common cause of a mass is a large thyroid goitre. Confirmation that a mass is in the thyroid can usually be obtained clinically by demonstrating that it moves when the patient swallows. Plain films of the thoracic inlet may show the mass and deviation of the trachea. Ultrasound will show whether the mass is solid or cystic and the extent of the mass. The ultrasound signs of a cystic structure are:

1 The structure contains no echoes (it is 'anechoic' or 'echo-free').

2 Ultrasound is conducted through the cyst and there is thus increased reflection of ultrasound from structures deep to the cyst (enhancement).

3 Doppler ultrasound will show no blood flow in a cyst thus distinguishing it from a vascular lesion such as an aneurysm or tortuous vessel.

If it is cystic, the surgeon may wish to 'needle' the cyst and aspirate the contents. The fluid is usually then sent for cytology and culture. Solid masses will usually be treated surgically.

When there is more clinical doubt as to the origin of the mass, computed tomography may be of assistance by showing the extent of the lesion and involvement of mediastinal structures. The radiodensity (attenuation) of the structure can be measured using CT, giving some indication as to the nature of the lesion. If there are signs or symptoms to suggest involvement of the oesophagus, or if the mass is clearly posterior, a barium swallow should be performed.

Case 94

Madeleine presented to her general practitioner with a swelling in the left side of her neck of a few weeks' duration. It was painless and on examination the mass moved upwards on swallowing. The patient was referred to the surgical outpatient clinic for further investigation and treatment. Radiographs of the thoracic inlet were performed (fig. 94a). An ultrasound scan was also done and is shown in figures 94b and 94c with a line drawing of the scan in figure 94d.

Figure 94a

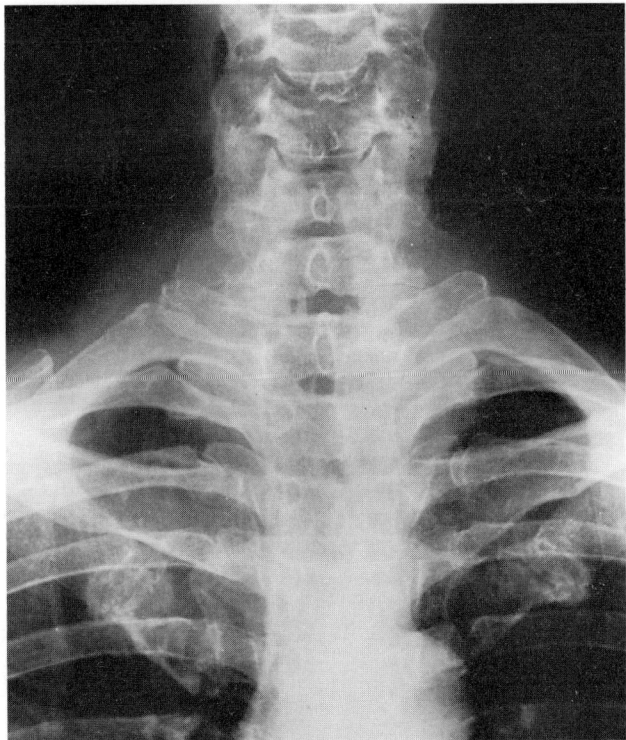

The plain radiograph of the thoracic inlet shows that the trachea is being compressed by a soft tissue mass in the left side of the neck.

The ultrasound scans are shown in figures 94b and 94c. Figure 94b is a longitudinal scan and figure 94c is a transverse scan of the patient's neck 4 cm above the sternal notch.

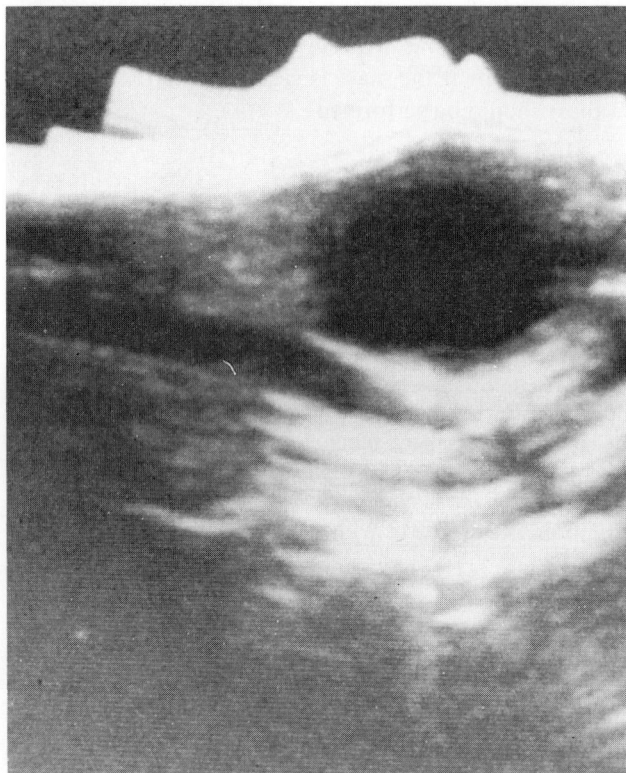

Figure 94b

Figure 94c

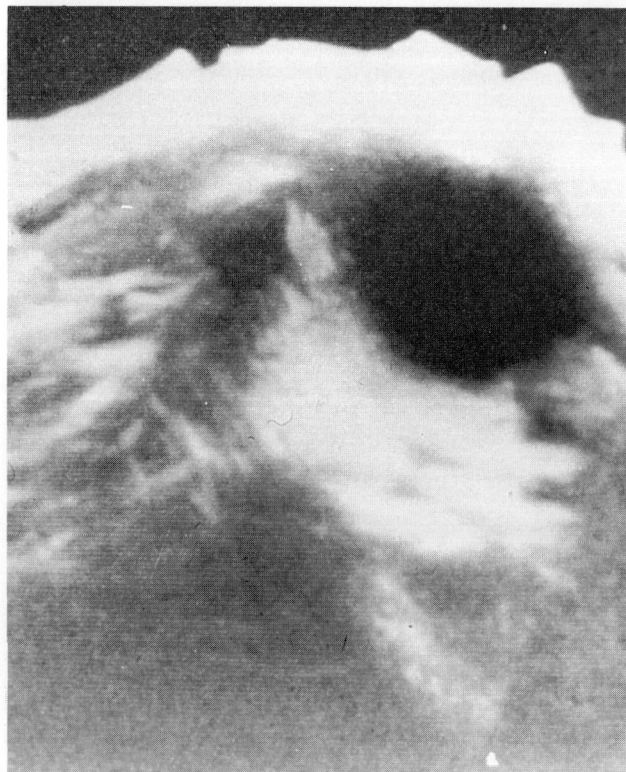

The right lobe of the thyroid is normal in appearance and labelled A. There is a large, echo-free area in the left lobe of the thyroid (labelled B) with an area of enhancement behind it (also labelled). It remained echo-free even when the power output of the ultrasound transducer was increased. All these signs are characteristic ultrasonographic features of a cyst.

A radioisotope scan of Madeleine's thyroid showed a photon-deficient 'cold' area in the left lobe. Aspiration was performed and cytology of the fluid obtained suggested a multi-nodular goitre. This was confirmed at operation, when a thick-walled colloid cyst was found lying within a benign, multinodular goitre.

When investigating a suspected thyroid swelling there are certain important questions which must be answered.

Does the mass indeed lie within the thyroid? This is usually determined by physical examination, the findings of which are easily confirmed by ultrasound.

Is the mass cystic or solid? This distinction is important in order to differentiate thyroid cysts from tumours or benign thyroid nodules. The difference between cystic and solid lesions is elegantly made by ultrasound.

Is the mass metabolically active? Radioisotope scanning of the thyroid may be helpful in making this distinction. Metabolically active lesions (adenomas, follicular carcinomas) show increased isotope uptake and appear as photon-dense 'hot' areas. Metabolically inactive lesions (cysts, papillary or anaplastic carcinomas) appear as photon-deficient 'cold' areas. The scan may also show additional lesions which have not been detected clinically. These include metastatic deposits from follicular thyroid tumours which may be shown in the lungs or skeleton.

Figure 94d

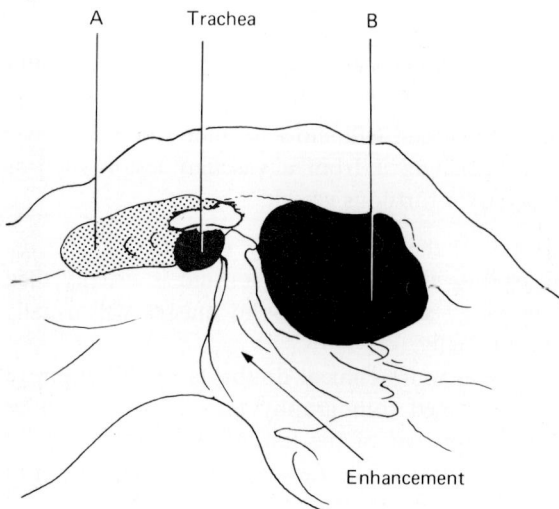

Does the mass extend retrosternally or compress the trachea? This point is important as tracheal compression or deviation is an indication for surgical management even if the lesion is thought on other grounds to be benign. Although ultrasound may show compression or deviation of the trachea in the neck, it cannot demonstrate the retrosternal area well. A radioisotope scan may show retrosternal extension of the thyroid mass but will not demonstrate whether it compresses the trachea. The plain radiograph of the thoracic inlet is still a good method of assessing this area and if, the results are equivocal, it may be necessary to proceed to linear tomography or computed tomography.

Case 95

A thyroid mass was detected clinically. The thoracic inlet radiograph and the cross-sectional ultrasound are shown.

As in the previous case there is deviation of the trachea shown on the plain film. The ultrasound shows the mass to be solid.

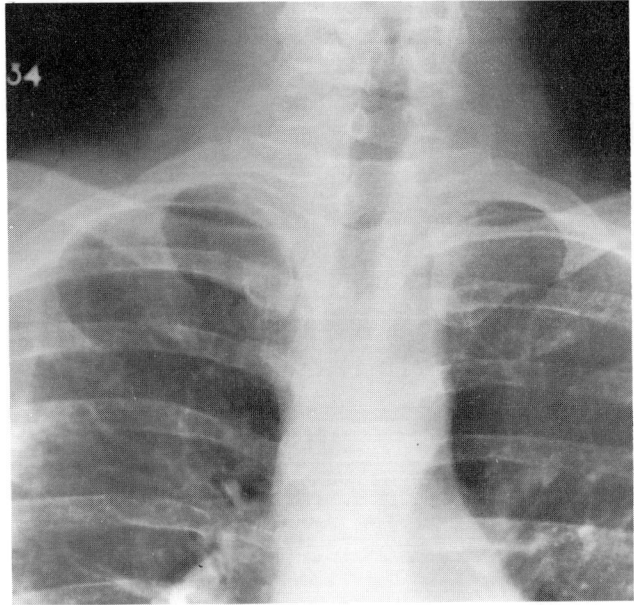

Figure 95a

Figure 95b

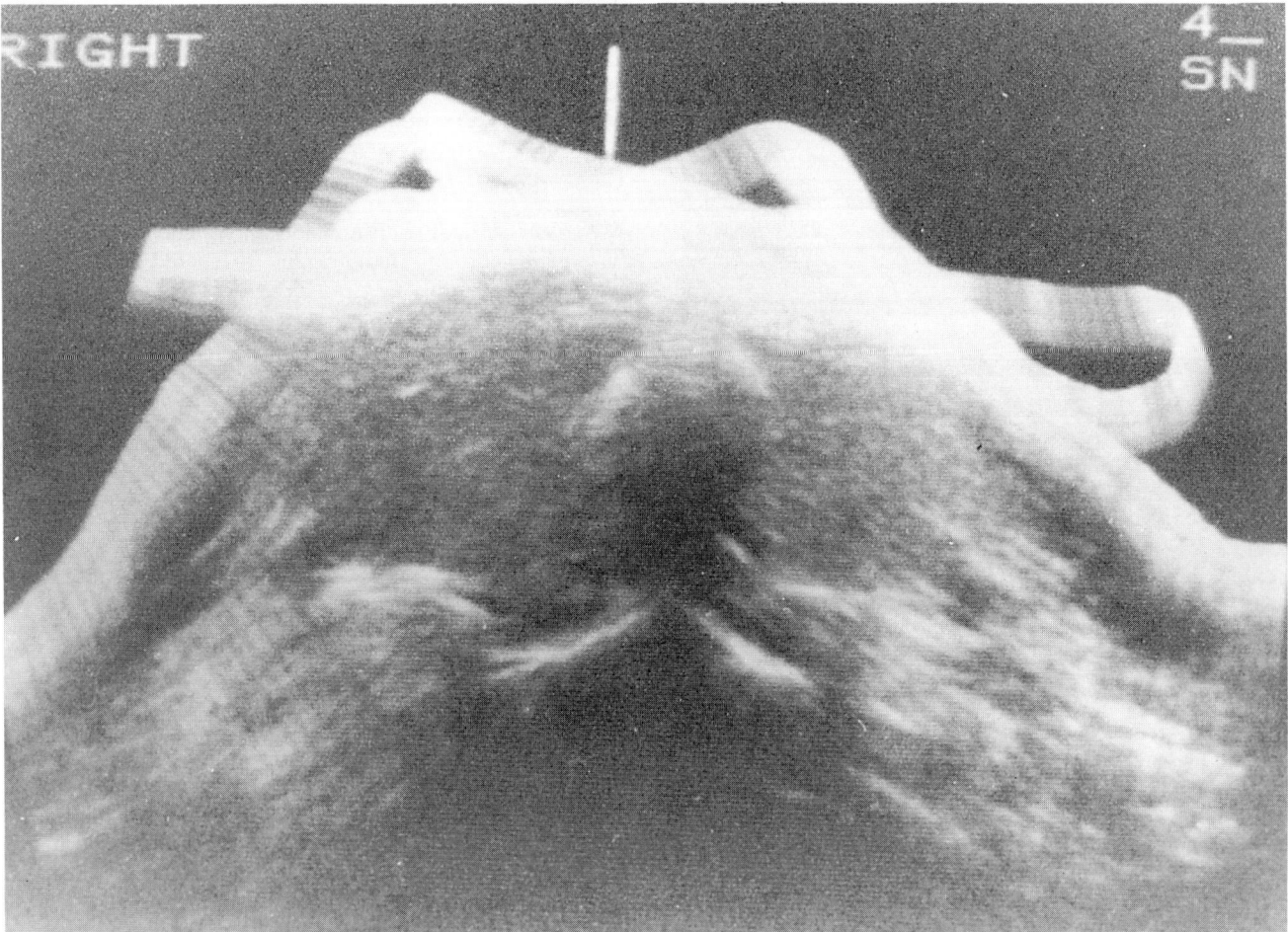

Case 96

An Italian lady presented with shortness of breath on exertion and raised blood pressure.

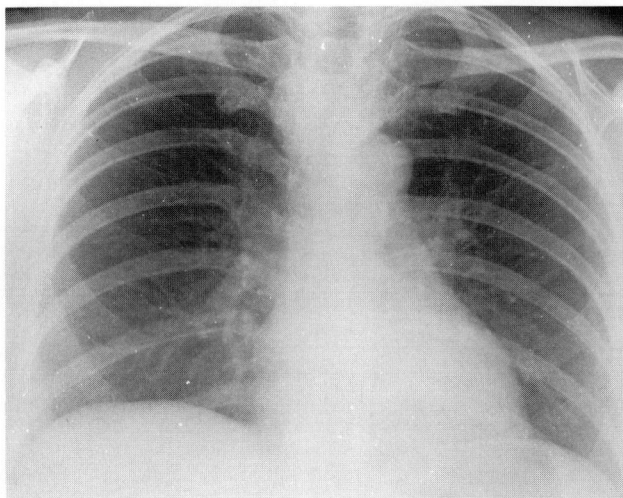

Figure 96a

Figure 96b

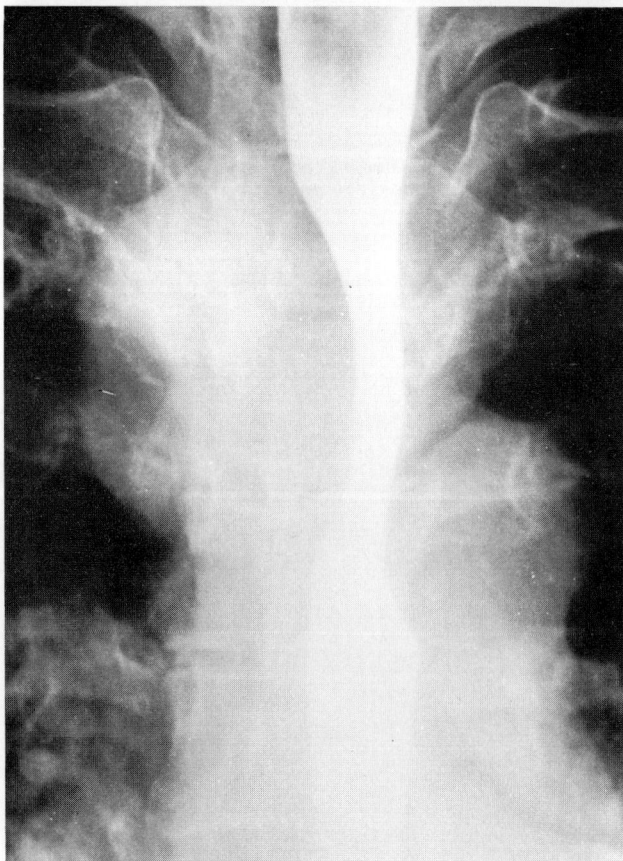

The plain films shows a mass to the right of the mediastinum at the level of the aortic arch. The barium swallow shows the mass to be posteriorly placed compressing but not invading the oesophagus. On CT the mass is seen to be separate from the great vessels and has a rounded shape, 'bulging' in a dependent direction. At surgery the lesion was found to be a foregut cyst.

Figure 96c

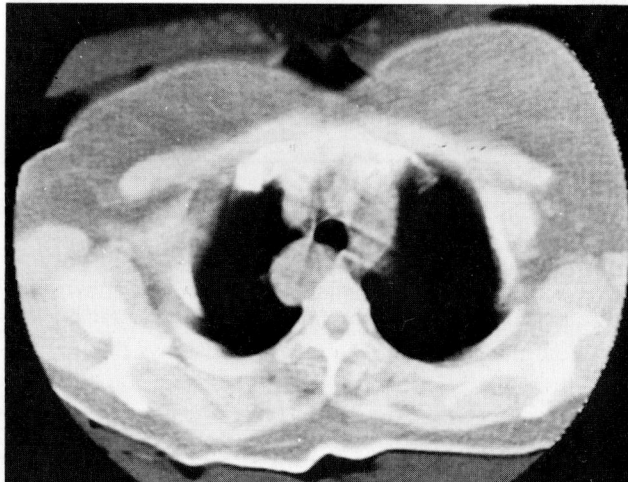

Case 97

A 64 year old lady with a history of carcinoma of the right breast treated with radiotherapy presented at follow-up with the following x-ray.

Figure 97a

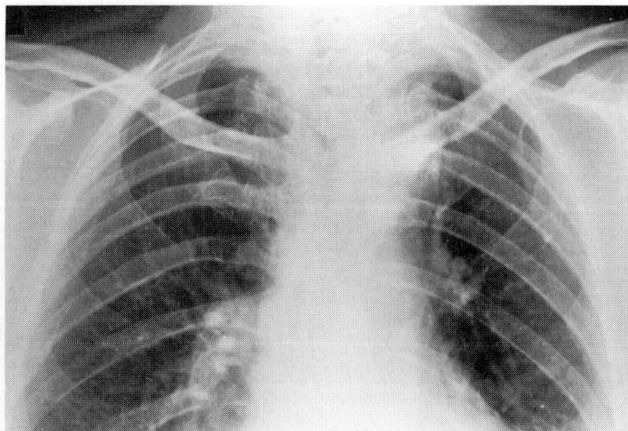

The chest radiograph showed an abnormal shape of the mediastinum with a bulge to the left superiorly. The aortic knuckle was obscured. CT was performed to determine whether or not there was enlargement of lymph nodes.

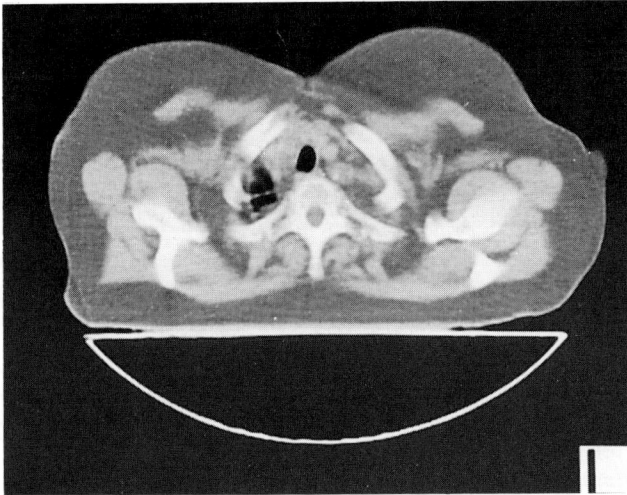

Figure 97b

Figure 97c

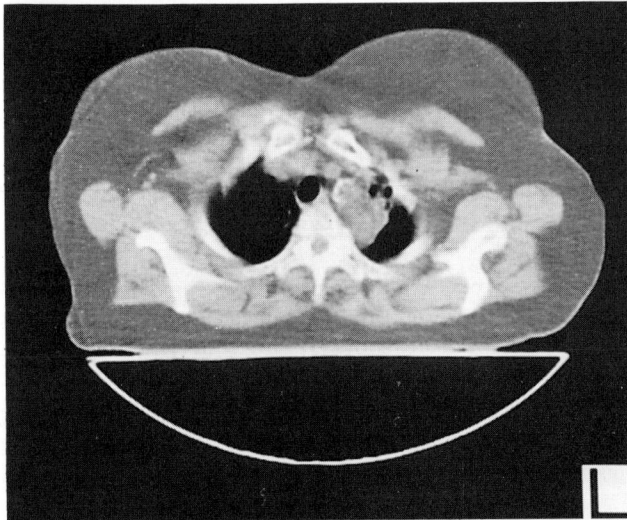

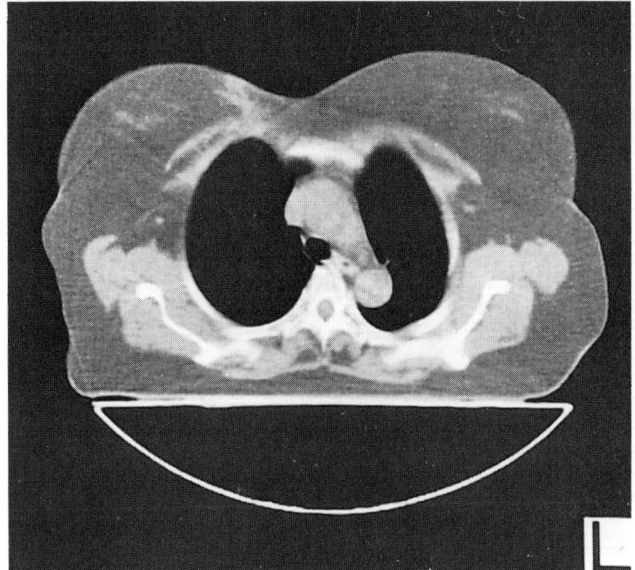

Figure 97e

Figure 97f

Figure 97d

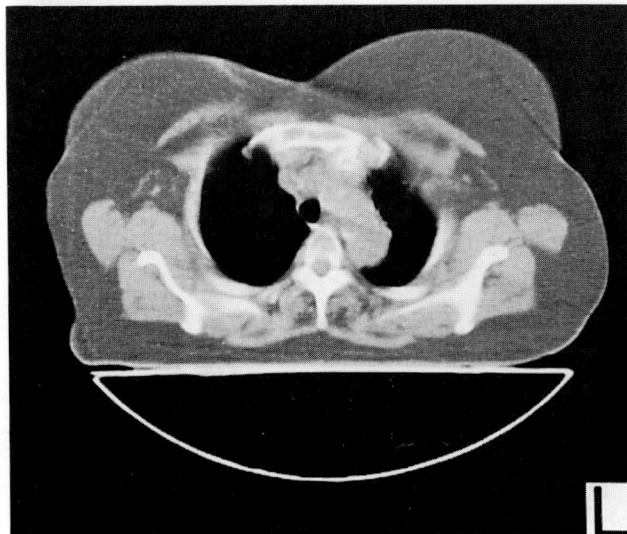

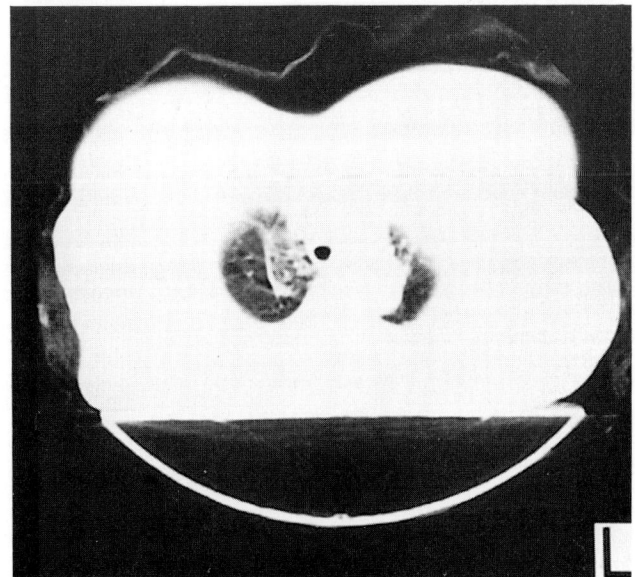

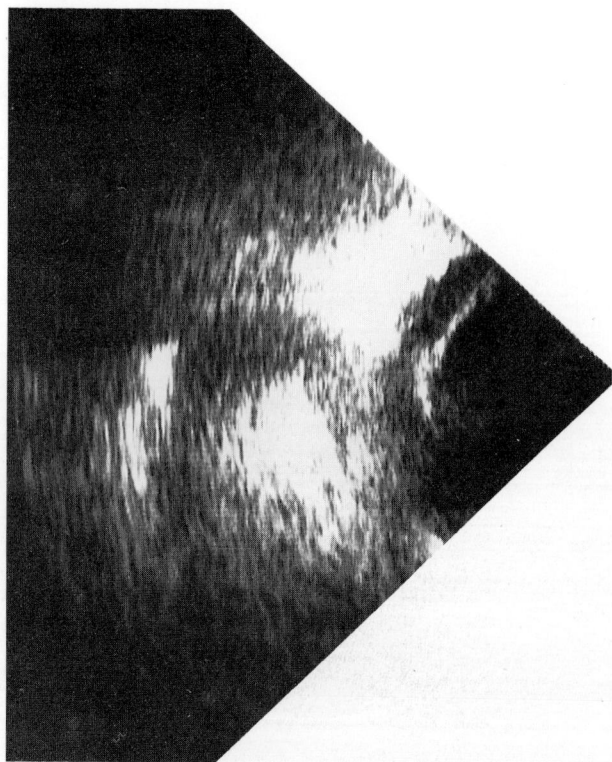

Figure 97g

Figure 97h

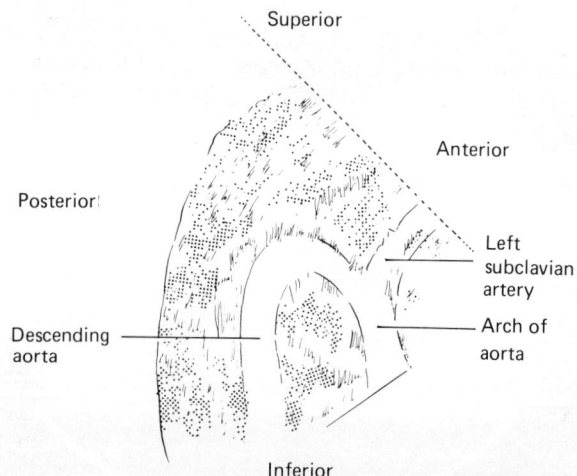

Pulmonary fibrosis was shown in both lung apices, no doubt due to the radiotherapy. There was calcification of the aorta and left subclavian artery and their position was distorted due to the fibrosis. Confirmation of the site of the aorta and subclavian was also obtained by real-time ultrasound which clearly showed the tortuous subclavian and the high position of the arch of the aorta.

Tracheal narrowing

Narrowing of the trachea can be due to lesions within the lumen, in the wall or outside the trachea.

Lesions in the lumen include foreign bodies, polyps, carcinoma of the larynx and trachea, tuberculosis and amyloidosis. Direct laryngoscopy and bronchoscopy are the investigations of choice but linear tomography or CT may help define the extent of the lesion.

Lesions affecting the wall again include tumours but also include abnormalities of the cartilage of the wall (relapsing polychondritis, tracheomalacia and tracheobronchomegaly). The latter can best be studied by fluoroscopy to show the effect on the trachea of inspiration and expiration. Fluoroscopy is also useful to study the tongue, epiglottis and larynx in patients with sleep apnoea syndrome.

Masses outside the trachea have been outlined in Table 18 and any of the masses that occur in the superior, middle or posterior mediastinum can compress the trachea if large enough.

Case 98

A baby boy of two months of age had dyspnoea and expiratory stridor from birth. The chest x-ray and spot films from fluoroscopy are shown (with a line-drawing of the fluoroscopic spot films).

Figure 98a

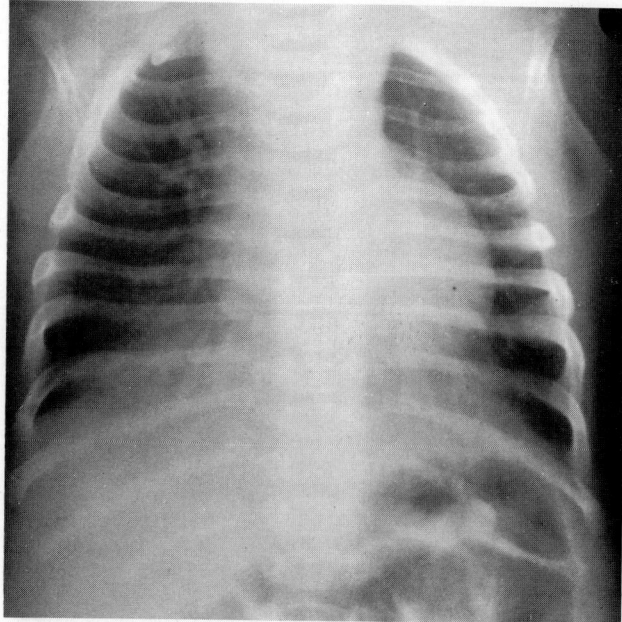

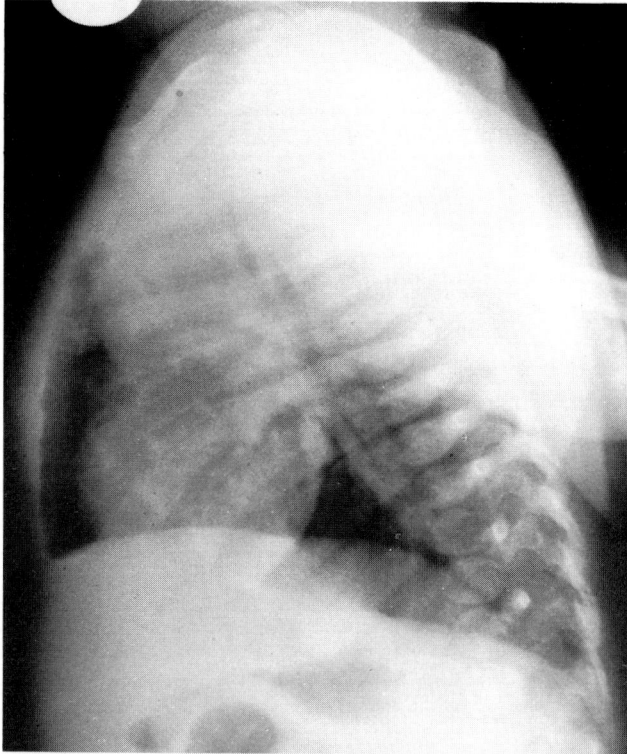

Figure 98b

The trachea is seen to collapse on expiration. These appearances are due to tracheomalacia.

Figure 98d

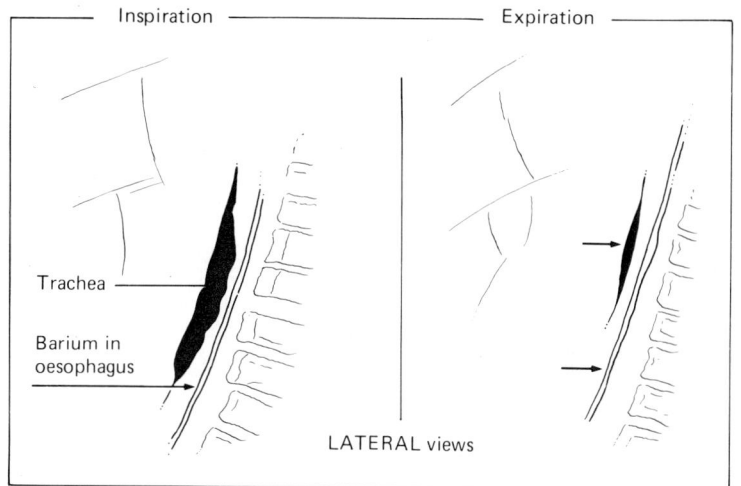

Inspiration — Expiration —

Trachea

Barium in oesophagus

LATERAL views

Figure 98c

Inspiration

Expiration

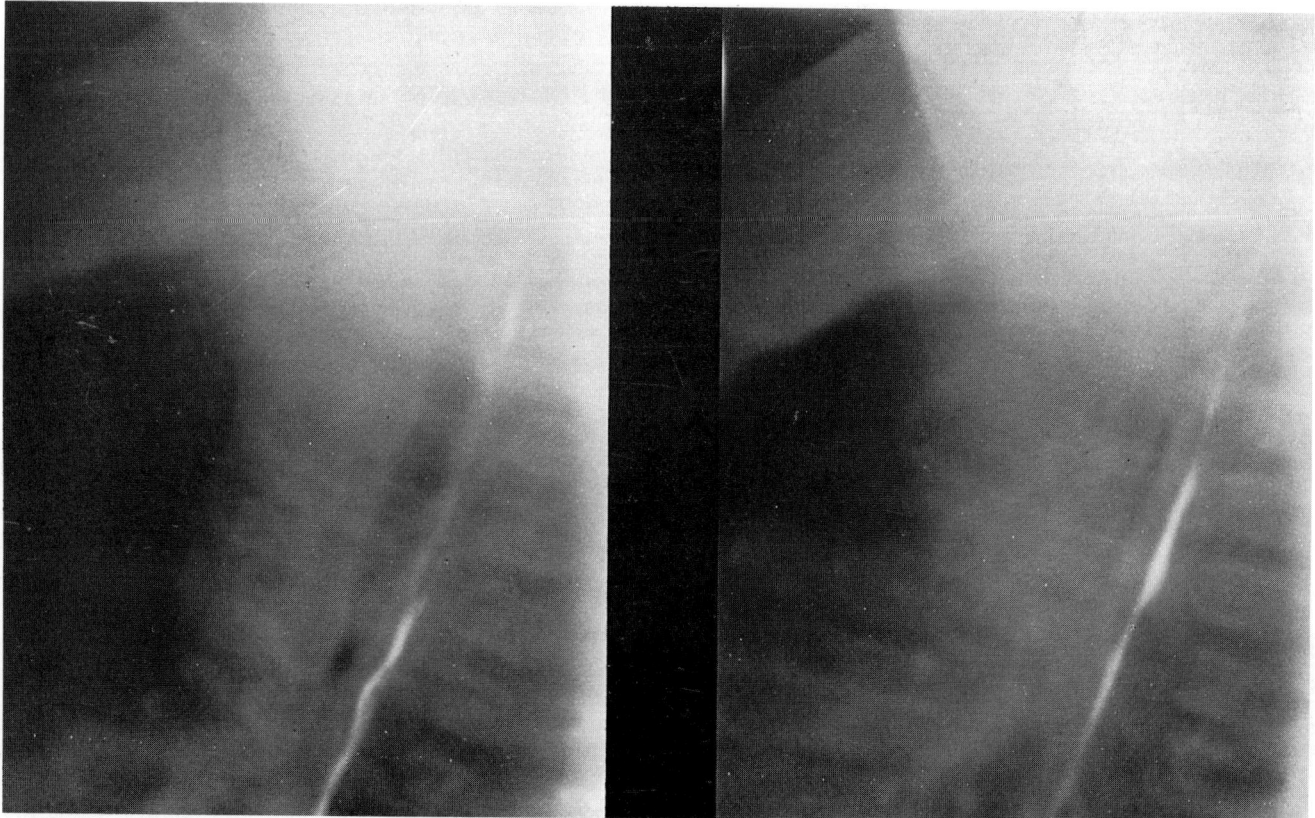

Case 99

A man aged 54 had a chest radiograph whilst being investigated for angina.

There is a large upper mediastinal mass with narrowing and displacement of the trachea. Clinical examination indicated that the mass extended into the neck.

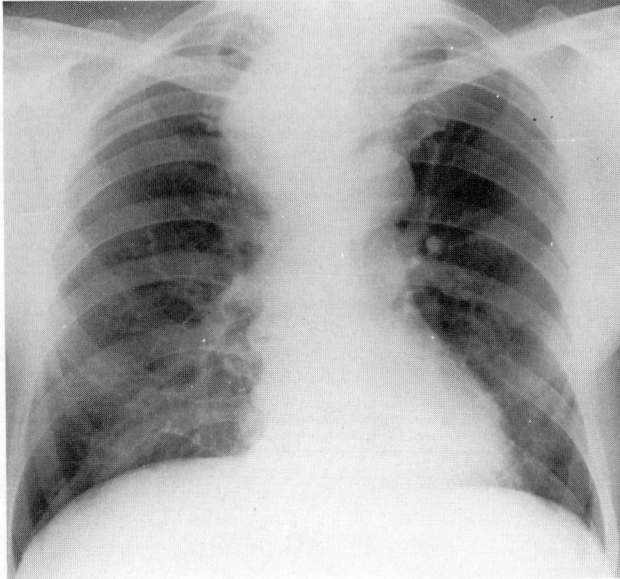

Figure 99a

Figure 99b

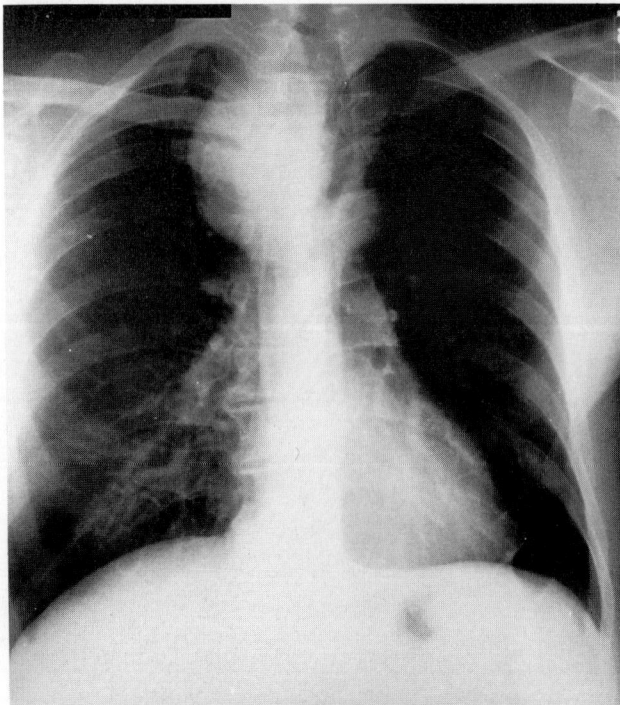

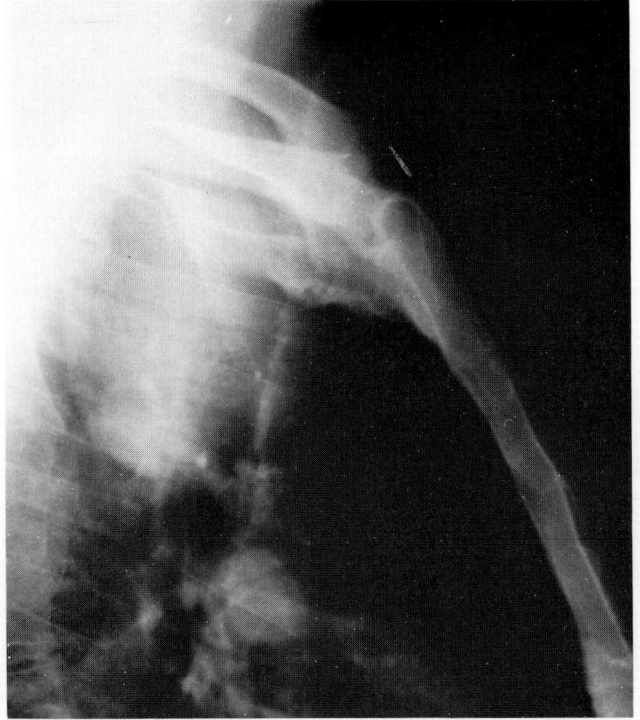

Figure 99c

The penetrated film shows displacement of the trachea but the compression is not definitely confirmed. The lateral view of the thoracic inlet shows posterior compression of the trachea.

The CT scans show the trachea to be narrowed with a crescentic cross section. The mass is posteriorly positioned in the lower part of the superior mediastinum but its origins in the thyroid are more easily shown on the higher scans (fig. 99d).

Figure 99d

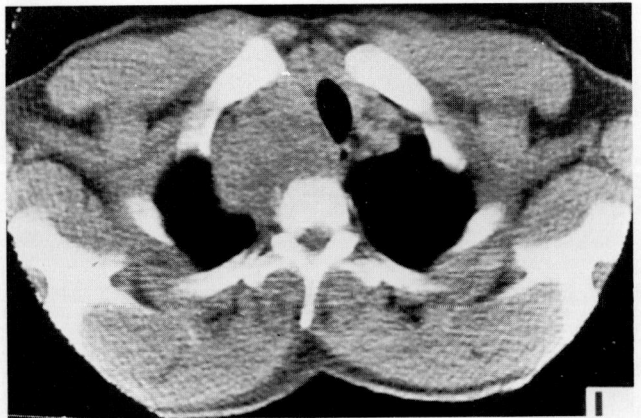

The histogram of attenuation values of the mass as shown by CT indicate that the mode and the mean are in the soft-tissue range. Notice that there is a distribution of values with a few high and a few low values—this is the

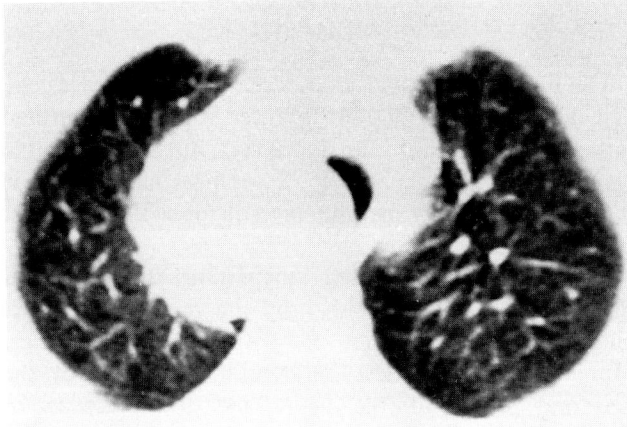

Figure 99e

Figure 99f

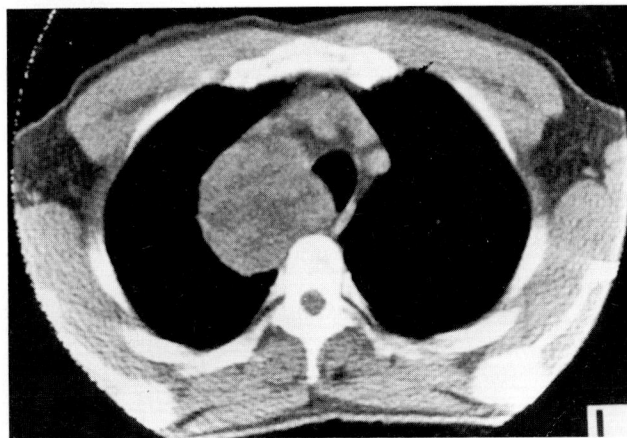

case with all masses measured by CT and it is the mode or the mean which can be used most easily for tissue differentiation. Diagnosis at surgery: large thyroid goitre.

Figure 99g

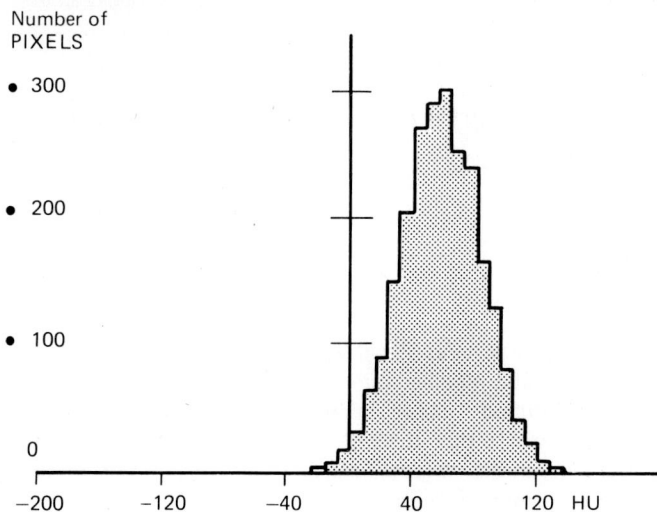

Number of PIXELS

Anterior and middle compartments of the mediastinum

In the anterior mediastinum, conditions that can give rise to a mass include a retrosternal thyroid, thymoma, thymic cyst, teratodermoid and lymphadenopathy. A certain degree of differentiation can again be made by computed tomography or ultrasound.

Ultrasound can be used to differentiate between vascular structures (such as aneurysms or tortuous arteries), cysts (e.g. thymic cysts), and solid masses (enlarged nodes, thymoma, teratodermoid). If the mass is fatty in nature, there may be increased echogenicity (lipoma, teratodermoid). Ultrasound can be used to make similar differentiation in the middle compartment of the mediastinum, although the extent to which lesions can be examined by ultrasound will depend on the shape of the patient and availability of an 'acoustic window'.

There are several catches when examining the chest with ultrasound. If the lesion being examined is at the furthest possible range of penetration of the ultrasound, it is difficult to distinguish between cysts and homogeneous tumour such as lymphoma. In all sites, if the ultrasound demonstrating a lesion shows it to be mainly transonic but containing a few echoes, it may be representing a cyst with semi-solid contents, an abscess, or a necrotic or homogeneous tumour. Fifty per cent of bronchogenic cysts, for example, have very thick turbid contents at surgery and some of these may appear to be semi-solid using ultrasound, and have soft tissue density on computed tomography.

Vascular structures can be distinguished from cysts by the presence of pulsation detectable on real-time scanning and blood flow detectable by Doppler studies. In particular it is possible to show the size of vessels and, therefore, to demonstrate the presence of aneurysmal dilatation, dissection, aberrant vessels and shunts and tortuous vessels. Ultrasound of the mediastinum is a valuable adjunct to plain chest films and may assist in the interpretation of computed tomography.

Computed tomography of the mediastinum can:

1 Show the site of a mass.

2 Show the extent of the lesion, particularly showing whether there is invasion of mediastinal structures, pleura, lungs or chest wall.

3 Demonstrate the radiodensity (attenuation) of the

lesion often allowing differentiation between fat, water (cysts), soft tissue and calcification.

4 By the use of intravenous contrast the great vessels can be clearly shown (see Cases 91 and 92).

5 Be used to guide percutaneous needle biopsy of a mediastinal mass.

If the mass is shown to be of soft tissue density, it may be important to proceed further for investigation. There may of course be other features that indicate the origin of the mass, for example, a known primary carcinoma, especially carcinoma of the breast or bronchus, or lymph nodes in the neck as in patients with lymphoma. If there are accessible nodes, they can be biopsied either by percutaneous needle biopsy or excision. There may be features on the CT scan that indicate a mass is malignant, for example, invasion of mediastinal structures or of the chest wall.

If the diagnosis cannot be made from other clinical details and the mass appears solid, it is often necessary to obtain a biopsy specimen either by surgery (e.g. mediastinotomy), by mediastinoscopy or by percutaneous needle biopsy. The latter can be undertaken with CT guidance.

In the middle compartment of the mediastinum the main structure is, of course, the heart and its pericardium. Many cardiac abnormalities cause enlargement of the heart shadow but particularly important are:

1 ischaemic heart disease,

2 valvular disease,

3 cardiomyopathies,

4 shunts,

5 pericardial effusion.

These conditions are to be covered in another book in this series covering the imaging of cardiovascular disease.

Other causes of a mass in the mid part of the mediastinum include enlarged lymph nodes, aneurysms, and lipoma. A specific abnormality arising near the trachea or bronchi is the bronchogenic cyst. A pulmonary mass, such as carcinoma of the bronchus, may arise adjacent to any part of the mediastinum and thus appear to be a mediastinal lesion.

Once again, if the patient presents with relatively few symptoms and few clinical pointers, computed tomography and/or ultrasound may be the best investigations following chest radiographs (PA and lateral). If cardiac disease is suspected, real-time ultrasound and Doppler studies may be indicated as the first line of investigation followed by either cardiac catheterization and angiography or radionuclide scanning of the heart. If a non-cardiac cause is suspected, CT may be the investigation that is most likely to give the answer.

There may be pointers suggesting that there is cardiovascular disease, either by the presence of heart failure, murmurs, cyanosis or other clinical findings. Moreover, on the chest radiograph, alteration of the size and shape of the heart and the presence of pulmonary oligaemia, pulmonary plethora or pulmonary oedema are pointers towards cardiovascular causes of mediastinal abnormality.

Case 100

Jane, now aged eight years, first developed cyanosis at the age of three months. ECG showed right ventricular strain and she had a systolic murmur. Her present chest x-ray is shown and the venous phase of a pulmonary arteriogram.

Figure 100a

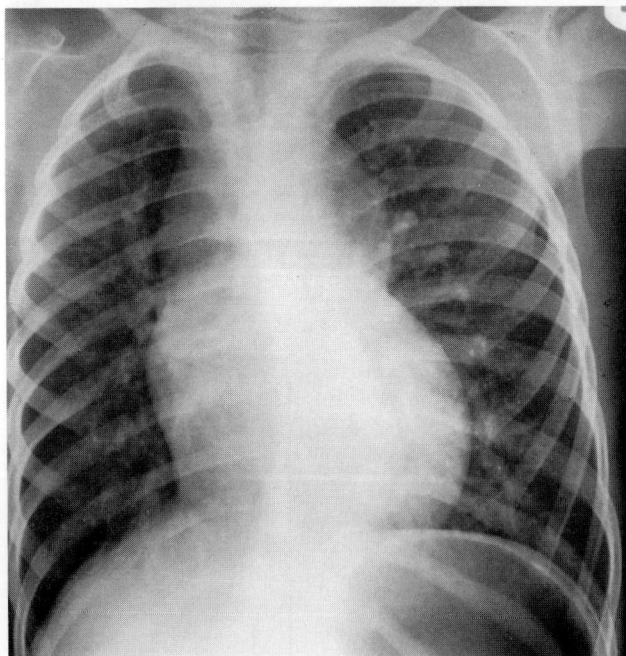

The striking radiological abnormality is the appearance of the heart and mediastinum. The heart is enlarged and there is a rounded 'mass' immediately superior to it. This appearance is due to total anomalous pulmonary venous drainage and is variously called a 'snowman' appearance, a figure of eight or a 'cottage loaf'.

THE MEDIASTINAL MASS 149

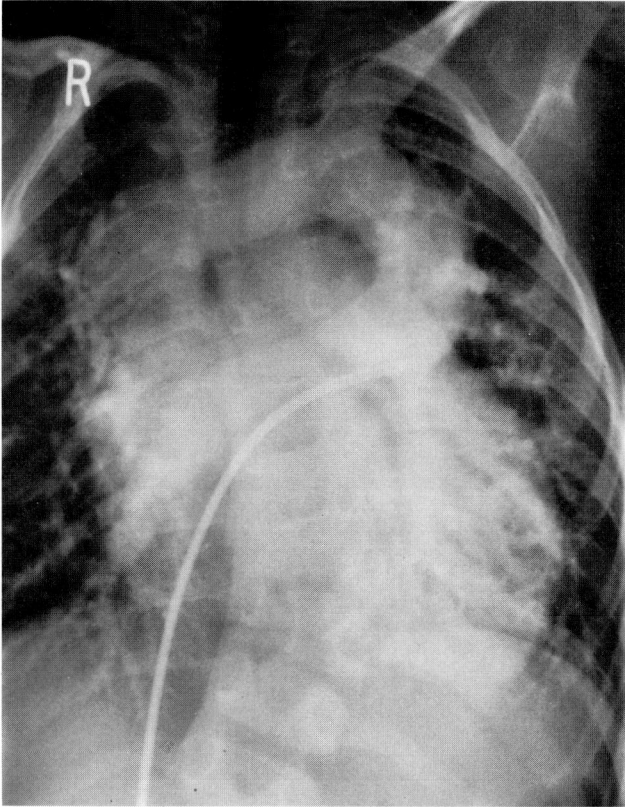

Figure 100b

The angiogram shows the venous phase—the contrast medium has been injected into the main pulmonary artery and at the time the radiograph was taken the pulmonary veins are opacified. There is abnormal drainage across the mediastinum from the right side into a persistent left superior vena cava. Total anomalous pulmonary venous drainage is a form of congenital heart disease in which all the pulmonary veins connect anomalously to the right atrium or one of its tributaries. Systemic and pulmonary venous blood both return to the right atrium where mixing occurs. In order for the patient to live, there must be a patent foramen ovale or atrial septal defect. The mixed venous blood passes into the systemic circulation via the atrial septal defect and through the tricuspid valve into the right ventricle and thence to the lungs. There is cyanosis due to the mixing effect and pulmonary arterial hypertension due to increased pulmonary flow.

Total anomalous pulmonary venous drainage is classified radiologically into four types.

(i) Supracardiac (commonest variety)

The pulmonary veins are either connected to a left superior vena cava (as in this case), or to a right superior vena cava or to the azygos vein.

(ii) Cardiac

The pulmonary veins connect directly to the right atrium or coronary sinus.

(iii) Infracardiac

The pulmonary veins connect to either the portal vein, the ductus venosus, inferior vena cava or hepatic vein. This often results in pulmonary oedema due to obstruction of the pulmonary veins (see Case 7 for an example of partial anomalous pulmonary venous drainage).

(iv) Mixed

A mixture of the above anomalous connections.

In Jane's case, as mentioned above, there is connection of the pulmonary veins to a vertical vein known as the left superior vena cava. This vein then joins the left innominate (brachiocephalic) vein and blood flows from this into the right superior vena cava and thus into the right atrium. The 'snowman' appearance is due to the dilatation of both superior vena cavae.

Case 101

A man, aged 39, presented with a mass to the right of his heart obscuring the right heart border. CT was performed.

Figure 101a

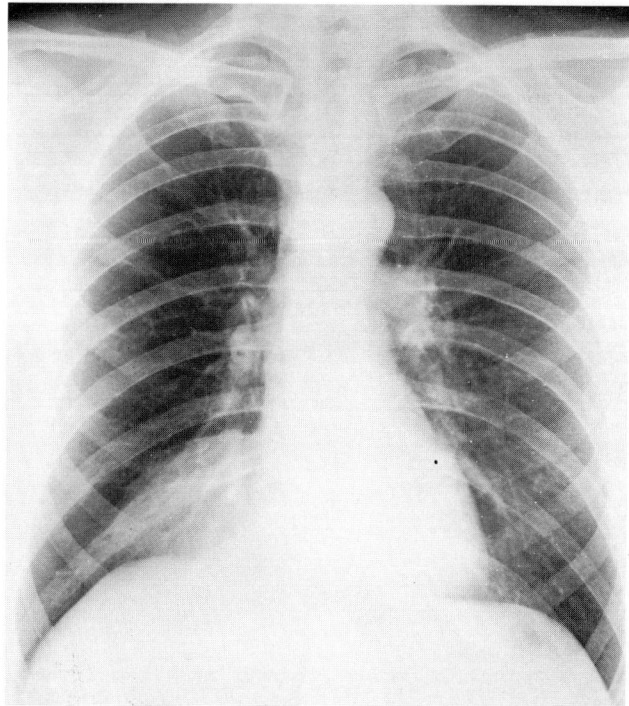

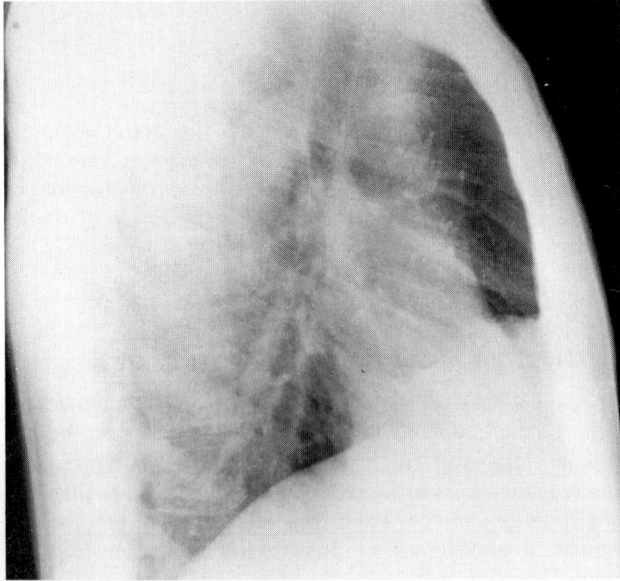

Figure 101b

Figure 101c

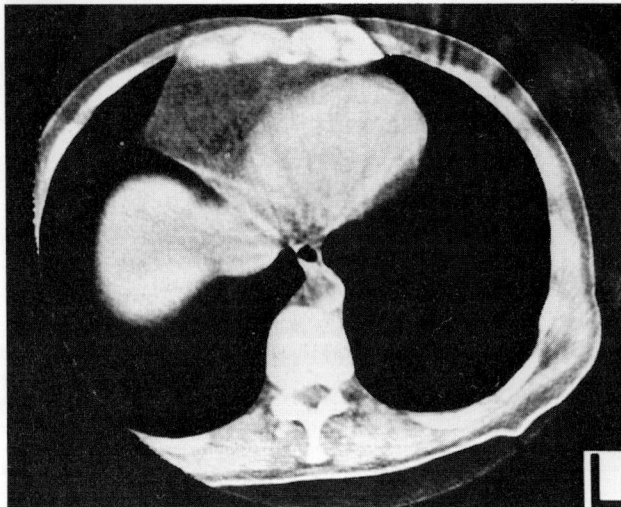

Figure 101d

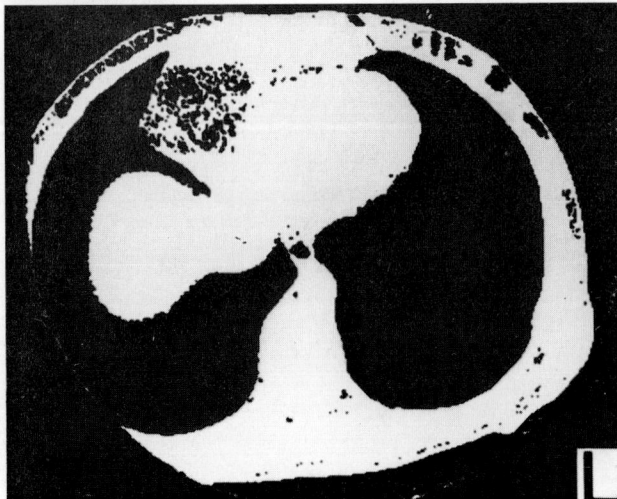

The mass was shown by CT to have a mean density of −90 HU which is the density of fat. In figure 101c the 'window' has been set on measure. Comparison with the subcutaneous fat also shows the lesion to be of the same density.

Conclusion: large fat pad or lipoma.

Case 102

Man, aged 40, with widened mediastinum and an opacity in the right upper zone. Sternotomy and biopsy showed malignant thymoma.

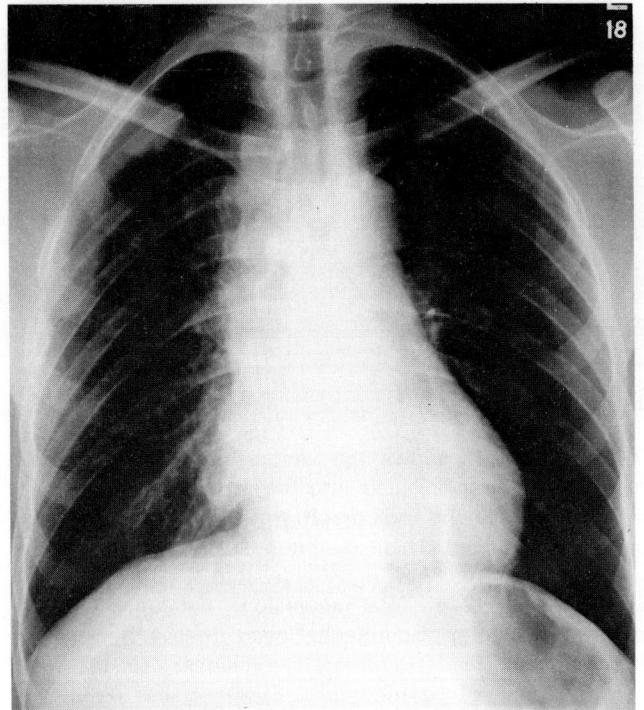

Figure 102a

CT was performed. This showed the mass in the mediastinum obliterating the outline of the great vessels and lobulated pleural thickening all around the right pleural space. Calcification is seen in the mediastinal mass.

Figure 102b

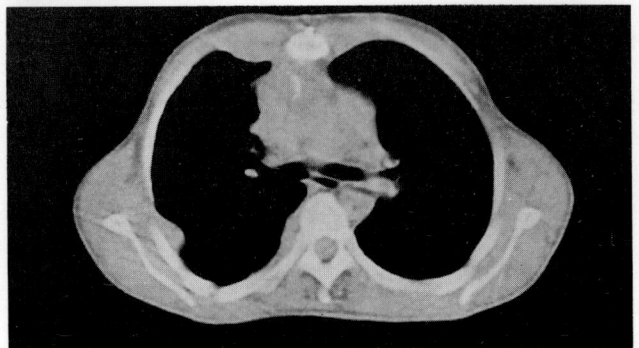

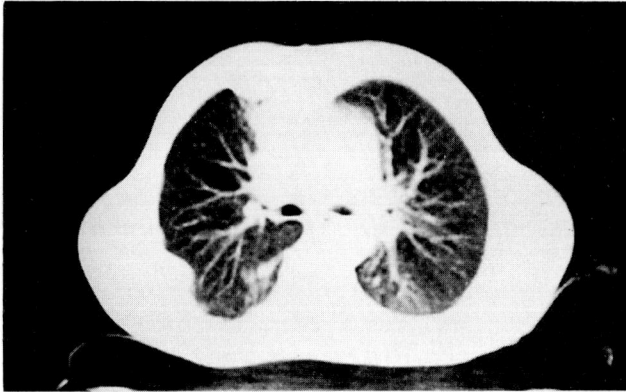

Figure 102c

Figure 102d

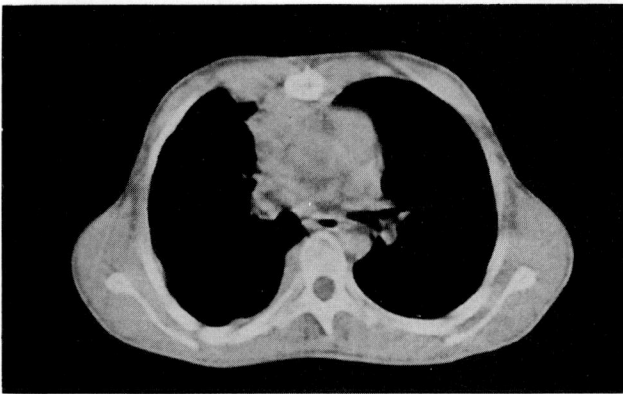

Figure 102e

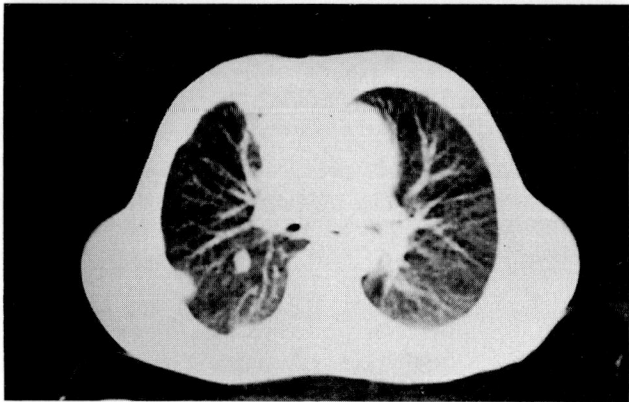

An opacity is also seen in the middle of the lung field. This lies in the oblique fissure. Malignant thymoma typically spreads locally by creeping around the pleura and mediastinum and 'invasive' may therefore be a better term than malignant [42].

Thymomas occur in 15 per cent of patients with myasthenia gravis. It is important to detect the tumours in these patients since 30 per cent of thymomas are invasive. Thus, if a lobulated mass is detected in the thymus or the gland is asymmetrically enlarged, its removal is mandatory.

Case 103 (A)

(With the permission of the Bristol Medico-Chirurgical Journal [73].)

A 57 year old publican was transferred to the chest physicians with a history of pyrexia, productive cough and purulent sputum. He gave a history of chronic productive cough with mucoid sputum since childhood and was a smoker of 40 cigarettes a day for many years. Investigation of his respiratory function at the time of referral showed a reduced peak flow rate of 155 litres/minute and an obstructive pattern on spirometry with FEV1 of 1.3 litres and FVC 3.15 litres. These results were not significantly changed following administration of a bronchodilator. His sputum grew *Haemophilus influenzae*.

His chest radiograph had shown an area of consolidation in the lingula which proved slow to resolve in spite of antibiotic treatment but had almost cleared when the PA chest x-ray (fig. 103a) was taken.

Figure 103a

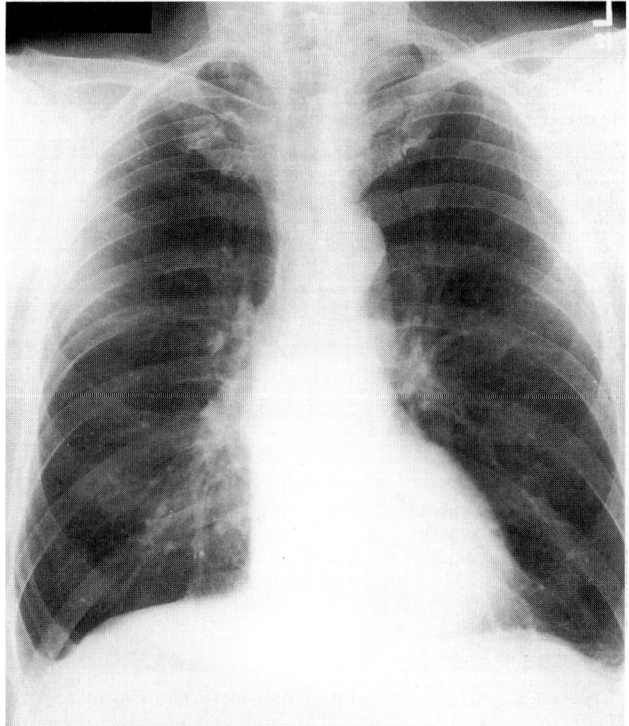

The lateral radiograph showed a well defined, rounded opacity posterior to the heart lying in or adjacent to the mediastinum (figs. 103a and 103b). A CT scan of the thorax showed opacification in the lingula due to a localized area of consolidation and a well defined, right paramediastinal opacity posterior to the right main bronchus which was thought to represent a neoplasm in the apical segment of the right lower lobe (fig. 103c). Bronchoscopy was accordingly performed and was normal.

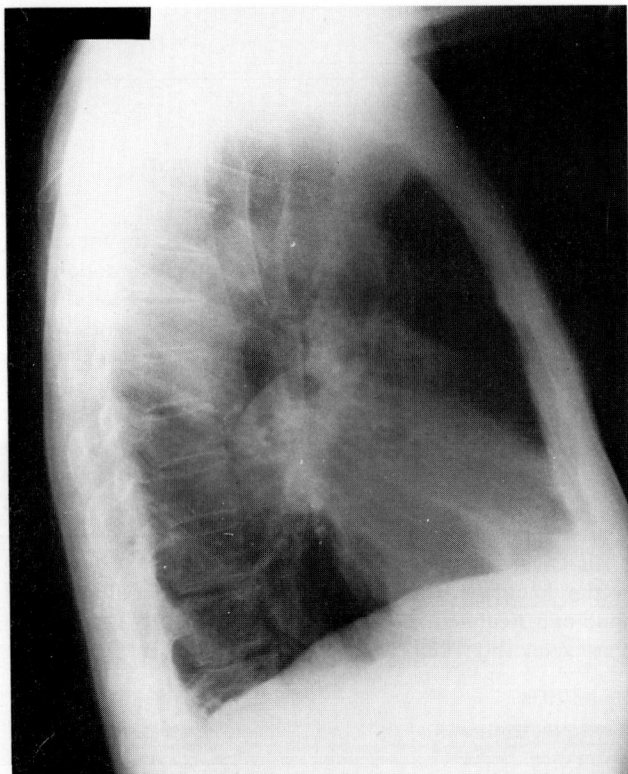

Figure 103b

Figure 103c

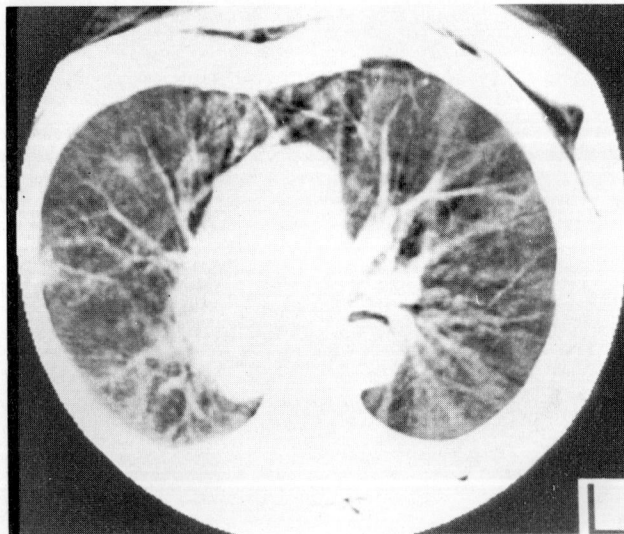

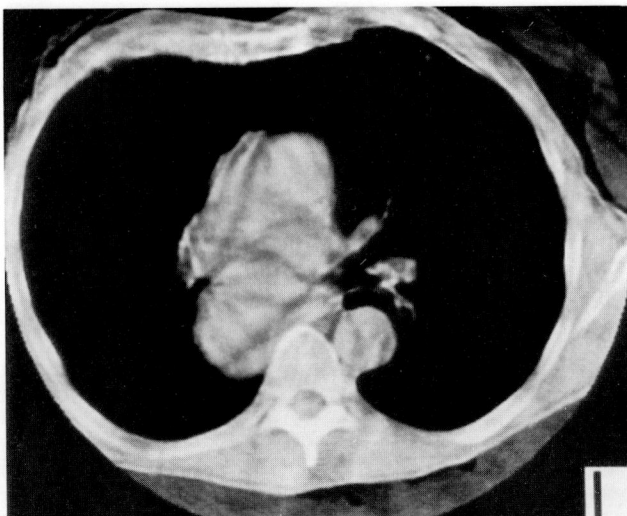

Figure 103d

Figure 103e

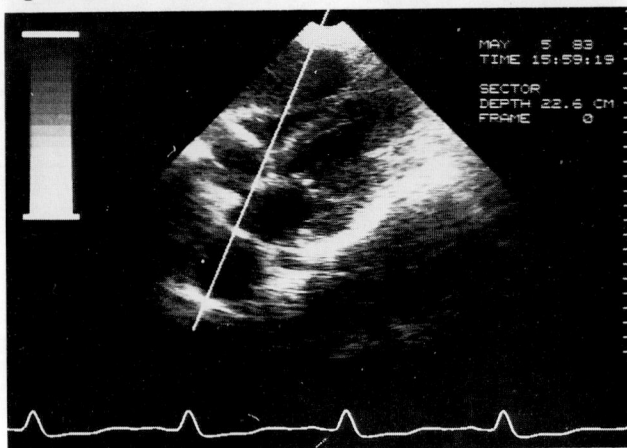

Figure 103f

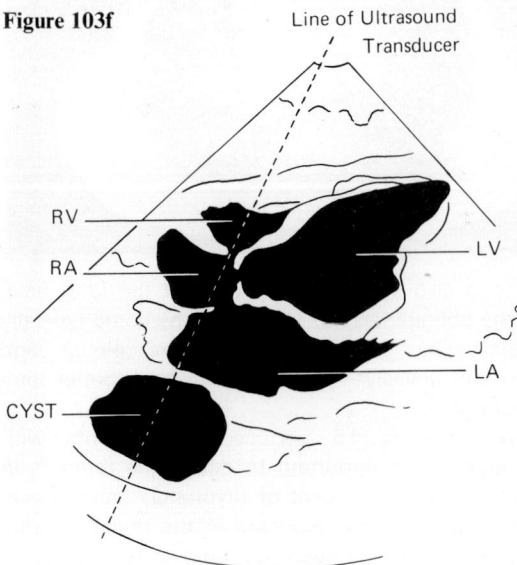

Because of the well defined nature of the lesion and the normal bronchoscopy the possibility of a benign lesion was raised. Two-dimensional ultrasound was then performed using the heart as an ultrasonic window.

This revealed a well defined echo-free structure immediately behind the left atrium consistent with a cyst (figs. 103d, 103e and 103f). Doppler showed no flow in the mass. A diagnosis of bronchogenic (bronchial) cyst was therefore made.

The ultrasound also showed myocardial function to be poor.

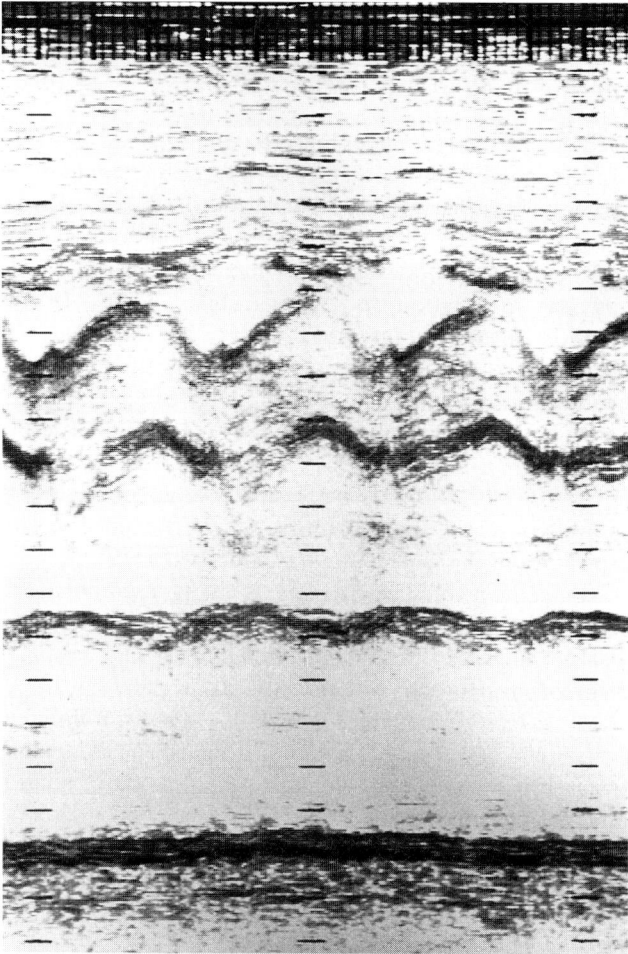

Figure 103g M-mode echocardiogram

Bronchogenic cysts are congenital and benign and those in the lungs are rarely symptomatic unless they become infected [74]. Those which occur in the mediastinum are more likely to be mucus-filled, opaque on chest radiograph and radiologically indistinguishable from other mediastinal tumours. Because of their position and proximity to the large bronchi, symptoms may arise as a result of compression or displacement of other mediastinal structures and include exertional dyspnoea, persistent cough or even symptoms of major airway obstruction [75, 76]. A cyst may become infected and behave like a chronic lung abscess, producing recurrent fever, productive cough or haemoptysis if rupture into the bronchial tree occurs. Atelectasis due to a mediastinal bronchogenic cyst is a rare but well recognized hazard in infants which has also been reported in adults (77, 78).

Case 103 (B)

The CT scan of the thorax in another patient with a bronchogenic cyst is shown in figure 103h. In this case the cyst was found to be of water density by measurement of the pixel values within the small square region of interest. The great vessels were opacified by contrast medium administered intravenously. The diagnosis was confirmed at surgery (*courtesy of Dr Clive Perry*).

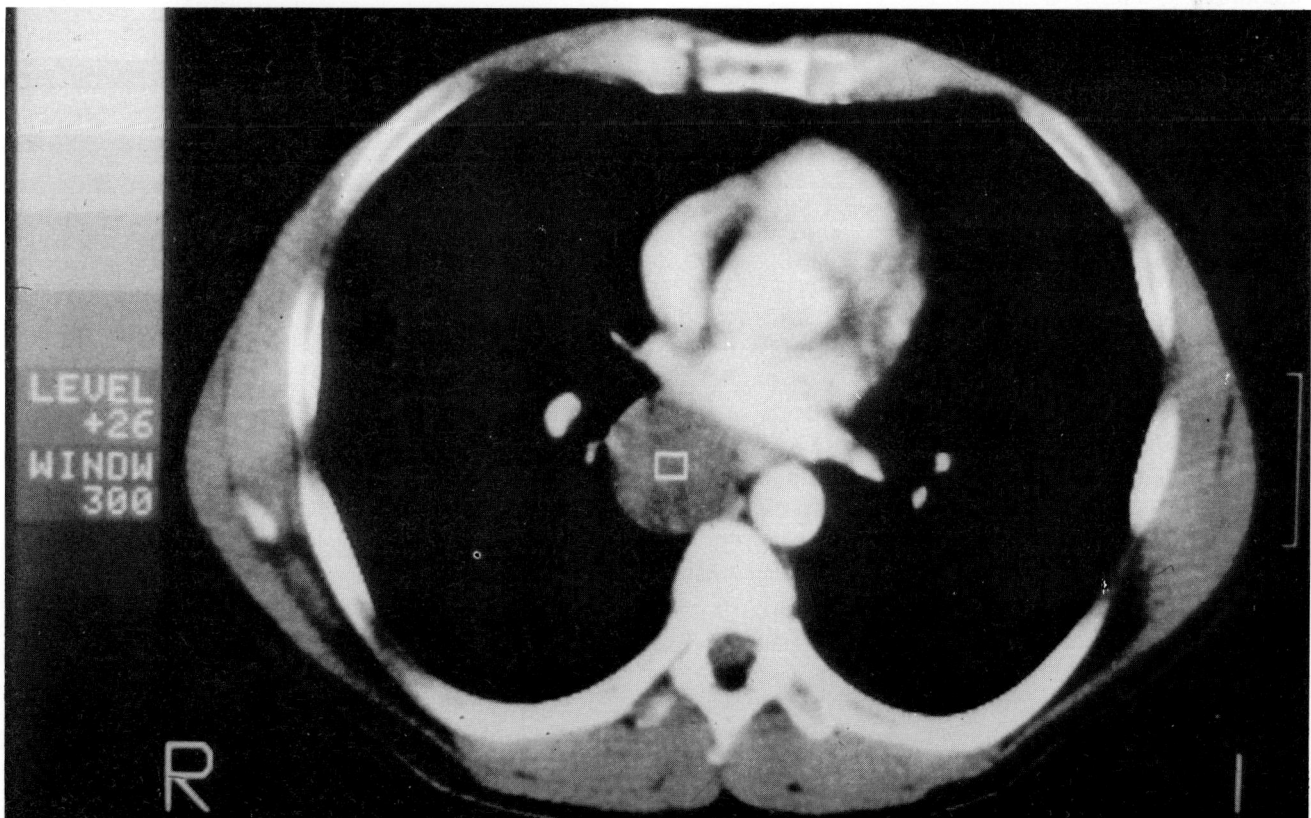

Posterior mediastinum

Again the main differentiation is between the solid, cystic or vascular lesions. In the posterior mediastinum common causes of a swelling include aortic aneurysm, oesophageal abnormality, various reduplication and bronchogenic cysts, lymph node masses and tumours of neurogenic origin. In any site in the mediastinum it is possible to have an abscess and in the posterior mediastinum these may be associated with spinal abnormalities, particularly tuberculosis, or pyogenic.

Depending on the clinical condition and the plain x-ray appearances a number of different investigations may be undertaken. If the patient presents with gastrointestinal complaints or dysphagia, a *barium* examination may provide the answer. Oesophageal abnormalities that may present with mediastinal widening include hiatus hernia, carcinoma of the oesophagus, achalasia, scleroderma and associated conditions such as reduplication cysts.

If there are any neurological symptoms, either *computed tomography* or linear tomography, depending upon availability, and *myelography* are the investigations that may give the diagnosis. Possible causes include neurofibroma, ganglioneuroma and lateral thoracic meningoceles. Abnormalities may arise from the vertebral column itself and these include metastatic deposits, primary malignant and benign bone tumours.

Ultrasound of the posterior mediastinum can only be performed if the lesion is large or can be visualized behind the heart or from below the xiphisternum. Subject to certain reservations, discussed on page 147, it is possible to demonstrate aortic aneurysms, cysts and solid masses.

The most common vascular cause of a large mass in the posterior mediastinum is, of course, an aortic aneurysm. This is best investigated by *aortography*. *Digital vascular imaging* can also be used in order to show whether or not there is a fusiform aneurysm or a dissection.

Carcinoma of the bronchus sometimes occurs in the periphery of the lung and may abut the mediastinum. It is thus not always possible to tell between a pulmonary lesion abutting the mediastinum or a mediastinal lesion that is projecting out into the lung. If there is a possibility of a lesion being pulmonary rather than mediastinal, the investigations for diagnosis of a pulmonary mass should be undertaken as discussed in Chapter 2. If bronchogenic carcinoma is suspected, sputum should be sent for cytology and bronchoscopy may be necessary.

Mediastinal lymph nodes

Mediastinal lymph nodes may be enlarged in any part of the mediastinum (superior, anterior, middle or posterior compartments). They are discussed also in Chapter 2 (Case 9) in reference to a pulmonary mass and mediastinal nodes and in Chapter 12 (Cases 83, 84 and 88) in relation to enlarged hilar nodes. In the anterior mediastinum they may be sampled by mediastinotomy. In the middle compartment of the mediastinum, lymph node sampling can usually be performed by mediastinoscopy particularly in order to sample the free tracheal nodes. In the posterior mediastinum biopsy is usually undertaken at thoracotomy. In many centres now CT-guided needle aspiration of the mediastinum is undertaken [19].

Magnetic resonance imaging is being used in a few centres now for studying mediastinal abnormalities [79]. Using magnetic resonance imaging it is easy to distinguish between vascular structures and causes of masses. The particular T1 and T2 times of different tissues enable fat to be easily distinguished and results from early experiments with spectroscopy using nuclear magnetic resonance indicate that it may be possible to determine parameters indicating whether a mass is malignant or benign.

Case 104

A woman aged 55 underwent coronary artery bypass grafting for angina. In the post-operative period she suffered from dysphagia and had one episode of inhalation of food. Chest radiographs are shown.

Figure 104a

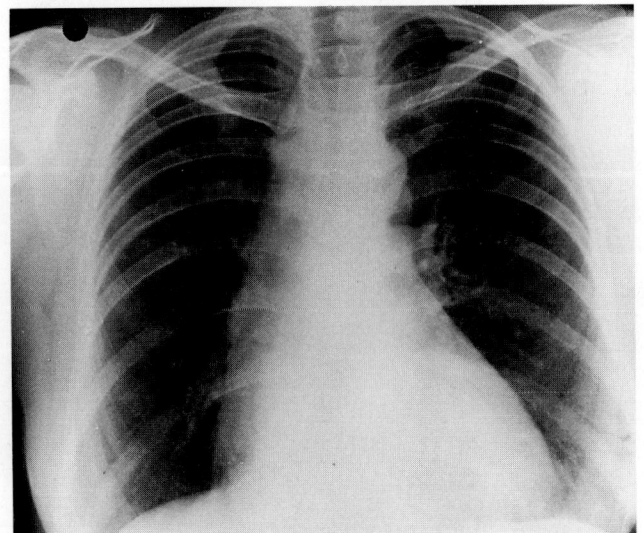

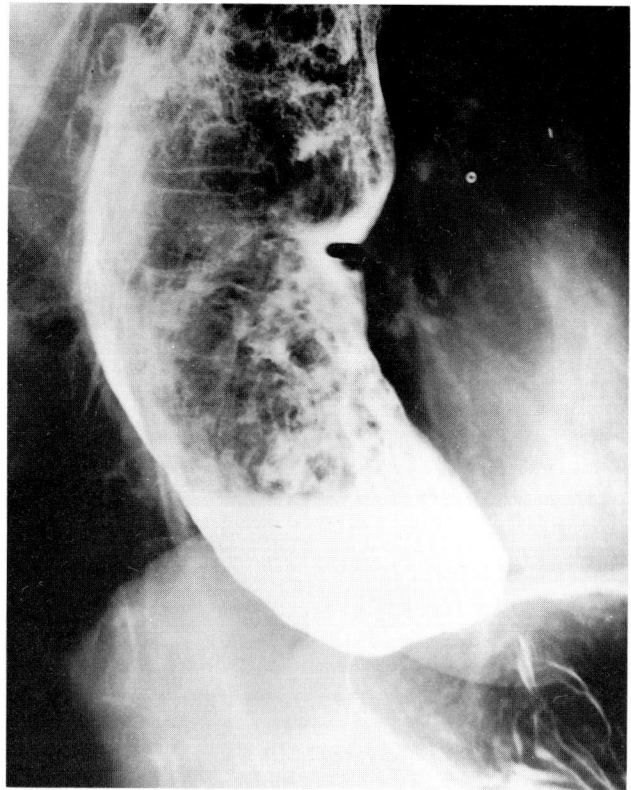

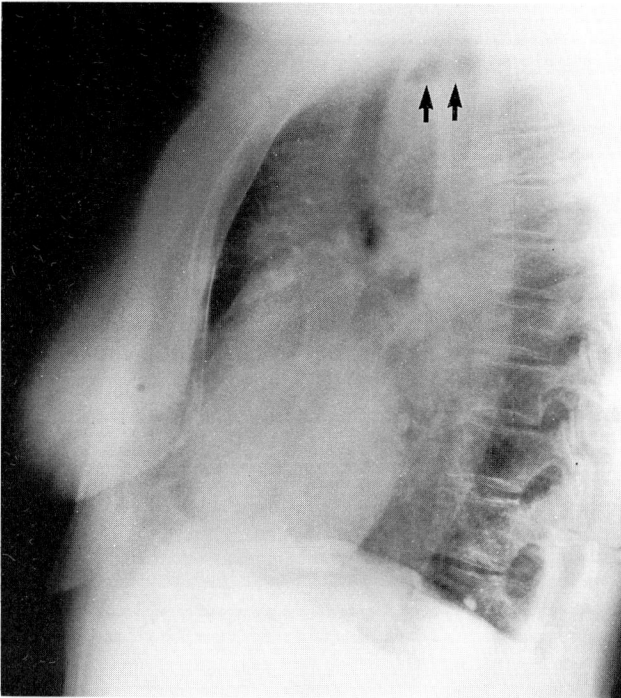

Figure 104b

Figure 104c

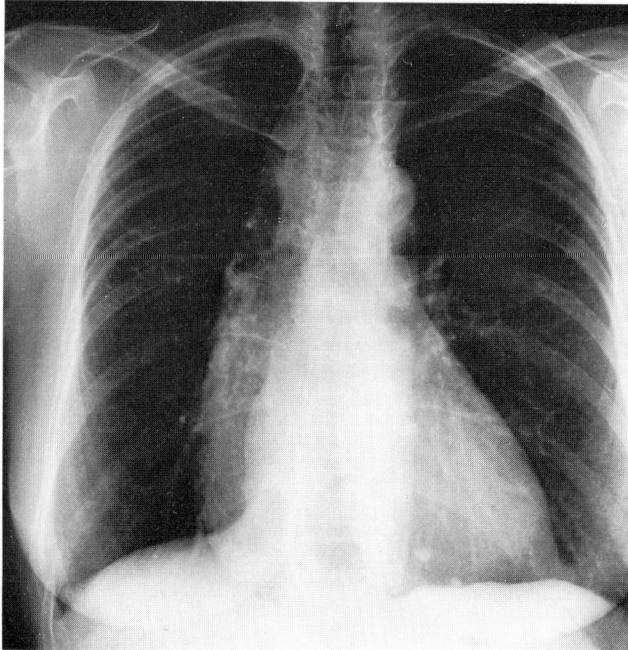

The PA and penetrated chest films show widening of the mediastinum with a double shadow and a patchy opacification. On the lateral there is a small fluid level (*arrowed*).

Barium swallow confirmed the suspected diagnosis of achalasia. (*This case courtesy of Dr J Virjee.*)

Figure 104d

Case 105

A man of 55 presented with hoarseness of the voice. The PA chest radiograph and linear tomography are shown.

The PA chest x-ray showed an unusual mass adjacent to

Figure 105a

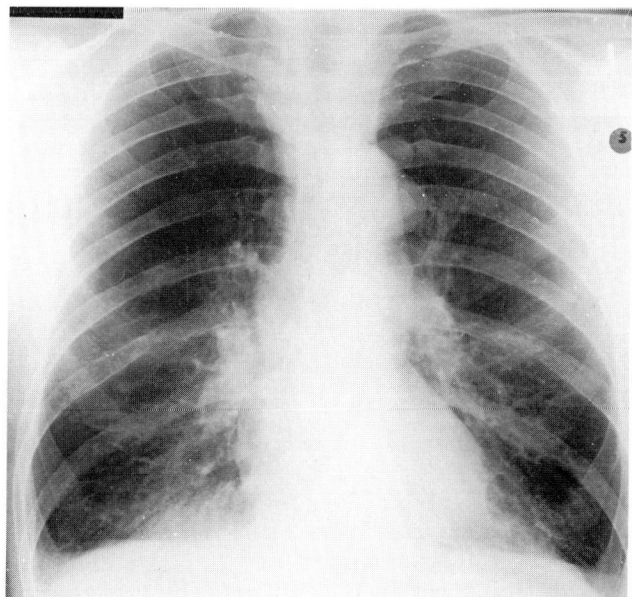

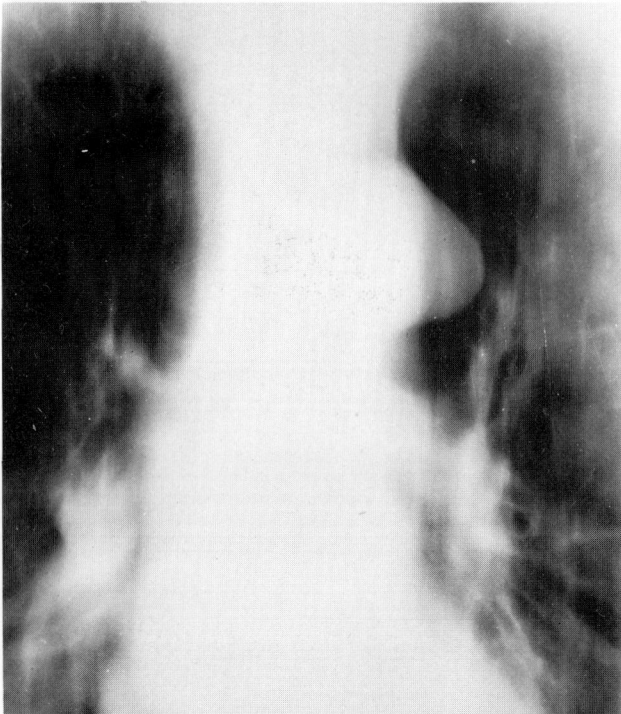

Figure 105b

the aortic knuckle and the site of the abnormality at the aortic knuckle was confirmed by linear tomography.

Computed tomography shows a bulge from the arch of the aorta and there is calcification in the wall of the abnormality. The appearances are those of a traumatic aortic aneurysm and on close questioning the patient admitted to having a road traffic accident immediately before the onset of the hoarseness of the voice.

Of particular interest, in addition to the traumatic aortic aneurysm, were the pulmonary changes. The CT settings to show the lungs (figs. 105b–g) show gross emphysema throughout both lung fields and some fibrosis. This had not been suspected from the chest radiograph, although in

Figure 105c

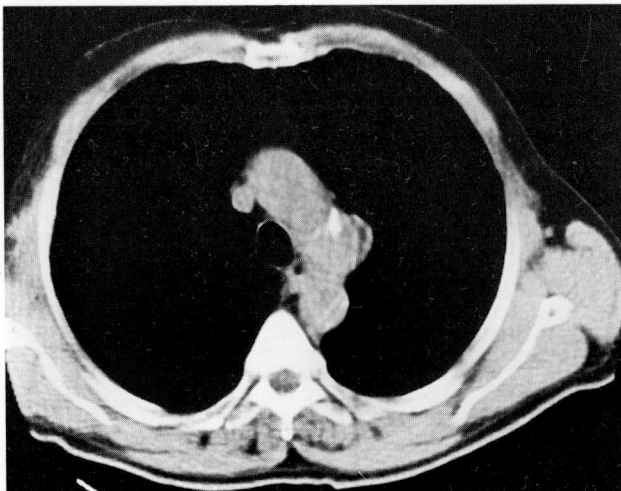

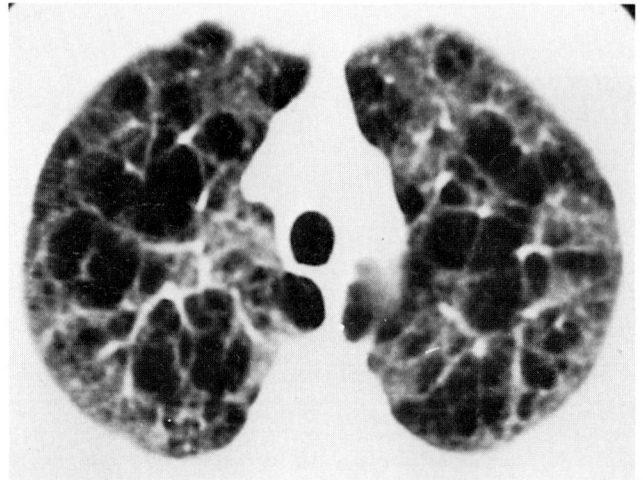

Figure 105d
Figure 105e

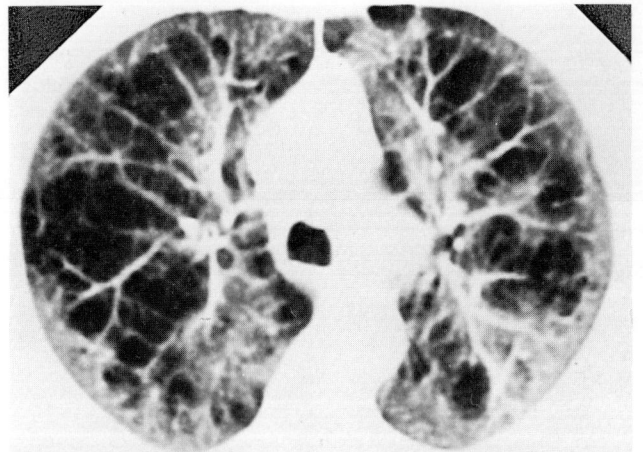

Figure 105f

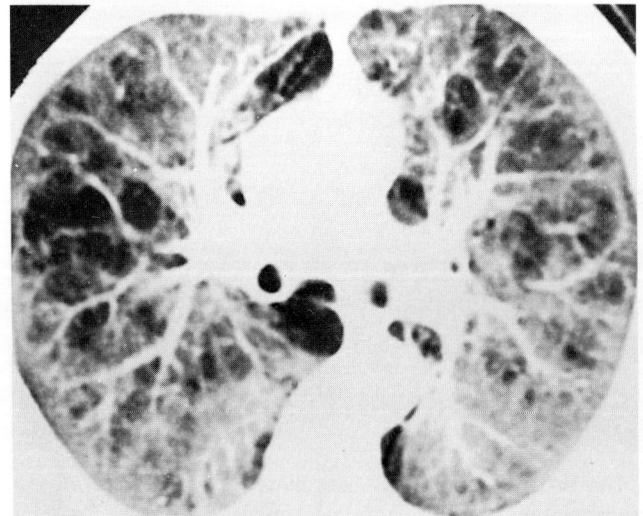

retrospect it is clear that there is slight over-expansion and abnormality of pulmonary vascularity on the chest x-ray. The patient had an arch aortogram and subsequent successful surgery to the aorta.

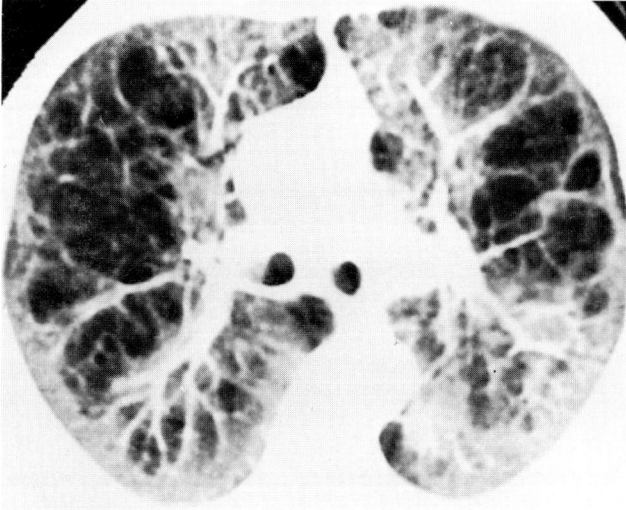

Figure 105g

This case illustrates a golden rule: 'Whenever the CT of the chest is being performed, pictures must be obtained to show both mediastinal and soft tissues, and the lung fields.' It is always best to report the films and to view them on the viewing console. This is not, however, always possible and in practice it is important to obtain good hard copies. When looking at the lung fields it is best not to use too wide a window setting or the lung parenchyma will not be visible. In Bristol a level of around −750 and a window of 400 or 800 (HU) are the usual settings.

Case 106

A man aged 38 with a history of previous thymoma presented with further chest pain. A chest x-ray and penetrated coned view are shown.

Figure 106a

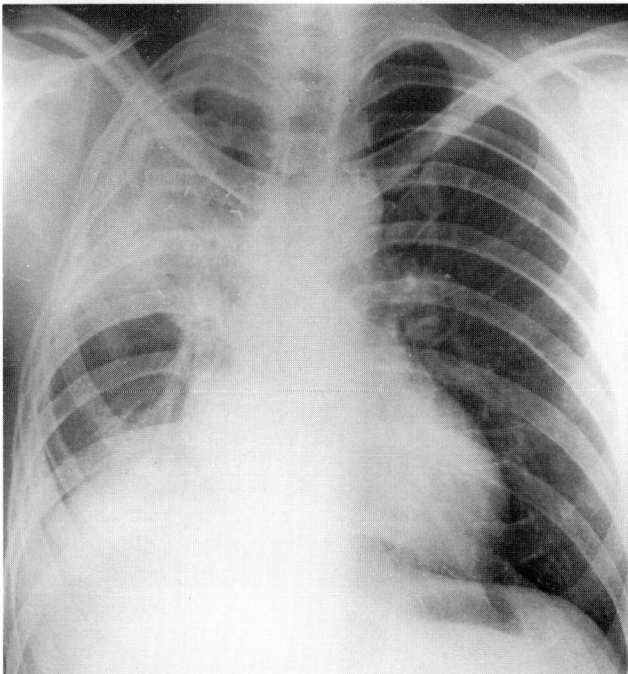

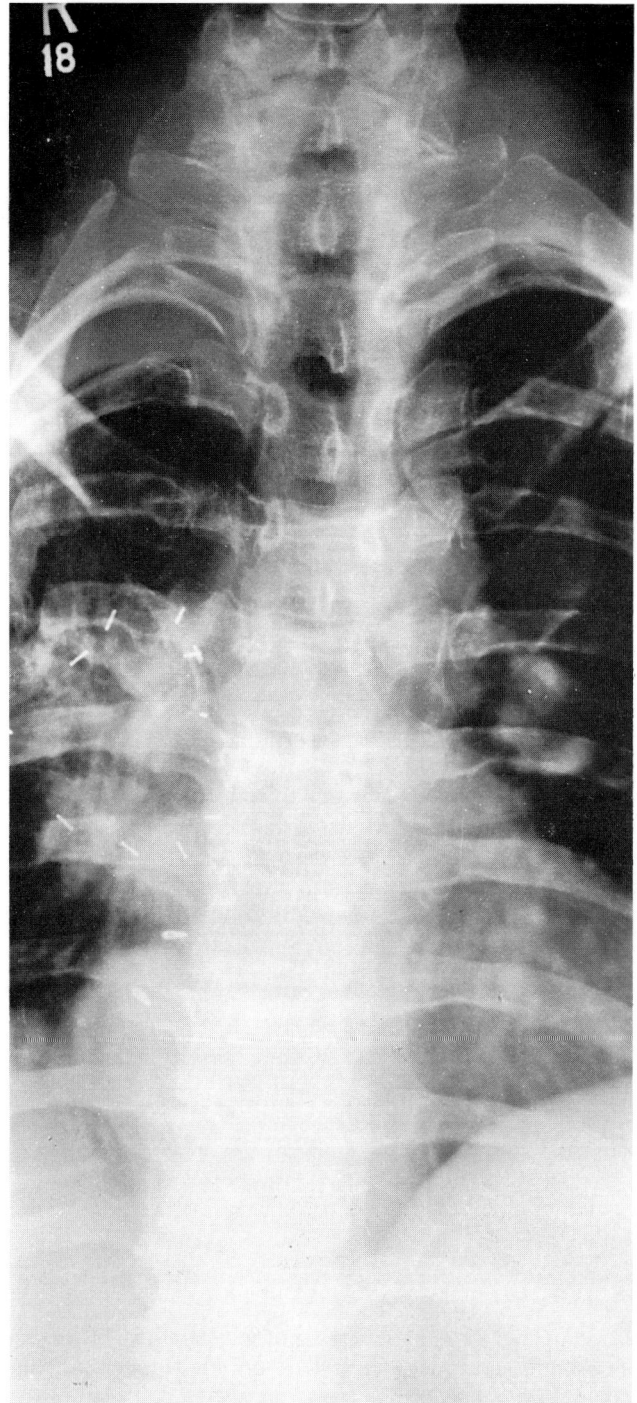

Figure 106b

There is a rounded opacity visible in the right cardiophrenic angle. Ultrasound, CT and gallium scanning were performed.

The rounded mass is seen posteriorly positioned in the mediastinum on CT (fig. 106c) extending down

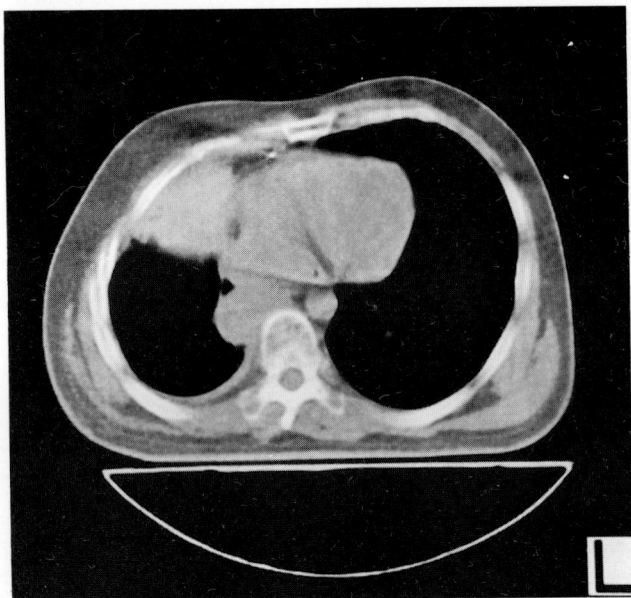

Figure 106c

Figure 106d

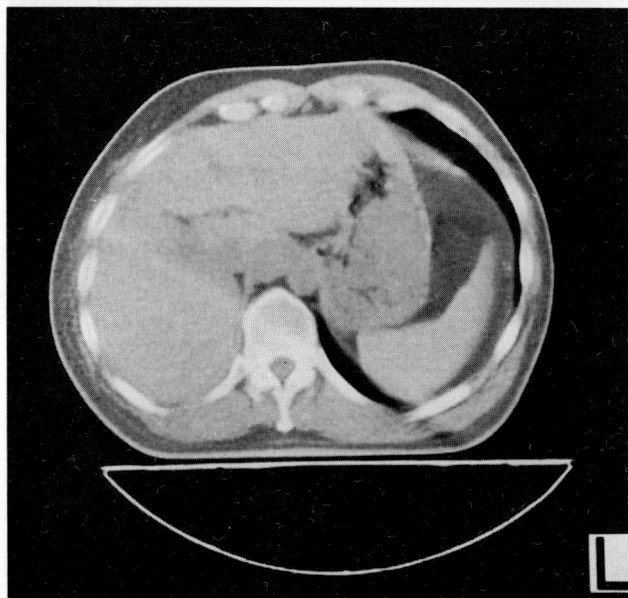

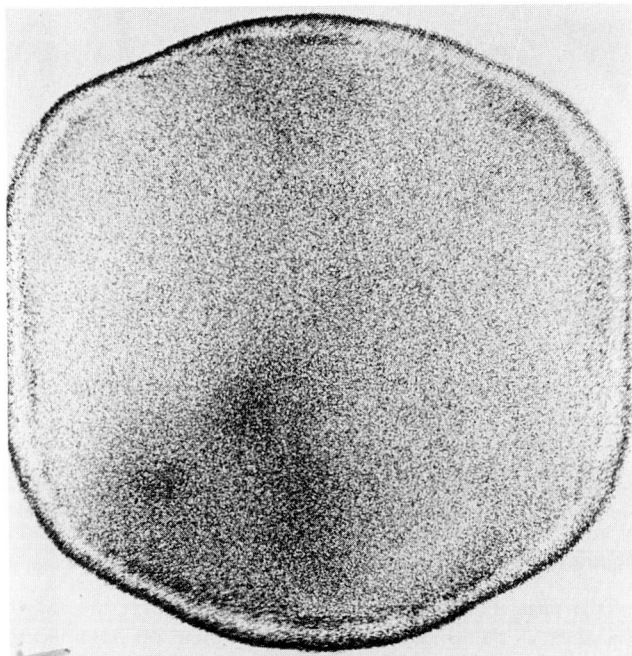

Figure 106e

Case 107

A man aged 70 presented with a history of dysphagia. A barium swallow was performed.

This showed a smooth stricture which changed in shape due to peristalsis. These were features typical of an extrinsic

Figure 107a

retrocrurally. It was shown to be of low echogenicity on the ultrasound and to take up gallium on the isotope scan (fig. 106e). The appearances were consistent with an active mass, either recurrence of thymoma or an abscess. Thoracotomy was performed and demonstrated recurrence of the thymoma. This case was very similar to Case 102 in that the mass had initially started in the anterior mediastinum, had spread by invasion around the pleura and to the mediastinum posteriorly. Gallium scanning and CT also showed the mass to extend inferiorly through the diaphragm adjacent to the aorta.

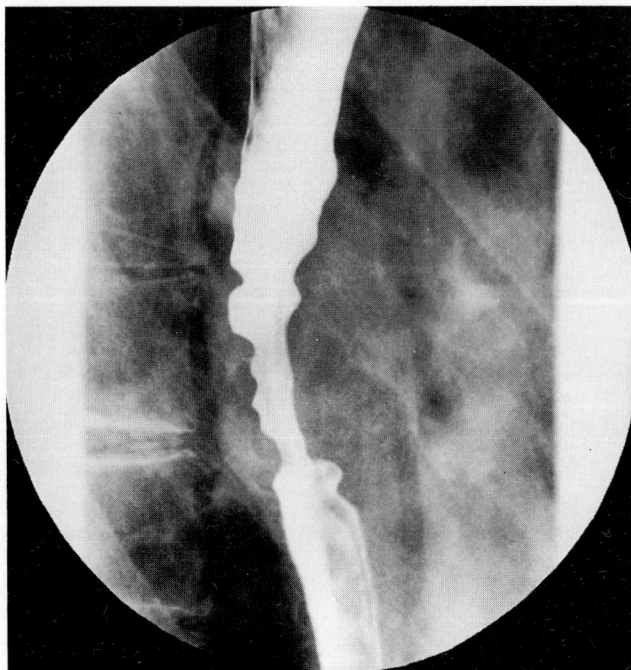

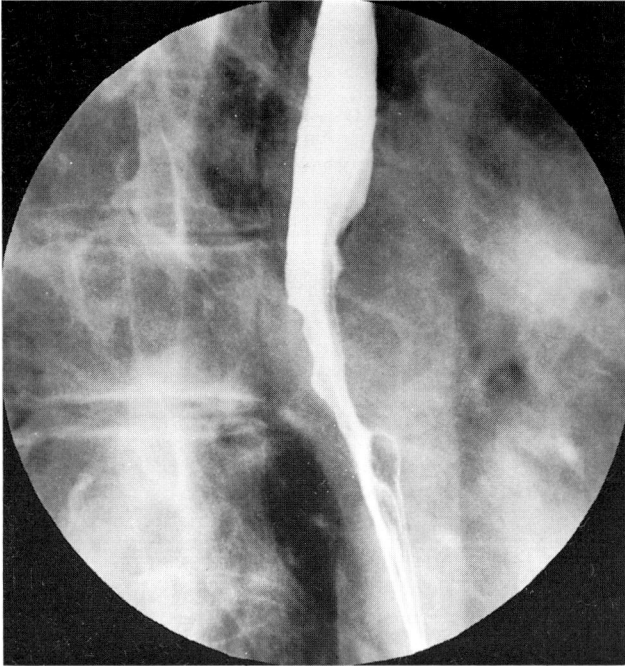

Figure 107b

mass compressing the oesophagus. Chest x-ray at this time was considered to be normal. No abnormality was seen on endoscopy. After a repeat barium swallow had again shown an extrinsic mass a repeat chest x-ray and CT of the chest were performed.

The chest x-ray shows left lower lobe consolidation. CT shows the consolidation to be confined to the left lateral basal segment (fig. 107g) — suggestive of an endobronchial lesion. There was a large mass posteriorly in the

Figure 107c

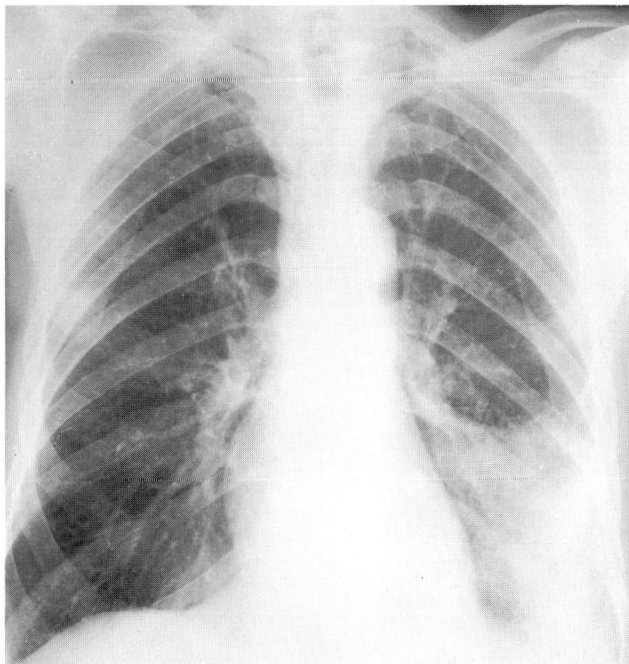

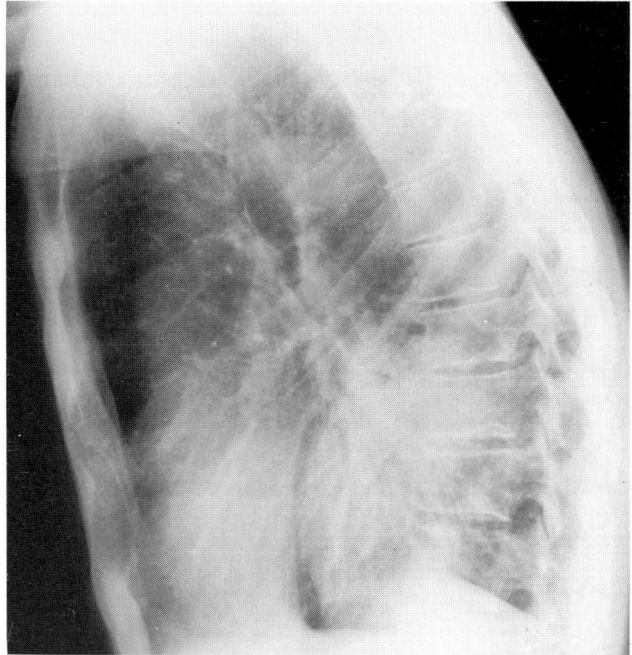

Figure 107d

Figure 107e

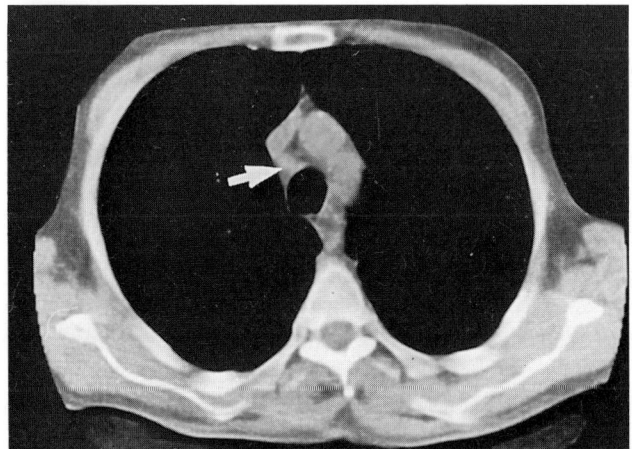

Figure 107f

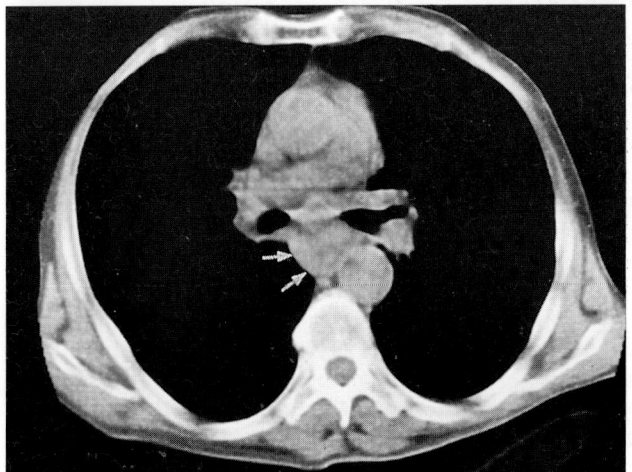

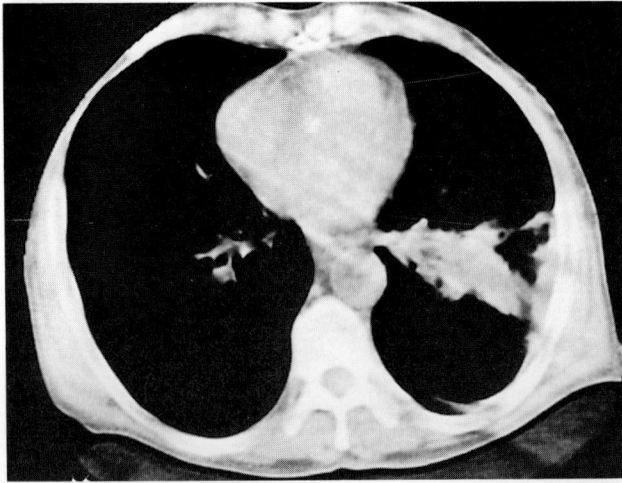

Figure 107g

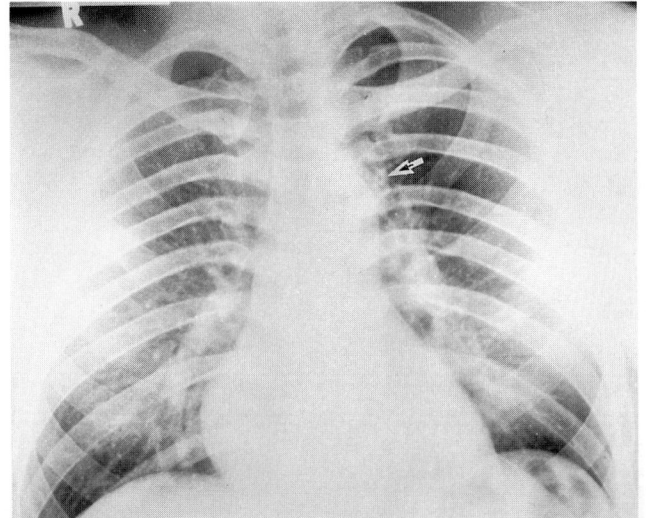

Figure 108a
Figure 108b

mediastinum (*arrowed*, fig. 107f) and a further enlarged node anterior to the trachea (*arrowed*, fig. 107e).

Bronchoscopy was performed and showed a bronchogenic carcinoma in the left lower lobe bronchus obstructing the orifice of the lateral basal segment bronchus.

This case is similar to Cases 43 and 83.

The anatomy of the pulmonary lymphatic system helps to explain why the particular lymph node groups become involved with tumour. The posterior mediastinal lymph nodes are behind the pericardium, close to the oesophagus and descending thoracic aorta. They receive afferents from the diaphragm, oesophagus and pericardium and also from the mediastinal and diaphragmatic pleura. Their efferents mostly end in the thoracic duct but some join the tracheobronchial nodes [80].

Case 108 (*Courtesy of Mr G K Tutton*)

An Italian man aged 23 presented with profound weakness in his legs and a past history of swelling of his bones. His chest x-ray is shown with a penetrated film and lateral tomography.

The chest x-ray revealed an opacity adjacent to the aortic knuckle (*arrowed*, fig. 108a). The penetrated film and lateral tomography showed a calcified opacity adjacent to and eroding into the 5th thoracic vertebra. A well defined sclerotic margin was apparent.

The myelogram showed complete obstruction at the level of the mass. X-rays of his limbs were performed because of the history of swellings of his bones.

Multiple exostoses are demonstrated (diaphyseal aclasia). The neurosurgeon removed almost all the calcified tumour but left a small lateral remnant (marked

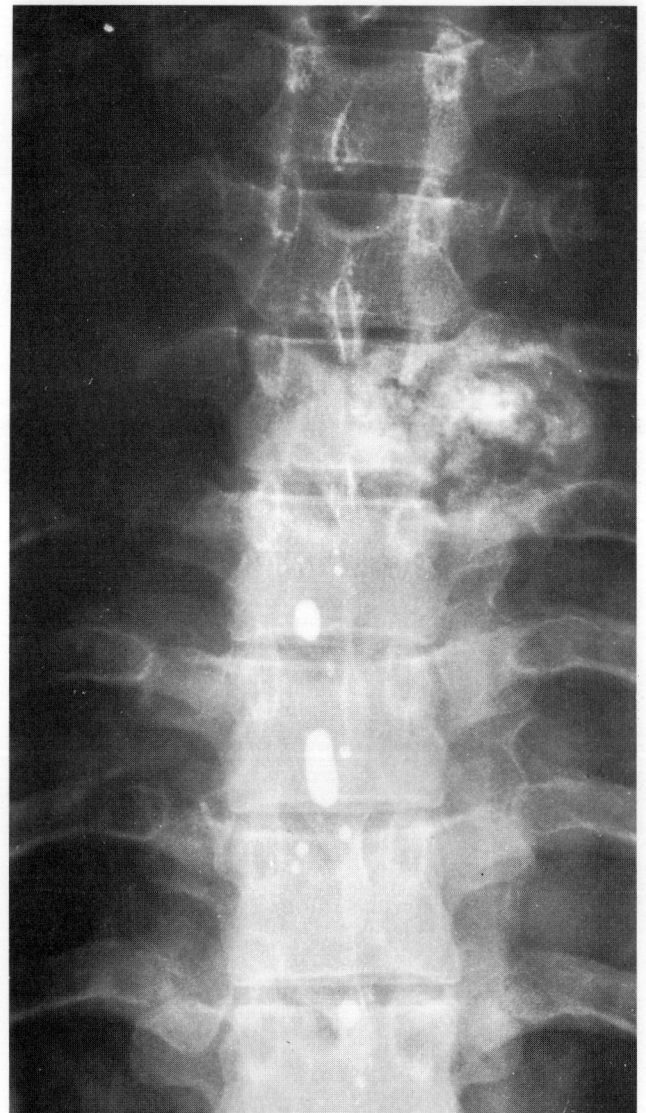

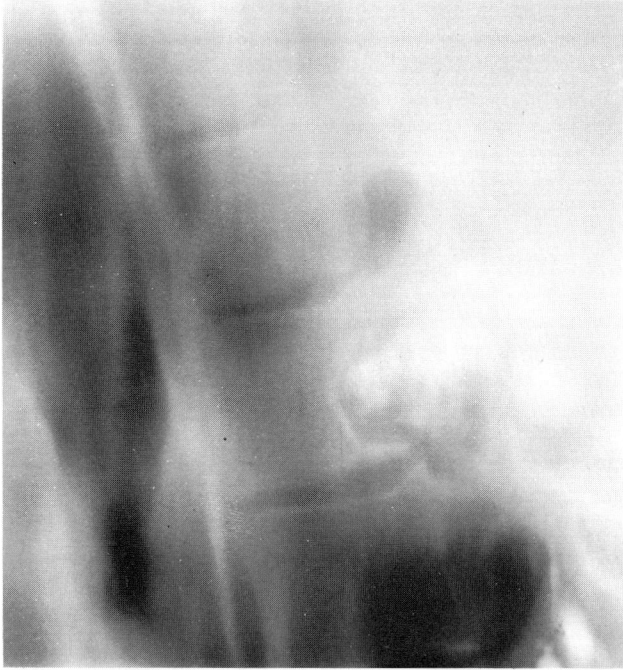

Figure 108c
Figure 108d

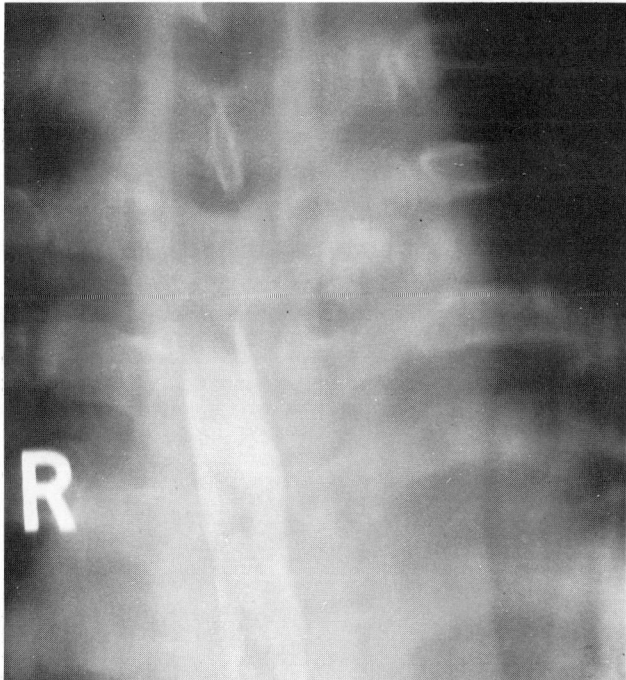

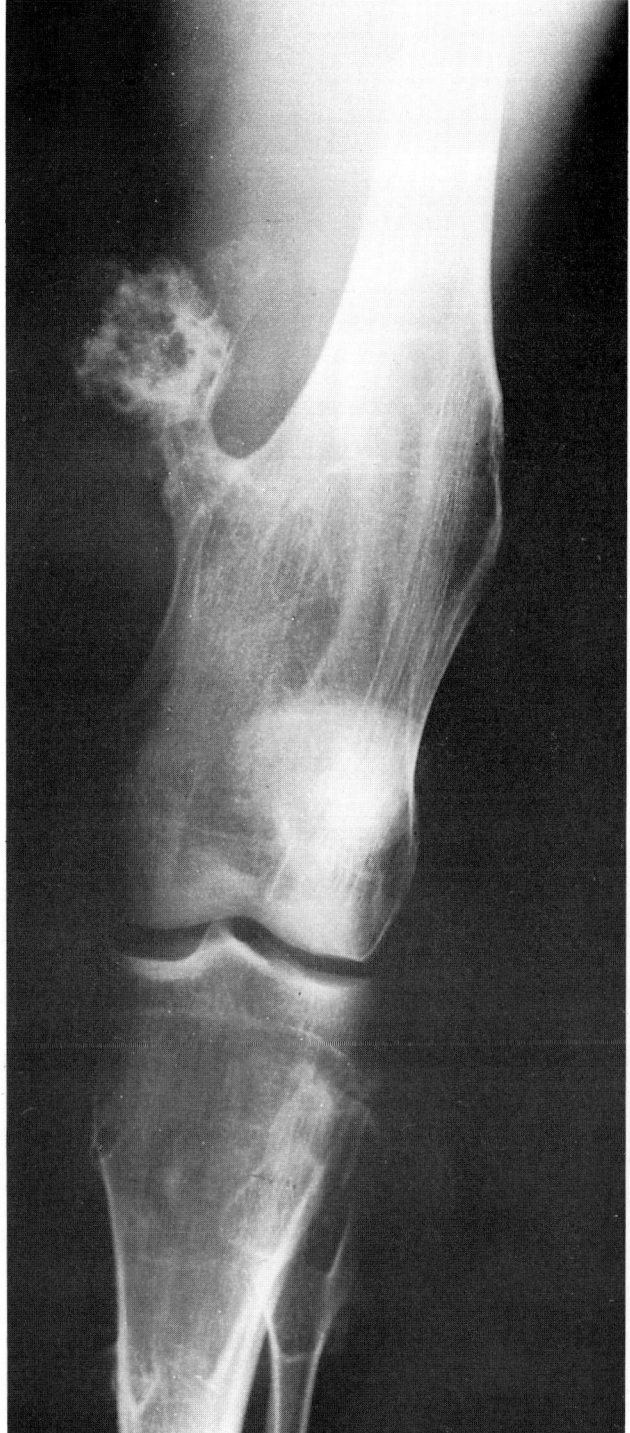

Figure 108e

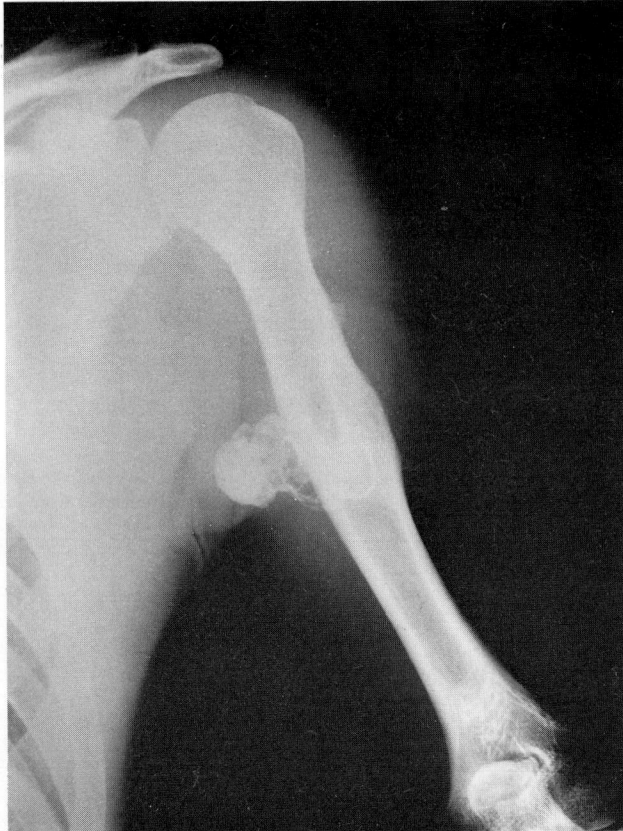

Figure 108f

Figure 108g

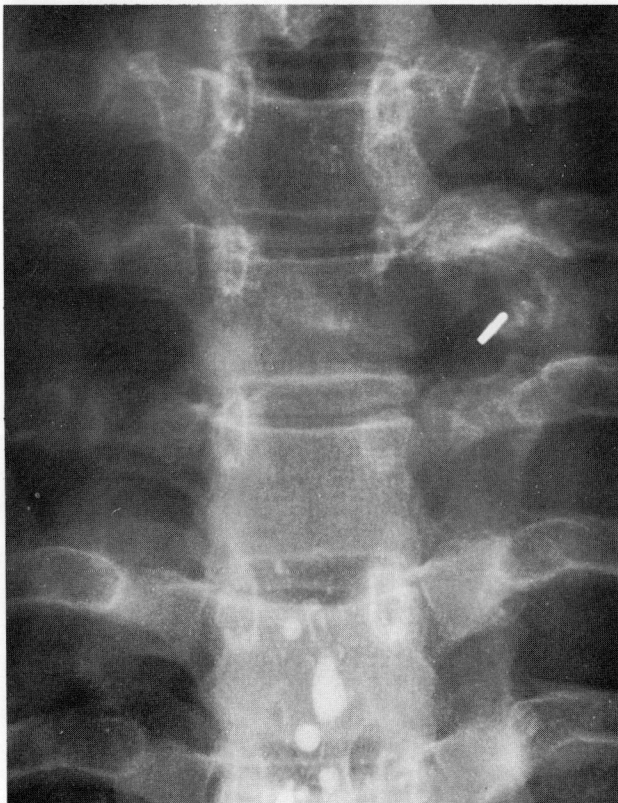

with a clip in fig. 108g). This small remnant was left because discretion was considered to be the better part of valour. Pulsation was visible and the immediate anterior relationship was, of course, the aorta! Histology showed the tumour to be a chondroma with no evidence of malignant change. The man is now fit and with full use of his legs.

Case 109

A woman with endometrial carcinoma presented with weakness of her legs and an opacity in the region of the right hilum on chest x-rays. A CT scan of her thorax is shown.

Figure 109a

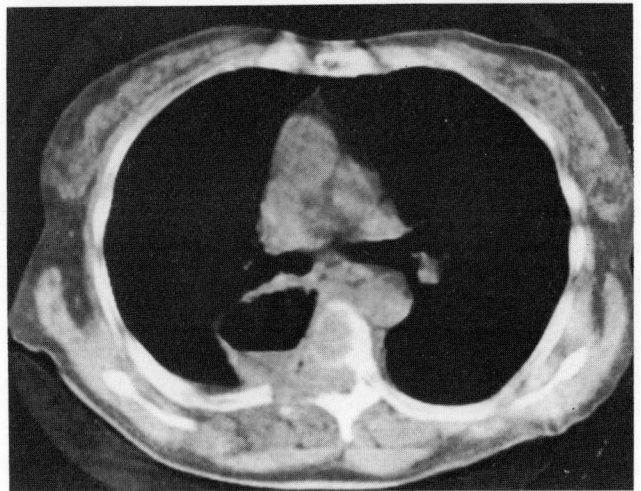

There is a thick-walled, cavitating neoplastic mass eroding and invading the thoracic spine. A fluid level is seen within the necrotic centre of the secondary deposit.

Figure 109b

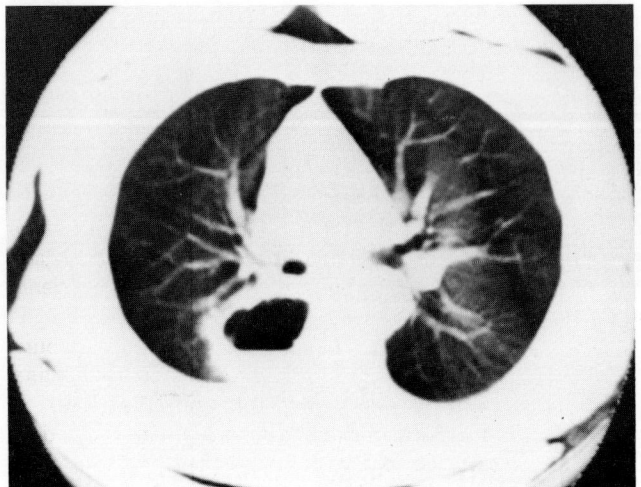

Superior vena cava obstruction

In many patients presenting with symptoms due to superior vena cava obstruction the chest radiograph will show a mediastinal mass and there is a history of a malignant disease. A lateral radiograph and views of the thoracic inlet may be of value in placing the lesion and determining whether or not the trachea is compressed, but otherwise little is required in the way of diagnostic imaging before the instigation of treatment.

If there is a mediastinal mass and no known primary tumour, the lesion should be investigated, with some urgency, in the same way as any other mediastinal mass.

If the initial plain chest films appear normal or are in any way equivocal, venography may be considered as the next investigation in order to demonstrate the site of obstruction. The venogram will show whether the obstruction is in the lumen, in the wall, or external to the superior vena cava. CT, with intravenous contrast medium, would in some centres be performed rather than venography. CT can, in any case, be performed next to evaluate whether or not a mass is present and what form the mass takes. It is important to remember that SVC obstruction can occur due to non-malignant conditions. For example, an aortic aneurysm may compress the superior vena cava — such a case is shown on page 137. If no mass is seen on the CT and venography shows extrinsic impression but no intraluminal embolus and no thrombus, the obstruction may be due to fibrosis. In some cases of idiopathic mediastinal fibrosis causing SVC obstruction there may be a mass due to the fibrosis. If a mass is present, biopsy is indicated. (See also gallium scanning in fibrosing mediastinitis, page 96.)

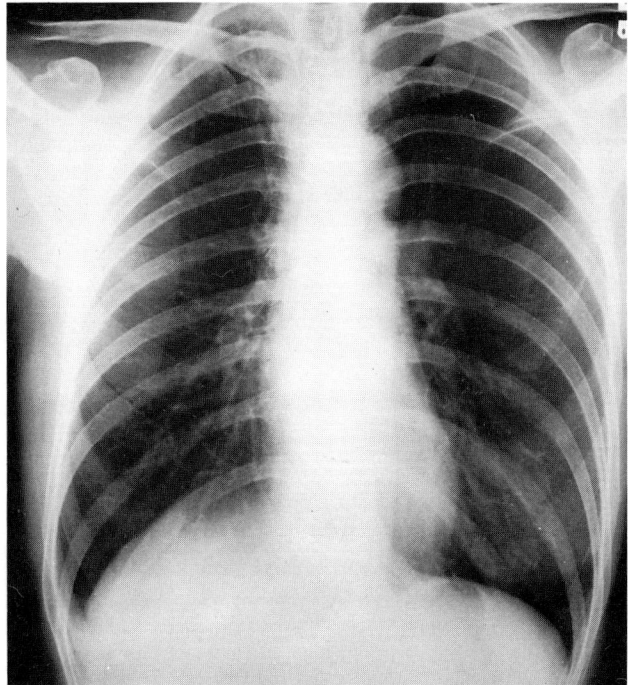

Figure 110a

Figure 110b

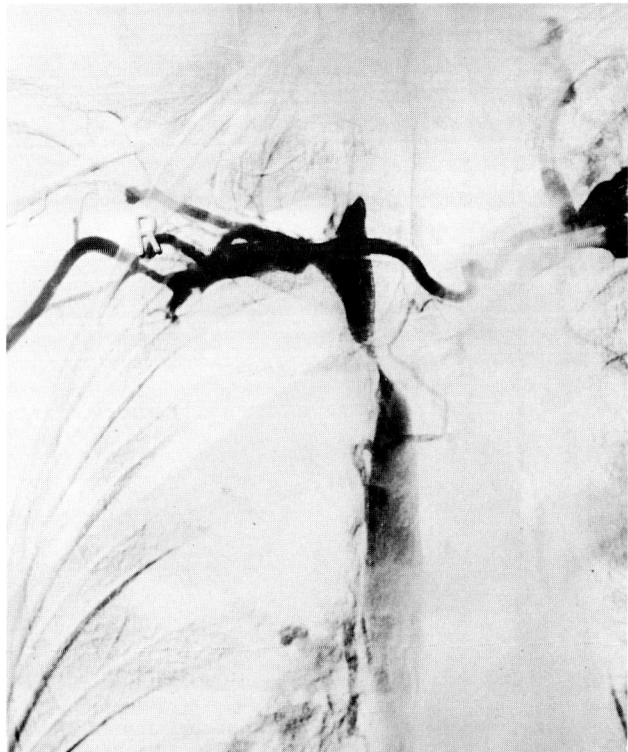

Case 110

A female patient, aged 46, with a previous history of carcinoma of the right breast treated with mastectomy and radiotherapy, presented with mild symptoms of superior vena cava obstruction (SVCO).

Chest x-ray (see fig. 110a) showed slight pleural thickening in the right apex but no obvious mediastinal lesion. Venography was performed and the level of obstruction was shown to be where the left and right brachiocephalic veins join to form the superior vena cava (see fig. 110b). The stenosis was smooth and tapering and had the appearances of an abnormality external to the vein. Computed tomography was performed before and during intravenous contrast medium injection.

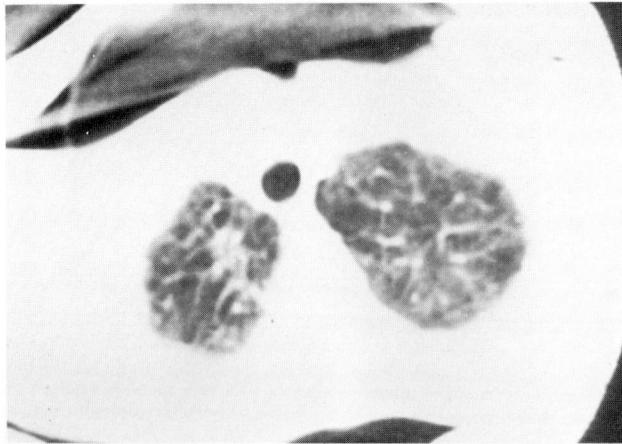

Figure 110c

Figure 110d

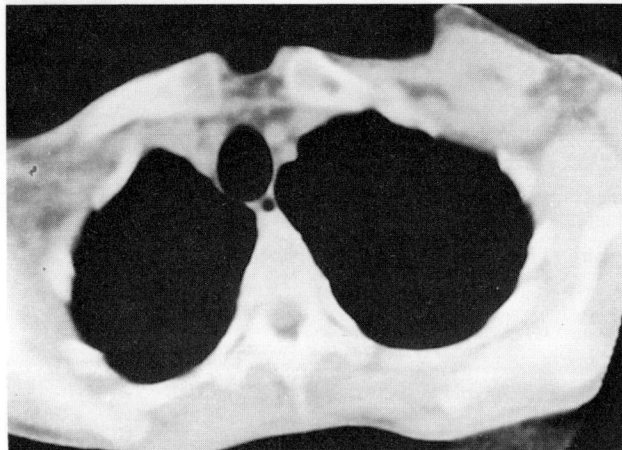

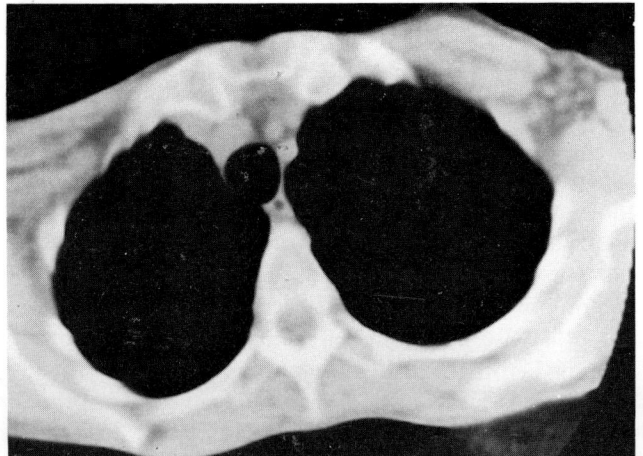

Figure 110f

Figure 110g

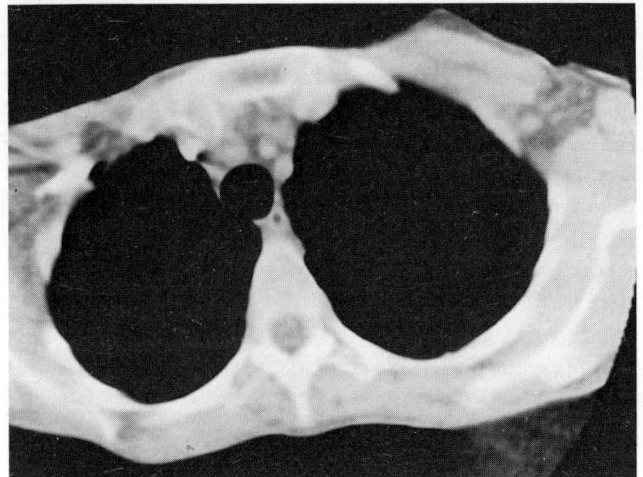

Figure 110e

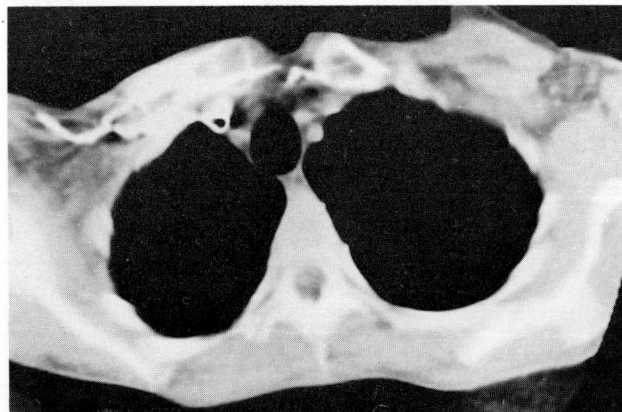

Figure 110h

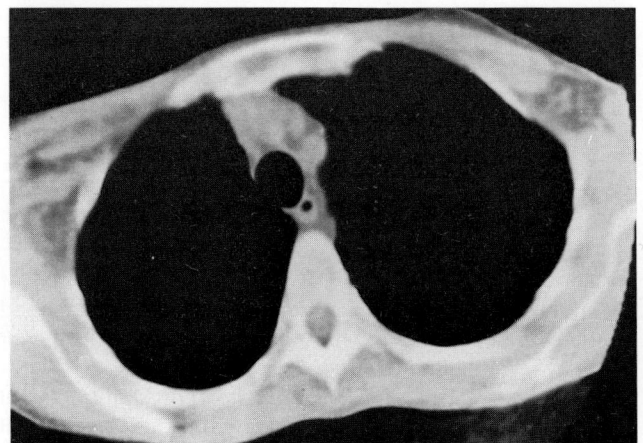

No mass was demonstrated in the mediastinum at the site of the obstruction. Opacification of the apex of the right upper lobe was present due to the radiotherapy pneumonitis. The cause of the SVCO was therefore assumed, by exclusion, to be mediastinal fibrosis due to

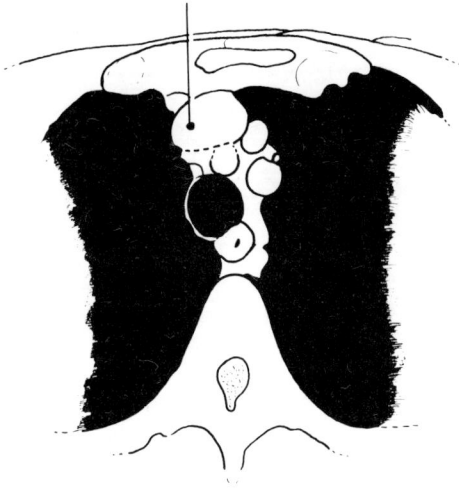

Arch of (L) brachiocephalic vein distended

Figure 110i

radiotherapy. Per-catheter balloon dilatation of the SVC was attempted but was unsuccessful. The patient was referred to the thoracic surgeons who declined to perform surgery at that stage. Close follow-up by chest radiography and CT was undertaken with no further change in symptoms or radiological signs one year after presentation.

Mediastinal fibrosis can occur with no known cause but can also result from radiation therapy or as a side effect of some drugs (e.g. methysergide). Various chronic infections can cause fibrosing mediastinitis but especially histoplasmosis in the USA and tuberculosis in Great Britain. Acute infections are an unusual cause of mediastinitis but can occur due to oesophageal rupture and less commonly tracheal rupture. In acute cases the neck should also be x-rayed in order to look for a retropharyngeal abscess.

Case 111

A 54 year old woman presented with symptoms of superior vena cava obstruction. The chest x-ray and venography are shown in figures 111a and 111b respectively.

The chest x-ray shows no definite abnormality. Venography (via both arms) shows obstruction at the junction of the brachiocephalic veins.

Computed tomography showed a mass anteriorly in the mediastinum (fig. 111c) but also demonstrated an opacity posterior to the oesophagus (fig. 111d). Barium swallow was done to further evaluate the posterior mediastinal mass.

The barium swallow showed a smooth external band-like filling defect passing obliquely behind the oesophagus.

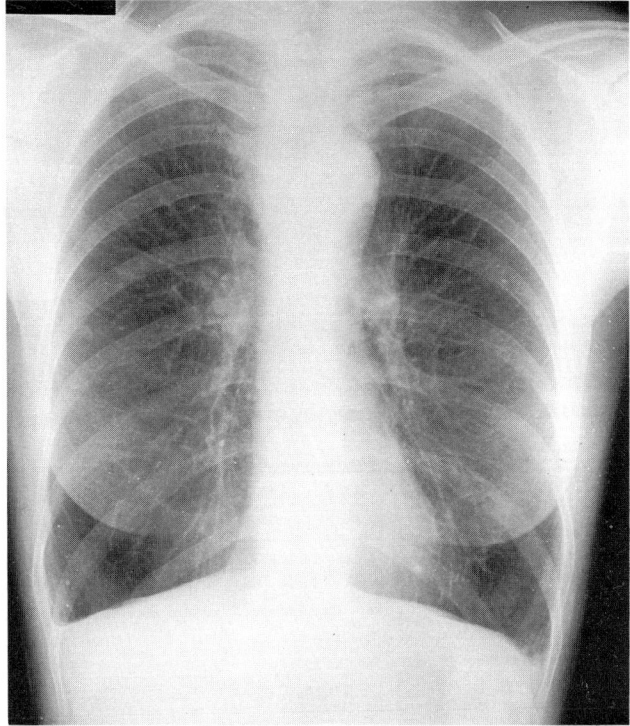

Figure 111a

Figure 111b

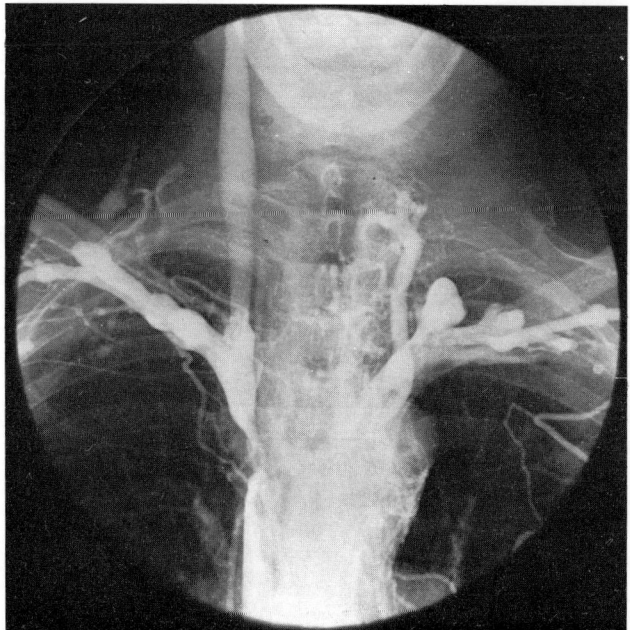

These were the typical features of an aberrant right subclavian artery, the anatomy of which is shown in the line drawing (fig. 111f). The anterior mass causing the SVCO was shown at mediastinotomy to be poorly differentiated adenocarcinoma.

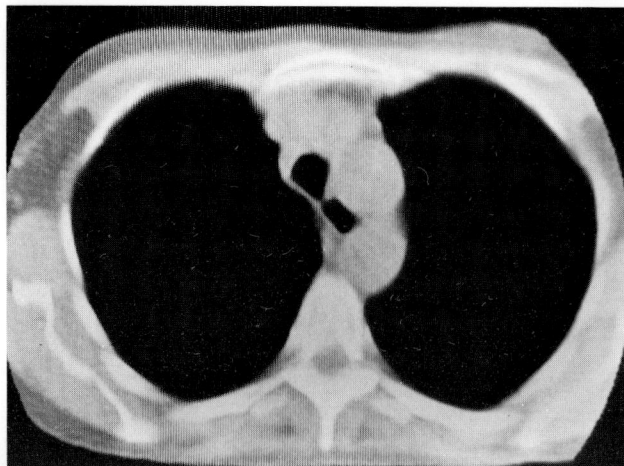

Figure 111c

Figure 111d

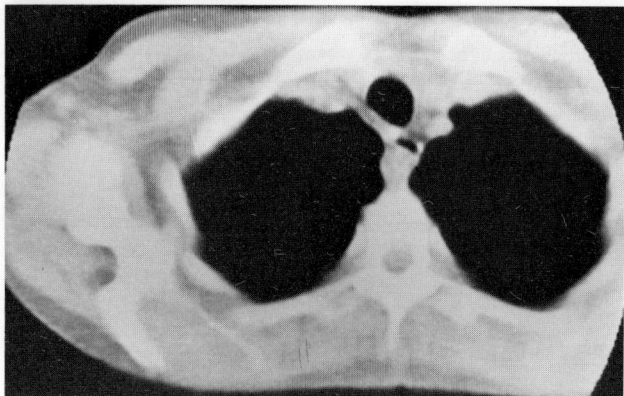

Figure 111e

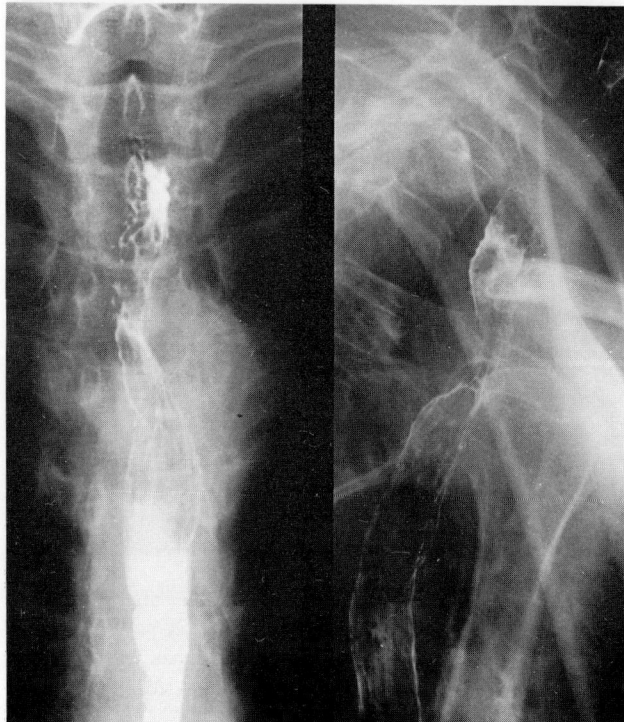

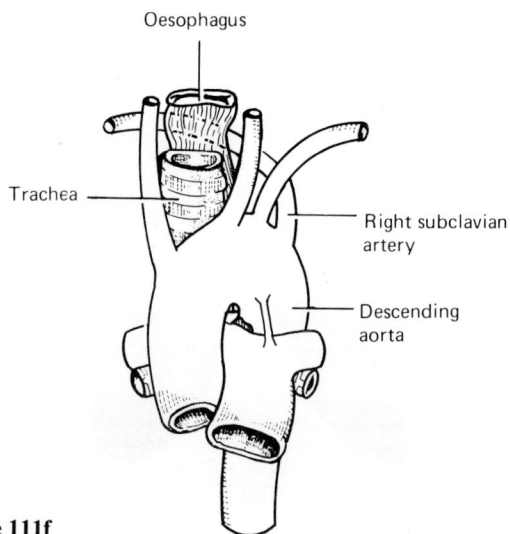

Figure 111f

Vascular anomalies are common in the mediastinum and a thorough knowledge of the anatomy and common variants is essential when interpreting the appearances of the mediastinum. (*This case was provided courtesy of Mr Forrester Wood and the diagnostic imaging was undertaken at Frenchay Hospital.*)

Summary: mediastinal mass

The investigative procedures undertaken in a patient with mediastinal lesion will depend largely on the nature of the presentation, signs and symptoms. As usual it is important to review any previous chest x-rays and to perform a lateral to help place the lesion.

If the symptoms are suggestive of an acute vascular lesion, some form of angiography may be necessary. This is usually performed by the transfemoral route, but the use of digital vascular imaging and of computed tomography is increasing.

If the patient presents with dysphagia or other symptoms referable to the oesophagus, a barium swallow may provide the answer.

If there is a mass on the chest x-ray but no particular distinguishing features, two investigations that may prove of value are computed tomography and ultrasound. CT is probably the best method of analysing masses in the mediastinum and can determine the exact position of the mass, its radiodensity and relationship to surrounding structures. Ultrasound is a useful adjunct to CT since lesions may appear solid on CT but can be demonstrated as cystic by ultrasound.

Masses in the mediastinum may be biopsied by a variety of methods. Retrosternal lesions can be sampled by CT guided needle biopsy or by mediastinotomy, lesions near the trachea can be sampled by mediastinoscopy and posterior lesions may also be sampled either by CT guided needle biopsy or by surgery. Magnetic resonance imaging is a technique that is rapidly gaining a place in the investigation of mediastinal masses and can be used to complement or replace CT or ultrasound.

When a patient presents with superior vena cava obstruction, if there is a large mediastinal mass and a known diagnosis, little further imaging is necessary. If, however, on the chest radiograph there is no obvious mass, it may be important to determine whether the cause of the obstruction is intraluminal, in the wall of the vessel, or due to external compression. Superior vena cavography can be performed by simultaneous bilateral injection of contrast media into antecubital veins. Again it is possible to use digital vascular imaging to obtain subtraction films and in some centres computed tomography would be performed as the procedure of choice.

Bibliography

1 Wilkins and Fraser (1975) *Applied Radiology, Vol 4*, p 41. Brentwood Publishing Corporation, Los Angeles

2 Schaner E G, Chang A E, Doppman J L, Conkle D M, Wayne M, Rosenberg F (1978) Comparison of computed tomography and conventional whole lung tomography in detecting pulmonary nodules. *Am J Roentgenol*, **131**, 51–54

3 Jost R G, Sagel S S, Stanley R J, Levitt R G (1978) CT of the thorax. *Radiology*, **126**(1), 125–136

4 Muhm J R, Brown L R, Crowe J K (1977) Detection of pulmonary nodules by computed tomography. *Am J Roentgenol*, **128**, 267–270

5 Husband J E, Reckham M J, MacDonald J S, Hendry W F (1979) The role of computed tomography in the management of testicular teratoma. *Clin Radiol*, **30**, 243–252

6 Katz D, Fasianos S (1981) Computed tomography in the radiology of testicular teratomas. *Clin Radiol*, **32**, 679–682

7 Goddard P (1982) *CT of the Lungs*. MD Thesis, University of Bristol, England

8 Chakraborty D P, Breatnach E, Fraser R G, Barnes G T (1983) Digital vs. conventional chest images in the detection of nodules: a modified ROC study. *Radiology*, **194**(P), 64. Presented at the RSNA meeting

9 Eastham R D (1983) *A Laboratory Guide to Clinical Diagnosis*, pp 67–68. John Wright and Sons Ltd, Bristol

10 Goddard P R, Nicholson E M, Laszlo G, Watt I (1982) Computed tomography in pulmonary emphysema. *Clin Radiol*, **33**, 379–387

11 Siegelman S S, Zerhouni E A, Leo F P, Khouri N F, Stitik F P (1980) CT of the solitary pulmonary nodule. *Am J Roentgenol*, **135**, 1–13

12 Proto A V (1983) CT analysis of the pulmonary nodule. *Radiology*, **149**(P), 42. Presented at the RSNA meeting

13 Maile C W, Rodan B A, Godwin J D, Chen J T T, Rvin C E (1982) Calcification in pulmonary metastases. *Br J Radiol*, **55**, 108–113

14 Jefferson K, Rees S (1975) *Clinical Cardiac Radiology*, p 142. Butterworths, London

15 Sagel S S (1983) *Radiology* **149**(P), 225. Presented at the RSNA meeting

16 Baron R L, Levitt R G, Segal S S et al (1982) CT in the preoperative evaluation of bronchogenic carcinoma. *Radiology*, **145**, 727–732

17 Schwartz E E (1984) Respiratory tract and mediastinum. In: *The Radiology of Complications in Medical Practice*, pp 53–57. University Park Press, Baltimore

18 Gobien R P, Vujic 1 (1983) Interventional radiology of the thorax: advanced techniques. *Radiology*, **149**(P), 151

19 Fink I, Gamsu G, Harter L P (1982) CT-guided aspiration biopsy of the thorax. *J Comput Assist Tomogr*, **6**(5), 958–962

20 Walls W J, Thornbury J R, Naylor B (1974) Pulmonary needle biopsy in the diagnosis of Pancoast tumors. *Radiology*, **111**, 99–102

21 Stein H L, Evans J A (1966) Percutaneous transthoracic lung biopsy utilizing image amplification. *Radiology*, **87**, 350

22 Coleman R, Driver M, Gishen P (1982) Percutaneous lung biopsy: experiences during the first 54 biopsies. *Cardiovasc Intervent Radiol*, **5**, 61–63

23 Nordenstrom B, Sinner W N (1978) Needle biopsies of pulmonary lesions. Precautions and management of complications. *ROEFO*, **129**, 414–418

24 Wandtke J C, Plewes D B (1983) Raster scan radiography with regional exposure control: preliminary clinical experience. *Radiology*, **149**(P), 290. Presented at the RSNA meeting

25 Plewes D B (1983) A scanning system for chest radiography with regional exposure control: theoretical considerations. *Med Phys*, **10**(5), 646–654

26 Plewes D B, Vogelstein E (1983) A scanning system for chest radiography with regional exposure control: practical implementation. *Med Phys*, **10**(5), 655–663

27 Cooke N T (1984) The lungs and rheumatoid arthritis. In: *Respiratory Disease in Practice, Vol 2*, No. 13, pp 20–25

28 Studdy P R, Rudd R M, Gellert A R, Uthayakumar S, Sinha G, Geddef D M (1984) Bronchoalveolar lavage in the diagnosis of the diffuse pulmonary shadowing. *Br J Dis Chest*, **78**, 46–54

29 Sorsdahl O A, Powell J W (1965) Cavitary pulmonary lesions following non-penetrating chest trauma in children. *Am J Roentgenol*, **95**, 118

30 Pitcher D, Wood P, Goddard P, Russell Rees J (1984) Fulminating aspergillus pneumonia complicating radiation fibrosis. *Bristol Med Chir J*, July, 84–87

31 Bodey G P (1966) Fungal infections complicating acute leukaemia. *J Chronic Dis*, 667–687

32 Meyer R D, Young L S, Armstrong D, Yu B (1973) Aspergillosis complicating neoplastic disease. *Am J Med*, **54**, 6–15

33 Daly B D (1983) Successful treatment of invasive pulmonary aspergillosis in a patient with acute leukaemia. *Ir J Med Sci*, **152**, 103–105

34 McLeod D T, Milne L J R, Seaton A (1982) Successful treatment of invasive pulmonary aspergillosis complicating influenza. *Br Med J*, **285**, 1166–1167

35 Fraser R G, Pare J A (1970) Bronchopulmonary sequestration. In: *Diagnosis of Diseases of the Chest*, pp 577–581. W B Saunders Co., Philadelphia

36 Eastham R D (1983) *A Laboratory Guide to Clinical Diagnosis, 5th edn*, p 208. John Wright and Sons Ltd, Bristol

37 Cooper T J, Tinker J (1984) The adult respiratory distress syndrome. *Hospital Update Vol 10*, No. 10, pp 849–859

38 Basran G S, Byrne A J, Hardy J E (1983) Monitoring lung vascular permeability in health and ARDS in man. *Proceedings of the British Thoracic Society, Winter Meeting, Thorax*

39 Fraser R G, Pare J A (1977) *Diagnosis of Diseases of the Chest, Vol I*, p 344. W B Saunders Co, Philadelphia

40 Felson B (1973) *Chest Roentgenology*. W B Saunders Co, Philadelphia

41 Roswit B, White D C (1977) Severe radiation of the lung. *Am J Roentgenol*, **129**(i), 127–136

42 Naidich D P et al (1984) *Computed Tomography of the Thorax*. Raven Press, New York

43 Coddington R, Mera S L, Goddard P R, Bradfield J W S (1982) Pathological evaluation of computed tomography images of the lungs. *J Clin Pathol*, **35**, 536–540

44 Crofton J, Douglas A (1981) *Respiratory Diseases, 3rd edn*, p 758. Blackwell Scientific, Oxford

45 Fraser R G, Pare J A (1970) Unilateral emphysema (Swyer-James syndrome). In: *Diagnosis of Diseases of the Chest, Vol II*, p 1037, W B Saunders Co, Philadelphia

46 Breatnach E, Kerr I (1982) The radiology of cryptogenic obliterative bronchiolitis. *Clin Radiol*, **33**, 657–661

47 Frank P (1984) Chest pain in general practice. *Respiratory Disease in Practice, Vol 2*, No. 11, pp 23–26

48 Eastham R D (1983) *A Laboratory Guide to Clinical Diagnosis*, p 213. John Wright and Sons Ltd, Bristol

49 Hoffer P B, Gottschalk A, Zaret B L (1982) *The Year Book of Nuclear Medicine*, p 109. Year Book Publishers Inc., Chicago

50 Donaldson R M, Kahn O, Raphael M J, Jarritt P H, Ell P J (1982) Emission tomography in embolic lung disease: angiographic correlations. *Clin Radiol*, **33**, 389–393

51 Fraser J R, Lansdown M, Goddard P (1984) An unusual pulmonary embolus. *Bristol Med Chir J*, January, 8–10

52 Li D K, Seltzer S E, McNeil B J (1978) V/Q mismatches unassociated with pulmonary embolism: case report and a review of the literature. *J Nucl Med*, **19**(12), 1331–1333

53 Park H M, Jay S J, Brandt M H, Holden R W (1981) Pulmonary scintigraphy in fibrosing mediastinitis due to histoplasmosis. *J Nucl Med*, **22**(4), 349–351

54 Gamsu G, Hirji M, Moore E H, Webb W R, Brito A (1984) Experimental pulmonary emboli detected using magnetic resonance. *Radiology*, **153**(2), 467–470

55 Moore E H, Gamsu G, Webb W R, Stulberg M S (1984) Pulmonary embolus: detection and follow-up using magnetic resonance. *Radiology*, **153**, 471–472

56 McMillan P, Jackson P, Davies E R, Goddard P (1983) Emission and transmission pulmonary computed tomography. *Br J Radiol*, **56**, 991–992

57 Goddard P, Bullimore J A, Coutts I I, Davies E R, Mitchelmore A (1984) Pulmonary transmission and emission CT in patients becoming breathless after radiotherapy. *Thorax*, **39**, No. 9 Sept, 688

58 Fraser R G, Pare J A (1970) *Diagnosis of Diseases of the Chest, Vol II*, p 1220. W B Saunders Co, Philadelphia

59 Khan A, Gould D A (1984) The primary role of ultrasound in evaluating right-sided diaphragmatic masses. *Clin Radiol*, **35**, 413–418

60 Fataar S (1979) Diagnosis of diaphragmatic tears. *Br J Radiol*, **52**, 375–381

61 Doust B D, Baum J K, Maklad N F, Doust V L (1975) Ultrasonic evaluation of pleural opacities. *Radiology*, **114**, 135–140

62 Sandweiss D A, Hanson J C, Gosink B B, Moser K M (1975) Ultrasound in diagnosis, localization and treatment of loculated pleural emphysema. *Ann Intern Med*, **82,** 50–53

63 Laing F C, Filly R A (1978) Problems in the application of ultrasonography for the evaluation of pleural opacities. *Radiology*, **126,** 211–214

64 Hirsch J H, Carter S J, Chikos P M, Colacurcio C (1978) Ultrasonic evaluation of radiographic opacities of the chest. *Am J Roentgenol*, **130,** 1153–1156

65 Cunningham J J (1978) Gray scale echography of the lung and pleural space. Current applications of oncologic interest. *Cancer*, **41,** 1329–1339

66 Miller J H, Reid B S, Kemberling C R (1984) Water-path ultrasound of chest disease in childhood. *Radiology*, **152,** 401–408

67 Lipscomb D J, Flower C D R, Hadfield J W (1981) Ultrasound of pleura: an assessment of its clinical value. *Clin Radiol*, **32,** 289–290

68 Aldridge S, Goddard P (1984) *Hospital Doctor Vol C4*, No. 43, p 15

69 Bell J, Goddard P (1984) *Hospital Doctor Vol C4*, No. 27, p 13

70 Beaumont D, Herry J Y, Sapene M, Bourguet P, Largul J J, De Labarthe B (1982) Gallium 67 in the evaluation of sarcoidosis. *Thorax*, January, **37**(1), 11–16

71 Symbas P N, Tyras D H, Ware R E et al (1973) Rupture of the aorta: a diagnostic triad. *Ann Thorac Surg*, **15,** 405

72 Fisher R G, Hadlock F, Ben-Menachem Y (1981) Laceration of the thoracic aorta and brachiocephalic arteries by blunt trauma. *Radiol Clin North Am*, **19**(1), 91–110

73 Bell J, O'Reilly J, Laszlo G, Wilde P, Goddard P (1983) Imaging techniques in the diagnosis of a mediastinal mass. *Bristol Med Chir J*, October, 176–178

74 Haller J A, Golladay E S, Pickard L R, Tepas J J III, Shorter N A, Shermeta D W (1972) Surgical management of lung bud anomalies. *Ann Thorac Surg*, **14,** 434–439

75 Ochsner J L, Ochsner S F (1966) Congenital cyst of the mediastinum, 20 years experience with 42 cases. *Ann Surg*, **163,** 909–920

76 Delarue N C, Pearson F G, Cooper J D, Todd T R J, Ilves R, Sanders D E (1981) Developmental bronchopulmonary disease in adults—practical clinical consideration. *Can J Surg*, **24,** 23–31

77 Stoner J, Kiragus C (1957) Considerations on an unrecognised mediastinal cyst. *J Pediatr*, **51,** 194–196

78 Ikard R W (1972) Bronchogenic cyst causing repeated left lung atelectasis in an adult. *Ann Thorac Surg*, **14,** 434–439

79 Gamsu G, Webb W R, Sheldon P, Kaufman L, Crooks L, Birnberg F A, Goodman P, Hinchcliffe W A, Hedgecock M (1983) Nuclear magnetic resonance imaging of the thorax. *Radiology*, **147,** 473–480

80 Gray H (1973) Lymphatic drainage of the thorax. In: *Gray's Anatomy, 35th edn* (Warwick R, Williams P L eds), pp 743–744. Longman, Edinburgh

Index